Learning Disabilities Sourcebook, 3rd Edition
Leukemia Sourcebook
Liver Disorders Sourcebook
Lung Disorders Sourcebook
Medical Tests Sourcebook, 3rd Edition
Men's Health Concerns Sourcebook, 2nd Edition
Mental Health Disorders Sourcebook, 4th Edition
Mental Retardation Sourcebook
Movement Disorders Sourcebook, 2nd Edition
Multiple Sclerosis Sourcebook
Muscular Dystrophy Sourcebook
Obesity Sourcebook
Osteoporosis Sourcebook
Pain Sourcebook, 3rd Edition
Pediatric Cancer Sourcebook
Physical & Mental Issues in Aging Sourcebook
Podiatry Sourcebook, 2nd Edition
Pregnancy & Birth Sourcebook, 2nd Edition
Prostate Cancer Sourcebook
Prostate & Urological Disorders Sourcebook
Reconstructive & Cosmetic Surgery Sourcebook
Rehabilitation Sourcebook
Respiratory Disorders Sourcebook, 2nd Edition
Sexually Transmitted Diseases Sourcebook, 3rd Edition
Sleep Disorders Sourcebook, 2nd Edition
Smoking Concerns Sourcebook
Sports Injuries Sourcebook, 3rd Edition
Stress-Related Disorders Sourcebook, 2nd Edition
Stroke Sourcebook, 2nd Edition
Surgery Sourcebook, 2nd Edition
Thyroid Disorders Sourcebook
Transplantation Sourcebook
Traveler's Health Sourcebook
Urinary Tract & Kidney Diseases & Disorders Sourcebook, 2nd Edition

Workplace Health & Safety Sourcebook
Worldwide Health Sourcebook

Teen Health Series

Abuse & Violence Information for Teens
Accident & Safety Information for Teens
Alcohol Information for Teens, 2nd Edition
Allergy Information for Teens
Asthma Information for Teens
Body Information for Teens
Cancer Information for Teens
Complementary & Alternative Medicine Information for Teens
Diabetes Information for Teens
Diet Information for Teens, 2nd Edition
Drug Information for Teens, 2nd Edition
Eating Disorders Information for Teens, 2nd Edition
Fitness Information for Teens, 2nd Edition
Learning Disabilities Information for Teens
Mental Health Information for Teens, 2nd Edition
Pregnancy Information for Teens
Sexual Health Information for Teens, 2nd Edition
Skin Health Information for Teens, 2nd Edition
Sleep Information for Teens
Sports Injuries Information for Teens, 2nd Edition
Stress Information for Teens
Suicide Information for Teens
Tobacco Information for Teens

3/25/11

Men's Health Concerns SOURCEBOOK

Third Edition

Health Reference Series

Third Edition

Men's Health Concerns SOURCEBOOK

Basic Consumer Health Information about Wellness in Men and Gender-Related Differences in Health, Including Facts about Heart Disease, Cancer, Traumatic Injury, Other Leading Causes of Death in Men, Reproductive Concerns, Sexual Dysfunction, Disorders of the Prostate, Penis, and Testes, Sex-Linked Genetic Disorders, and Other Medical and Mental Concerns of Men

Along with Statistical Data, a Glossary of Related Terms, and a Directory of Resources for Additional Information

Edited by
Sandra J. Judd

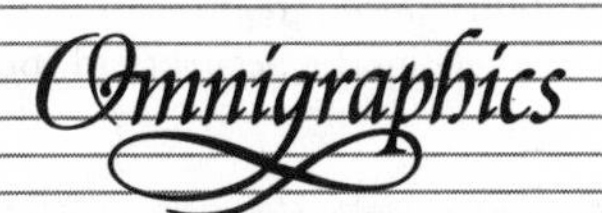

P.O. Box 31-1640, Detroit, MI 48231

Bibliographic Note

Because this page cannot legibly accommodate all the copyright notices, the Bibliographic Note portion of the Preface constitutes an extension of the copyright notice.

Edited by Sandra J. Judd

Health Reference Series

Karen Bellenir, *Managing Editor*
David A. Cooke, MD, FACP, *Medical Consultant*
Elizabeth Collins, *Research and Permissions Coordinator*
Cherry Edwards, *Permissions Assistant*
EdIndex, Services for Publishers, *Indexers*

* * *

Omnigraphics, Inc.
Matthew P. Barbour, *Senior Vice President*
Kevin M. Hayes, *Operations Manager*

* * *

Peter E. Ruffner, *Publisher*

ISBN 978-0-7808-1033-4

Library of Congress Cataloging-in-Publication Data

Men's health concerns sourcebook : basic consumer health information about wellness in men and gender-related differences in health, including facts about heart disease, cancer, traumatic injury, other leading causes of death in men, reproductive concerns, sexual dysfunction, disorders of the prostate, penis, and testes, sex-linked genetic disorders, and other medical and mental concerns of men ; along with statistical data, a glossary of related terms, and a directory of resources for additional information / edited by Sandra J. Judd. -- 3rd ed.

p. cm.

Previous ed. edited by Robert Aquinas McNally.

Summary: "Provides basic consumer health information about health conditions of concern to men, along with tips for maintaining physical and mental wellness. Includes index, glossary of related terms, and other resources"--Provided by publisher.

Includes bibliographical references and index.

ISBN 978-0-7808-1033-4 (hardcover : alk. paper) 1. Men--Health and hygiene--Popular works. I. Judd, Sandra J.

RA776.5.M457 2009

613'.04234--dc22

2009024973

∞

This book is printed on acid-free paper meeting the ANSI Z39.48 Standard. The infinity symbol that appears above indicates that the paper in this book meets that standard.

Printed in the United States

Table of Contents

Visit www.healthreferenceseries.com to view *A Contents Guide to the Health Reference Series*, a listing of more than 15,000 topics and the volumes in which they are covered.

Part II: Leading Causes of Death in Men

Part III: Reproductive and Sexual Concerns

Part IV: Other Common Health Concerns in Men

Part V: Additional Help and Information

Preface

About This Book

American men face a staggering array of health concerns. According to the Centers for Disease Control and Prevention, 70 percent of American men are overweight, a key predictor of future health problems. Almost 25 percent smoke, another key risk factor. One in five American men has heart disease, and 29 percent aged twenty and older suffer from hypertension. More than 11 percent of men face a limitation in their usual activities due to chronic health conditions. In addition, the medical concerns men face often differ from those of most concern to women. Compared with women, nearly twice as many men die of heart disease, and 50 percent more die of cancer. Men are also much more likely to commit suicide or to be victims of accidents and injuries or homicide.

Men's Health Sourcebook, Third Edition, provides up-to-date information on the health conditions of most significance to men. It includes guidelines for maintaining wellness with facts about recommended screenings, checkups, and vaccinations. It discusses heart disease, cancer, and other leading causes of death in men, and it offers information about sexual dysfunction and disorders of the prostate, penis, and testes. Mental health concerns and sex-linked genetic disorders are also described, and the book concludes with a glossary of related terms and a directory of additional resources.

How to Use This Book

This book is divided into parts and chapters. Parts focus on broad areas of interest. Chapters are devoted to single topics within a part.

Part I: Overview of Men's Health and Wellness summarizes male healthcare fundamentals. It discusses the differences in men's and women's life expectancies, includes guidelines for maintaining wellness, and offers tips for avoiding common risk factors. It details the screenings, checkups, vaccinations, and self-examinations recommended for men. Information about maintaining a healthy diet, avoiding obesity, and remaining physically active is also included.

Part II: Leading Causes of Death in Men provides facts about the most common causes of death in men, including heart disease, cancer, accidents and injuries, diabetes, and lung disease. It includes tips for avoiding these problems as well as guidelines for their diagnosis and treatment.

Part III: Reproductive and Sexual Concerns describes the most common reproductive and sexual disorders among men, including sexually transmitted diseases, infertility, sexual dysfunction, and disorders affecting the prostate, penis, and testes. A discussion of how the male reproductive system works, along with details about preventing pregnancy, is also included.

Part IV: Other Common Health Concerns in Men discusses a number of health concerns of special interest to men, including mental illness in men, male pattern baldness, sex-linked genetic disorders, and violence. A chapter is also included that addresses the unique concerns men face with disorders that may more frequently be associated with women, such as body image issues and osteoporosis.

Part V: Additional Help and Information includes a glossary of terms related to men's health and a directory of organizations able to provide additional help and support.

Bibliographic Note

This volume contains documents and excerpts from publications issued by the following U.S. government agencies: Agency for Healthcare Research and Quality (AHRQ); Bureau of Labor Statistics;

Centers for Disease Control and Prevention (CDC); National Cancer Institute (NCI); National Heart, Lung, and Blood Institute (NHLBI); National Highway Transportation Safety Administration (NHTSA); National Human Genome Research Institute (NHGRI); National Institute of Arthritis and Musculoskeletal and Skin Diseases (NIAMS); National Institute of Child Health and Human Development (NICHD); National Institute of Diabetes and Digestive and Kidney Diseases (NIDDK); National Institute of Mental Health (NIMH); National Institute of Neurological Disorders and Stroke (NINDS); National Institute on Aging (NIA); National Institute on Drug Abuse (NIDA); National Kidney Disease Education Program (NKDEP); National Women's Health Information Center (NWHIC); NIH Senior Health; Substance Abuse and Mental Health Services Administration (SAMHSA); U.S. Department of Health and Human Services; U.S. Department of Justice; and the U.S. Food and Drug Administration (FDA).

In addition, this volume contains copyrighted documents from the following organizations: A.D.A.M., Inc.; American Chemical Society; Optometric Association; American Osteopathic Association; American Urological Association; Andrology Australia; Cleveland Clinic; Domestic Abuse Helpline for Men and Women; Home Safety Council; Hormone Foundation; Men Can Stop Rape; National Foundation for Infectious Diseases; National Safety Council; National Sleep Foundation; Nemours Foundation; PsychCentral; Royal College of Psychiatrists; Skin Cancer Foundation; Sudden Cardiac Arrest Association; University of Iowa Hospitals and Clinics; University of Michigan Health System; and the University of Michigan News Service.

Acknowledgements

Thanks go to the many organizations, agencies, and individuals who have contributed materials for this *Sourcebook* and to medical consultant Dr. David Cooke and document engineer Bruce Bellenir. Special thanks go to managing editor Karen Bellenir and permissions coordinator Liz Collins for their help and support.

About the Health Reference Series

The *Health Reference Series* is designed to provide basic medical information for patients, families, caregivers, and the general public. Each volume takes a particular topic and provides comprehensive coverage. This is especially important for people who may be dealing with a newly diagnosed disease or a chronic disorder in themselves or in a family member. People looking for preventive guidance, information about disease warning signs, medical statistics, and risk factors for health problems will also find answers to their questions in the *Health Reference Series*. The *Series*, however, is not intended to serve as a tool for diagnosing illness, in prescribing treatments, or as a substitute for the physician/patient relationship. All people concerned about medical symptoms or the possibility of disease are encouraged to seek professional care from an appropriate healthcare provider.

A Note about Spelling and Style

Health Reference Series editors use *Stedman's Medical Dictionary* as an authority for questions related to the spelling of medical terms and the *Chicago Manual of Style* for questions related to grammatical structures, punctuation, and other editorial concerns. Consistent adherence is not always possible, however, because the individual volumes within the *Series* include many documents from a wide variety of different producers and copyright holders, and the editor's primary goal is to present material from each source as accurately as is possible following the terms specified by each document's producer. This sometimes means that information in different chapters or sections may follow other guidelines and alternate spelling authorities. For example, occasionally a copyright holder may require that eponymous terms be shown in possessive forms (Crohn's disease *vs.* Crohn disease) or that British spelling norms be retained (leukaemia *vs.* leukemia).

Locating Information within the Health Reference Series

The *Health Reference Series* contains a wealth of information about a wide variety of medical topics. Ensuring easy access to all the fact sheets, research reports, in-depth discussions, and other material contained within the individual books of the series remains one of our highest priorities. As the *Series* continues to grow in size and scope, however, locating the precise information needed by a reader may become more challenging.

A Contents Guide to the Health Reference Series was developed to direct readers to the specific volumes that address their concerns. It presents an extensive list of diseases, treatments, and other topics of general interest compiled from the Tables of Contents and major index headings. To access *A Contents Guide to the Health Reference Series*, visit www.healthreferenceseries.com.

Medical Consultant

Medical consultation services are provided to the *Health Reference Series* editors by David A. Cooke, MD, FACP. Dr. Cooke is a graduate of Brandeis University, and he received his M.D. degree from the University of Michigan. He completed residency training at the University of Wisconsin Hospital and Clinics. He is board-certified in Internal Medicine. Dr. Cooke currently works as part of the University of Michigan Health System and practices in Ann Arbor, MI. In his free time, he enjoys writing, science fiction, and spending time with his family.

Our Advisory Board

We would like to thank the following board members for providing guidance to the development of this series:

Dr. Lynda Baker, Associate Professor of Library and Information Science, Wayne State University, Detroit, MI

Nancy Bulgarelli, William Beaumont Hospital Library, Royal Oak, MI

Karen Imarisio, Bloomfield Township Public Library, Bloomfield Township, MI

Karen Morgan, Mardigian Library, University of Michigan-Dearborn, Dearborn, MI

Rosemary Orlando, St. Clair Shores Public Library, St. Clair Shores, MI

Health Reference Series *Update Policy*

The inaugural book in the *Health Reference Series* was the first edition of *Cancer Sourcebook* published in 1989. Since then, the *Series* has been enthusiastically received by librarians and in the medical community. In order to maintain the standard of providing high-quality health information for the layperson the editorial staff at Omnigraphics felt it was necessary to implement a policy of updating volumes when warranted.

Medical researchers have been making tremendous strides, and it is the purpose of the *Health Reference Series* to stay current with the most recent advances. Each decision to update a volume is made on an individual basis. Some of the considerations include how much new information is available and the feedback we receive from people who use the books. If there is a topic you would like to see added to the update list, or an area of medical concern you feel has not been adequately addressed, please write to:

Editor
Health Reference Series
Omnigraphics, Inc.
P.O. Box 31-1640
Detroit, MI 48231
E-mail: editorial@omnigraphics.com

Part One

Overview of Men's Health and Wellness

Chapter 1

Men and Life Expectancy

Chapter Contents

Section 1.1

Evolutionary Forces behind Lower Male Life Expectancy

Despite research efforts to find modern factors that would explain the different life expectancies of men and women, the gap is actually ancient and universal, according to University of Michigan researchers.

"Women live longer in almost every country, and the sex difference in lifespan has been recognized since at least the mid-eighteenth century," said Daniel J. Kruger, a research scientist in the U-M School of Public Health and the Institute for Social Research. "It isn't a recent trend; it originates from our deep evolutionary history."

This skewed mortality isn't even unique to our species; the men come up short in common chimps and many other species, Kruger added.

Kruger and co-author Randolph Nesse, a professor of psychology and psychiatry and director of the Evolution and Human Adaptation Program, argue that the difference in life expectancy stems from the biological imperative of attracting mates.

"This whole pattern is a result of sexual selection and the roles that males and females play in reproduction," Kruger said, "Females generally invest more in offspring than males and are more limited in offspring quantity, thus males typically compete with each other to attract and retain female partners."

For example, in common chimps, the greatest difference in mortality rates for males and females occurs at about thirteen years of age, when the males are just entering the breeding scene and competing aggressively for social status and females.

From the tail of the peacock to the blinged-out sport utility vehicle, males compete aggressively for female attention, and that costs them something. In nature, it means riskier physiology and behavior for the males, such as putting more resources into flashy plumage or engaging in physical sparring.

And even in modern life, where most dueling is a form of entertainment, male behavior and physiology is shortening their life spans relative to women, Kruger said. In fact, modern lifestyles are actually exacerbating the gap between male and female life expectancies.

Male physiology, shaped by eons of sexual competition, is putting the guys at a disadvantage in longevity. Male immune systems are somewhat weaker, and their bodies are less able to process the fat they eat, Kruger said. And behavioral causes—smoking, overeating, reckless driving, violence—set men apart from most women. "Because mortality rates in general are going down, behavioral causes of death are ever more prevalent," Kruger said.

Looking at human mortality rates sliced by socioeconomic status shows that the gender gap is affected by social standing. Human males in lower socioeconomic levels tend to have higher mortality rates than their higher-status peers. The impact of social standing is greater on male mortality than on female mortality, Kruger noted, partially because males who have a relatively lower status or lack a mate engage in a riskier pattern of behaviors in an attempt to get ahead, he said.

Section 1.2

Biological Forces May Aid Women's Longevity

Scientists in Spain and Italy have identified a group of proteins in laboratory rats that could help explain two enduring medical mysteries—why women live longer than men and why calorie restriction stands as the only proven method of extending longevity. Their study, which could help scientists understand the biochemical underpinnings of aging, is scheduled for the July 3, 2008, issue of the American Chemical Society (ACS)'s monthly *Journal of Proteome Research*.

In the study, Adamo Valle and colleagues point out that women, on average, live years longer than men. Previous studies also have shown that diets extremely low in calories consistently increase maximum life spans in a wide range of animals. Scientists have speculated that the explanation may involve hormones, stress, cardiovascular protection, and other factors.

Using lab rats as stand-ins for humans, the researchers found that the livers of both female rats and calorie-restricted rats produced different levels of twenty-seven proteins than male rats or those on a normal diet. The findings suggest that a previously unrecognized set of cellular pathways may be involved in the longevity boost from being female and eating a sparse diet, the study says, suggesting that these insights could lead to new ways of boosting human longevity.

Chapter 2

Does Gender Make a Difference in Health Risks?

When it comes to health risks, sex does matter. Women are twice as likely as men to get multiple sclerosis, rheumatoid arthritis, and migraines. They're also more likely to get cataracts, hepatitis, and thyroid disease. Women experience depression about twice as often as men. And irritable bowel syndrome (IBS) is thought to affect twice as many women as men. Although men have more heart attacks than women, more women die within a year after having a heart attack.

"Despite this increased susceptibility to so many diseases, females across the world have a longer lifespan," says Joseph Verbalis, M.D., clinical director of Georgetown University's Center for the Study of Sex Differences, in Washington, D.C. "We don't know why," says Verbalis, "but that's one of the things we're trying to find out."

Researchers are finding that men and women are different in ways that go beyond their reproductive systems, hormones, and bone structure. They get many of the same diseases, but they may have different symptoms, their diseases may progress differently, and they may respond differently to treatment. While researchers are working to discover the underlying causes of these differences, scientists and regulators at the Food and Drug Administration are working to ensure that drugs and medical devices are safe and effective for both men and women.

Just as one size doesn't fit all, one treatment or test doesn't fit all men or all women. It's important to test drugs and devices in both

---

Reprinted from "Does Sex Make a Difference?" U.S. Food and Drug Administration, July–August 2005.

women and men of different races and ethnicities in clinical trials, says Margaret Miller, Ph.D., manager of scientific programs in the U.S. Food and Drug Administration's (FDA's) Office of Women's Health (OWH).

The FDA has regulations and guidance in place to ensure that both sexes are represented in clinical trials, that study results are analyzed by gender, and that medical products are labeled to alert physicians and patients to any difference in the way men and women respond to a product. In addition, the agency is supporting research to identify gender differences that may affect the use of FDA-regulated products.

Gender as a Starting Point

Men and women are different in every organ of the body—even their skin, says Marianne J. Legato, M.D., a cardiologist and founder and director of Columbia University's Partnership for Gender-Specific Medicine. They are different at the cellular level, and these differences may influence the amount and type of medicine they need to treat a disease. "Dosage is not adjustable simply on the basis of body size anymore," says Legato. "I think we have to look at a whole variety of factors in prescribing dosages that are safe on the basis of gender."

"We know that different people, as individuals, respond to drugs differently," says Miller. "People routinely tell me, 'Oh, that drug doesn't do a thing for me.'" Some researchers place priority on studying differences in genetic makeup by individual, not gender, says Miller. They want to determine the exact sequence of DNA in a person's body in order to tailor treatments for that individual. "But even if the DNA is the same, men and women will express it differently," says Miller.

Researchers looking at DNA sequence may think that's a shortcut, says Legato, "which it obviously would be if we can take a slice of people's DNA and decide whether or not they would react appropriately to any medication to which they've not been previously exposed. That would be the ultimate, but I fear that that's years away. I think it would be nice to know the difference between men and women as a starting point."

In 2001, the Institute of Medicine (IOM), part of the National Academy of Sciences, published a report that supported studying potential gender differences during drug development. The IOM concluded that "sex matters"; that is, "being male or female is an important basic human variable that should be considered when designing and analyzing studies in all areas and at all levels of . . . health-related research." The IOM defined sex-based differences as biologically based differences in men and women, and described gender-based differences as distinctions shaped by the cultural and social environment. Generally, the FDA does not attempt to determine why men are different from women and refers to any identified difference as a "gender difference."

Drugs and Gender Differences

In 1998, the allergy drug Seldane® (terfenadine) was removed from the market when a safer alternative was approved. It had been discovered that Seldane could cause a life-threatening heart rhythm irregularity when used with certain other drugs. More women took Seldane, and more were reported to have had this heart arrhythmia, called torsade de pointes.

Researchers at the Georgetown Center for the Study of Sex Differences believe that the male hormone testosterone may protect the heart from some types of arrhythmia, says Verbalis. In addition, he says, research has shown that women are at greater risk for torsades de pointes because of their QT interval—the time it takes for the heart to relax after it contracts to pump out blood. Women often have a longer QT interval than men, and taking certain drugs can further lengthen this interval, thereby increasing the risk of the fatal arrhythmia more in women than in men.

Some drugs are approved to treat a disease based, in part, on patients' reporting of the relief of their symptoms. For example, Zelnorm® (tegaserod maleate) is approved only for women to relieve the symptoms of IBS. In clinical trials, more women taking Zelnorm reported relief of their symptoms than those taking an inactive pill (placebo).

IBS, which is found more commonly in women, produces a variety of symptoms. "The challenge in the evaluation of a drug for this disease is to determine if there is a gender difference in the patient's perception of symptoms and evaluation of relief of symptoms," says Joyce Korvick, M.D., acting director of the FDA's Division of Gastrointestinal and Coagulation Drug Products. "The perception of 'relief' of symptoms in men and women may be very different."

Because IBS is found more often in women, more women than men were enrolled in the clinical trials for Zelnorm. But for the nearly three hundred men with IBS enrolled in the trials, Zelnorm was not shown to be effective. "More research regarding men and women's perceptions of specific disease symptoms is needed to ensure that differences seen in clinical trials are meaningful to the gender being studied," says Korvick.

Another drug, Zoloft® (sertraline hydrochloride), is approved for both men and women to treat several conditions, including post-traumatic stress disorder (PTSD). This approval was based on clinical trials in which Zoloft showed little effect in men with PTSD, while the drug's benefit over a placebo was clear in the women studied.

"True gender differences in responsiveness may have been one explanation," says Thomas Laughren, M.D., team leader for the FDA's psychiatric drug products group. "However, it should also be noted that the types of PTSD differed in the two groups," he says. Many of the men in these trials had a long-lasting and treatment-resistant PTSD, based on military combat experience, compared to many of the women, who tended to have a more acute form of PTSD, based on recent physical abuse.

Scientists aren't sure why some drugs work better in one gender than in the other. But they do know that differences may occur in the way men and women absorb certain drugs into the bloodstream, distribute them to the body's tissues, break them down, and rid them from the body. The way the body handles a drug is known as pharmacokinetics (PK), and was the subject of an FDA study.

FDA researchers examined three hundred drug applications submitted to the agency between 1994 and 2000. More than half of these applications contained information on the effect of gender on PK. The PK was the same for 80 percent of the drugs in which PK was studied. But for the other 20 percent of the drugs, the PK was different.

"There must be some reason for this difference," says Miller. "That's where research comes in. We want to understand the biology and the mechanism enough to predict what's going to be in the 80 percent group and the 20 percent group. Then we can predict how a product's safety or effectiveness will be influenced in each gender."

Shiew-Mei Huang, Ph.D., deputy director for science in the FDA's Office of Clinical Pharmacology and Biopharmaceutics, says that drug metabolism plays an important role in the way men and women respond to drugs. An enzyme known as cytochrome CYP3A helps metabolize many drugs, and studies have shown that women have more cytochrome CYP3A in the liver, says Huang. Some drugs or dietary supplements, for example, St. John's wort, increase the activity of this enzyme, which makes the drugs break down faster. This rapid breakdown reduces the amount of the drug in the body, decreasing its effectiveness in women.

The reverse scenario may also occur: A drug could slow down enzyme activity, causing too much of the drug to build up in the body and resulting in more side effects.

But biology can't explain all the differences in the way men and women respond to drugs, cautions Huang. Other factors, such as medication use, must be considered. "A recent survey showed that women, in all age groups, tend to take more medications, including dietary supplements, than men," says Huang. This difference may put women at more risk for certain drug interactions than men.

Medical Devices and Gender Differences

Men and women may also respond differently to certain medical devices and the procedures in which they are used. Several FDA studies have focused on identifying some of these differences.

In 2003 and 2004, FDA researchers studied more than 150,000 people with suspected heart disease and found that women had about twice the risk of men for local complications after cardiac catheterization. In the catheterization procedure, a slender tube is inserted into a large artery in the leg (femoral artery) and is threaded up through the body to the heart to diagnose or treat narrowed heart arteries that block blood flow.

"The study was done to look at risks associated with hemostasis devices," says Dale Tavris, M.D., M.P.H., an FDA epidemiologist specializing in preventive medicine. These devices are used after cardiac catheterization to prevent continued bleeding of the femoral artery where the catheter is inserted.

We don't know why complications, such as hemorrhaging, occurred more in women, says Tavris. "There's speculation that it may be due to blood vessel size or hormonal differences. And the risk applies whether or not the hemostasis devices are used." Further information is needed to understand these occurrences, says Tavris, before we can determine whether any changes to the catheterization procedure or to hemostasis devices or their labeling are appropriate.

An FDA-sponsored study at Boston University involves men and women with diabetes who are using blood glucose monitors at home to test their blood several times a day. Researchers are looking for any differences in testing blood drawn from the fingertip or from another part of the body, since newer glucose monitors use blood samples from alternate body areas. "We found that the fingertip can have a different glucose value from an arm or leg, especially when sugar levels are changing rapidly, for example, after a meal or after exercise," says Jean

Cooper, D.V.M., director of the Division of Chemistry and Toxicology in the FDA's Center for Devices and Radiological Health. The study is continuing to determine whether gender might be a factor in this difference in glucose values.

The FDA now requires glucose monitors to carry a warning label cautioning against using alternate sites when glucose levels are changing rapidly. If a manufacturer can show in clinical trials that its device doesn't demonstrate this variance, the warning is not required.

Studies of Both Sexes

In 1977, an FDA guidance said that women able to become pregnant should not participate in the early phases of drug studies, with an exception for studies of potentially life-saving drugs. The exclusion reflected the concern that if a woman became pregnant, the baby might have birth defects.

Over more than two decades, the FDA has worked to ensure that both women and men are represented fairly in clinical trials involving drugs, biologics such as vaccines and blood products, and medical devices.

In 1988, the agency issued guidance to drug makers asking that the safety and effectiveness data in drug applications be analyzed according to gender, age, and race. And, in 1993, the agency issued its Guideline for the Study and Evaluation of Gender Differences in the Clinical Evaluation of Drugs, known as the gender guideline.

When the gender guideline was published, the FDA also revoked the 1977 restriction on women of childbearing age in early drug studies and reiterated the need to include patients of both sexes in the development of drugs, biologics, and medical devices. The guideline also recommended that drug companies analyze separately men's and women's responses to drugs.

Attention to potential gender differences became part of a larger agency effort to ensure that the safety and effectiveness of drugs are adequately studied in people who represent the full range of patients who could use the drugs when approved. In a 1998 regulation known as the Demographic Rule, the FDA again addressed the importance of collecting data on clinical trial volunteers by gender, race, and age. The regulation required companies to analyze the data to look for possible differences in effectiveness, safety, and dose-response and to submit this information in applications for new drugs. It also required reporting demographic data in annual reports during a drug's investigation phase.

A regulation in 1999 gave the agency the authority to halt studies of new drugs to treat life-threatening diseases if clinical trials excluded women solely because they could become pregnant.

"The Demographic Rule and gender guideline represent our commitment to looking at possible differences in various subgroups' response to drugs, whether men and women, black and white, old and young," says Robert Temple, M.D., director of the FDA's Office of Medical Policy. "The guidance tells drug sponsors what our expectation is and what we're looking for."

So far, a small number of differences have been found in the way men and women respond to drugs, says Temple. An FDA study reviewed gender-related labeling for 171 new drugs that were approved for both males and females from 1995 through 1999. Labeling for two-thirds of the drugs contained some statement about gender, although only 22 percent described actual gender differences and none of these differences were considered significant enough to recommend any change in dosage for one gender.

"But just knowing that is useful information," says Miller. "You know you can take these drugs without a higher risk because of your gender."

The FDA is also working to revise drug labeling so that both consumers and health care providers can better understand important information about a drug. A proposed FDA rule will require prescription drug labels to contain "highlights" in a prominent place. The highlights will discuss the more serious and common side effects and significant gender differences found in clinical trials.

Continuing Efforts

The FDA's Office of Women's Health is funding research within the agency to examine gender differences—particularly in the areas of heart disease, obesity, and human immunodeficiency virus (HIV)—that are important for the agency to consider in regulating medical products.

In one project funded by the OWH, scientists within the FDA's Center for Biologics Evaluation and Research are studying the replication of HIV, the virus that causes acquired immunodeficiency syndrome (AIDS), in human blood cells from male and female blood donors. By infecting the blood cells with HIV in a culture medium and then adding various sex hormones, scientists are learning more about the influence of gender on the concentration of the virus. They are also studying the effect of sex hormones on certain antiviral drugs used to treat HIV.

"Some of the things we're looking at may affect when treatment should be started in men and women," says Andrew Dayton, M.D., Ph.D., an FDA research medical officer. And it may give us preliminary insight into how gender might affect response to HIV treatments, he adds. This information may help in designing clinical trials to test the effectiveness of HIV treatments in men and women.

In another initiative, the OWH is developing an innovative knowledge management approach to make better assessments in groups of people (subpopulations) to protect patient safety. The Demographic Information and Data Repository (DIDR) was mandated by Congress in 2002 to monitor the inclusion of women in clinical trials and to study gender differences and variability in response to medical products.

Katherine Hollinger, D.V.M., M.P.H., a senior health promotions officer in the OWH, says the DIDR will help the agency to look at

Table 2.1. Gender Differences in Disease Risk

Disorder	Gender Differences
Heart attack	Men have more, but women are more likely to die within a year after a heart attack; women tend to get heart disease seven to ten years later than men
Stroke	Women have fewer strokes, but are more likely to die from them than men; women are generally older than men when they have a stroke
Depression	Twice as common in women
Migraine	Three times more common in women
Hearing loss	More common in men
Nearsightedness (myopia)	More common in women through age sixty
Irritable bowel syndrome	More common in women
Cancer	Cancer of the lungs, kidneys, bladder, and pancreas are more common in men; thyroid cancer is more common in women
Osteoporosis	More common in women
Rheumatoid arthritis	Two to three times more common in women
Gout	More common in men
Lupus	Nine times more common in women
Fibromyalgia	Nine times more common in women

Source: National Institutes of Health

groups of people—including groups characterized by gender, race and ethnicity, older people, and children—in a more informed way. "It will allow us to better look at subpopulation issues and differences in drug response that may affect safety and effectiveness," says Hollinger. "And it will allow us to not only track inclusion of women and other populations in clinical trials, but to monitor the types of trials women, children, or the elderly are participating in and identify patterns that are observed."

Other benefits of the agency-wide DIDR include helping the agency to design better studies for new products, enabling more efficient and informed reviews and approval decisions, and allowing better assessments of product labeling.

Part of the problem in looking at study data to determine subpopulation differences in response to medical products is the lack of standard approaches and terminology used in individual studies. The agency is working with the pharmaceutical industry and standards organizations to establish standardized approaches to labeling, study data, and study protocols that will be used in the DIDR to protect the safety of women, men, children, and older people of every race and ethnicity.

Men, Women, and Heart Disease

Heart disease is the leading cause of death in the United States for both men and women, according to the American Heart Association. "But the normal heart is different in men and women," says Marianne J. Legato, M.D., a cardiologist and founder and director of Columbia University's Partnership for Gender-Specific Medicine. "Women's hearts beat faster, even during sleep," she says. And women have different proteins in the heart cells.

"Some data suggest that the whole physiology of the coronary arteries and what keeps them open and what causes them to go into spasm might be significantly different in men and women," says Legato, adding that some women have had heart attacks without any of the fatty buildup of plaque seen in the coronary arteries in most people with heart attacks.

And the symptoms of a heart attack may be different. "Twenty percent of women will not have the 'typical symptoms' of chest pain radiating down the left arm," says Legato, "but will instead describe nausea, profound sweating, and shortness of breath and pain in the upper abdomen."

Chapter 3

Making Decisions about Health Care

Chapter Contents

Section 3.1

Choosing a Doctor

"Choosing a Doctor," Excerpted from *Your Guide to Choosing Quality Health Care*, AHRQ Publication No. 99-0012, July 2001, Agency for Healthcare Research and Quality, Rockville, MD. http://www.ahrq.gov/consumer/qnt/. Reviewed by David A. Cooke, M.D., March 2009.

It is important to choose your doctor with care, because quality varies. For example, the Pacific Business Group on Health asked patients of California doctors' groups how they rated their care. The results? More than 80 percent of the patients said they were satisfied with their care. But fewer than two-thirds were happy with the ease of getting that care.

This section can help you choose a primary care doctor who will meet your needs and give you quality care. The information also may be useful in choosing any specialists you might need. Primary care doctors are specially trained to serve as your main doctor over the long term. They provide your medical and health care, help you stay healthy, and help to manage your care. Your primary care doctor can refer you to specialists (doctors who treat only certain parts of the body, conditions, or age groups) if you need them.

Quick Check for Quality

Look for a doctor who:

- is rated to give quality care;
- has the training and background that meet your needs;
- takes steps to prevent illness—for example, talks to you about quitting smoking;
- has privileges at the hospital of your choice;
- is part of your health plan, unless you can you afford to pay extra;
- encourages you to ask questions;
- listens to you;

- explains things clearly;
- treats you with respect.

Doctors and Health Plans

If you already are in a health plan, your choices may be limited to doctors who participate in the plan. But if you have a choice of plans, you may want to first think about which doctor(s) you would like to use. Then, you may be able to choose a plan that has your choice of doctor(s).

Decide What You Want and Need in a Doctor

What is most important to you in a doctor? A few ideas are listed below. Add your own to create a list that will help you choose a doctor who is right for you:

- My doctor must be highly rated by a consumer or other group. You will want to find out who did the ratings. Is the information reliable? Who collected it? Does the group have something to gain from the ratings?
- My doctor needs to have experience with my condition(s). Research shows that doctors who have a lot of experience with a condition tend to have better success with it.
- I want a doctor who has privileges (is permitted to practice) at the hospital of my choice.
- My doctor must be part of my health plan.

Make a List of Doctors

- If you are in a managed care plan, check the plan's list of doctors first. Ask doctors or other health professionals who work with doctors, such as hospital nurses. Check the "Physician Select" service of the website of the American Medical Association. This can give you lists of doctors, by specialty, who practice near you. You can also check on training and board certification: http://www.ama-assn.org/aps/amahg.htm.
- Call a doctor referral service at a hospital. But keep in mind that these services usually refer you to any of the doctors on the staff of that hospital. The services do not have information on the quality of care these doctors provide.

- Some local medical societies offer lists of doctors who are members. Again, these lists do not have information on the quality of care these doctors provide.
- Ask family, friends, neighbors, and co-workers.

Check on Quality

Once you have a list of doctors, there are several ways to check on their skills and knowledge, and the quality of care they provide:

- Find out if a consumer or other group has rated doctors in the area where you live. Again you will want to find out how reliable the ratings are.
- Information on doctors in some states is available on the internet at http://www.docboard.org. This website is run by Administrators in Medicine—a group of state medical board directors.
- The American Board of Medical Specialties (800-733-2267) can tell you if the doctor is board certified. "Certified" means that the doctor has completed a training program in a specialty and has passed an exam (board) to assess his or her knowledge, skills, and experience to provide quality patient care in that specialty. Primary care doctors also may be certified as specialists. You can also check the Website at http://www.certifacts.org. (While board certification is a good measure of a doctor's knowledge, it is possible to receive quality care from doctors who are not board certified.)
- Call the American Medical Association (AMA) at 312-464-5000 for information on training, specialties, and board certification about many licensed doctors in the United States. This information also can be found in "Physician Select" at AMA's Website: http://www.ama-assn.org/aps/amahg.htm.

Contact the Doctors' Offices

When you have found a few names of doctors you might want to try, call their offices. The first thing to find out is whether the doctor is covered by your health plan and is taking new patients. If the doctor is not covered by your plan, are you prepared to pay the extra costs?

Below are some questions you might want to ask the office manager or other staff. You may have some additional questions. Note that some of these items might have more to do with the health plan than with the doctor's office.

Things to find out from the office staff:

- Which hospitals does the doctor use?
- What are the office hours (when is the doctor available and when can I speak to office staff)?
- Does the doctor or someone else in the office speak the language that I am most comfortable speaking?
- How many other doctors "cover" for the doctor when he or she is not available? Who are they?
- How long does it usually take to get a routine appointment?
- How long might I need to wait in the office before seeing the doctor?
- What happens if I need to cancel an appointment? Will I have to pay for it anyway?
- Does the office send reminders about prevention tests?
- What do I do if I need urgent care or have an emergency?
- Does the doctor (or a nurse or physician assistant) give advice over the phone for common medical problems?

You may also want to talk briefly with the doctor by phone or in person. Ask if you are able to do this and if there is a charge.

The next step is to schedule a visit with your top choice. During that first visit you will learn a lot about just how easy it is to talk with the doctor. You will also find out how well the doctor might meet your medical needs. Ask yourself, did the doctor:

- give me a chance to ask questions?
- really listen to my questions?
- answer in terms I understood?
- show respect for me?
- ask me questions?
- make me feel comfortable?
- address the health problem(s) I came with?
- ask me my preferences about different kinds of treatments?
- spend enough time with me?

Trust your own reactions when deciding whether this doctor is the right one for you. But you also may want to give the relationship some time to develop. It takes more than one visit for you and your doctor to get to know each other.

Once You Leave the Doctor's Office, Follow Up

- If you have questions, call.
- If your symptoms get worse, or if you have problems with your medicine, call.
- If you had tests and do not hear from your doctor, call for your test results.
- If your doctor said you need to have certain tests, make appointments at the lab or other offices to get them done.
- If your doctor said you should see a specialist, make an appointment.

Urgent or Emergency Care Centers

What if you get sick at night, on a holiday, or over the weekend? You can't get to your doctor, but you are not sick enough to go to the emergency room. There may be an "urgent" or "emergency" care center near you. These centers are open long hours every day to handle problems that are not life threatening. But they are no substitute for a regular primary care doctor.

To make sure an urgent or emergency care center provides quality care, call your health plan or visit the center to find out the following things:

- If your health plan will cover your care there.
- If it is licensed. Then check to see if it is accredited by a group such as the Joint Commission on Accreditation of Healthcare Organizations (telephone 630-792-5800; Website http://www.jcaho.org) or the Accreditation Association for Ambulatory Healthcare (telephone 847-853-6060; Website http://www.aaahc.org). The accreditation certificate should be posted in the facility.
- How well trained and experienced the center's health care professionals are.
- If the center is affiliated with a hospital. If it is not, find out how the center will handle any emergency that could happen during your visit.

Section 3.2

Tips for Using Medicines Safely

Reprinted from "Check Your Medicines: Tips for Using Medicines Safely," Agency for Healthcare Research and Quality, AHRQ Publication No. 08-M044-A, April 2008.

Take a List or a Bag with All Your Medicines When You Go to Your Doctor's Office, the Pharmacy, or the Hospital

Include all prescription and over-the-counter medicines, vitamins, and herbal supplements that you use. If your doctor prescribes a new medicine, ask if it is safe to use with your other medicines. Remind your doctor and pharmacist if you are allergic to any medicines.

Ask Questions about Your Medicines

Ask questions and make sure you understand the answers. Choose a pharmacist and doctor you feel comfortable talking with about your health and medicines. Take a relative or friend with you to ask questions and remind you about the answers later. Write down the answers.

Make Sure Your Medicine Is What the Doctor Ordered

Does the medicine seem different than what your doctor wrote on the prescription or look different than what you expected? Does a refill look like it is a different shape, color, or size than what you were given before? If something seems wrong, ask the pharmacist to double-check it. Most errors are first found by patients.

Ask How to Use the Medicine Correctly

Read the directions on the label and other information you get with your medicine. Have the pharmacist or doctor explain anything you do not understand. Are there other medicines, foods, or activities (such as driving, drinking alcohol, or using tobacco) that you should avoid while using the medicine? Ask if you need lab tests to check how the medicine is working or to make sure it doesn't cause harmful side effects.

Ask about Possible Side Effects

Side effects can occur with many medicines. Ask your doctor or pharmacist what side effects to expect and which ones are serious. Some side effects may bother you but will get better after you have been using the medicine for a while. Call your doctor right away if you have a serious side effect or if a side effect does not get better. A change in the medicine or the dose may be needed.

Section 3.3

How to Get a Second Opinion

Reprinted from "Tools to Help You Build a Healthier Life: How to Get a Second Opinion," National Women's Health Information Center, October 2006.

Even though doctors may get similar medical training, they can have their own opinions and thoughts about how to practice medicine. They can have different ideas about how to diagnose and treat conditions or diseases. Some doctors take a more conservative, or traditional, approach to treating their patients. Other doctors are more aggressive and use the newest tests and therapies. It seems like we learn about new advances in medicine almost every day.

Many doctors specialize in one area of medicine, such as cardiology or obstetrics or psychiatry. Not every doctor can be skilled in using all the latest technology. Getting a second opinion from a different doctor might give you a fresh perspective and new information. It could provide you with new options for treating your condition. Then you can make more informed choices. If you get similar opinions from two doctors, you can also talk with a third doctor.

Tips: What to Do

Ask your doctor for a recommendation: Ask for the name of another doctor or specialist, so you can get a second opinion. Don't worry about hurting your doctor's feelings. Most doctors welcome a second opinion, especially when surgery or long-term treatment is involved.

Ask someone you trust for a recommendation: If you don't feel comfortable asking your doctor for a referral, then call another doctor you trust. You can also call university teaching hospitals and medical societies in your area for the names of doctors. Some of this information is also available on the Internet.

Check with your health insurance provider: Call your insurance company before you get a second opinion. Ask if they will pay for this office visit. Many health insurance providers do. Ask if there are any special procedures you or your primary care doctor need to follow.

Ask to have medical records sent to the second doctor: Ask your primary care doctor to send your medical records to the new doctor. You need to give written permission to your current doctor to send any records or test results to a new doctor. You can also ask for a copy of your own medical records for your files. Your new doctor can then examine these records before your office visit.

Learn as much as you can: Ask your doctor for information you can read. Go to a local library. Search the Internet. Find a teaching hospital or university that has medical libraries open to the public. The information you find can be hard to understand, or just confusing. Make a list of your questions, and bring it with you when you see your new doctor.

Do not rely on the Internet or a telephone conversation: When you get a second opinion, you need to be seen by a doctor. That doctor will perform a physical examination and perhaps other tests. The doctor will also thoroughly review your medical records, ask you questions, and address your concerns.

Chapter 4

Recommended Screenings and Vaccinations for Men

Chapter Contents

Section 4.1

Stay Healthy at Any Age: Men's Checklist for Health

Excerpted from "Men: Stay Healthy at Any Age—Your Checklist for Health," Agency for Healthcare Research and Quality, AHRQ Publication No. 07-IP006-A, February 2007.

What can you do to stay healthy and prevent disease? You can get certain screening tests, take preventive medicine if you need it, and practice healthy behaviors.

Top health experts from the U.S. Preventive Services Task Force suggest that when you go for your next checkup, you should talk to your doctor or nurse about how you can stay healthy no matter what your age.

The most important things you can do to stay healthy are as follows:

- Get recommended screening tests.
- Be tobacco free.
- Be physically active.
- Eat a healthy diet.
- Stay at a healthy weight.
- Take preventive medicines if you need them.

Screening Tests for Men: What You Need and When

Screening tests can find diseases early, when they are easier to treat. Health experts from the U.S. Preventive Services Task Force have made recommendations, based on scientific evidence, about testing for the conditions below. Talk to your doctor about which ones apply to you and when and how often you should be tested.

Obesity: Have your body mass index (BMI) calculated to screen for obesity. (BMI is a measure of body fat based on height and weight.) You can also find your own BMI with the table in chapter 7.

High cholesterol: Have your cholesterol checked regularly starting at age thirty-five. If you are younger than thirty-five, talk to your doctor about whether to have your cholesterol checked if any of the following are true:

- You have diabetes.
- You have high blood pressure.
- Heart disease runs in your family.
- You smoke.

High blood pressure: Have your blood pressure checked at least every two years. High blood pressure is 140/90 or higher.

Colorectal cancer: Have a test for colorectal cancer starting at age fifty. Your doctor can help you decide which test is right for you. If you have a family history of colorectal cancer, you may need to be screened earlier.

Diabetes: Have a test for diabetes if you have high blood pressure or high cholesterol.

Depression: Your emotional health is as important as your physical health. If you have felt "down," sad, or hopeless over the last two weeks or have felt little interest or pleasure in doing things, you may be depressed. Talk to your doctor about being screened for depression.

Sexually transmitted infections: Talk to your doctor to see whether you should be tested for gonorrhea, syphilis, chlamydia, or other sexually transmitted infections.

Human immunodeficiency virus (HIV): HIV is the virus that can cause acquired immunodeficiency syndrome (AIDS). Talk to your doctor about HIV screening if any of the following are true:

- You have had sex with men since 1975.
- You have had unprotected sex with multiple partners.
- You have used or now use injection drugs.
- You exchange sex for money or drugs or have sex partners who do.
- You have past or present sex partners who are HIV-infected, are bisexual, or use injection drugs.

- You are being treated for sexually transmitted diseases.
- You had a blood transfusion between 1978 and 1985.

Abdominal aortic aneurysm: If you are between the ages of sixty-five and seventy-five and have ever smoked (one hundred or more cigarettes during your lifetime), you need to be screened once for abdominal aortic aneurysm, which is an abnormally large or swollen blood vessel in your abdomen.

Daily Steps to Health

Don't smoke: If you do smoke, talk to your doctor about quitting. Your doctor or nurse can help you. And, you can also help yourself. For tips on how to quit, go to chapter 10.

Be physically active: Walking briskly, mowing the lawn, dancing, swimming, and bicycling are just a few examples of moderate physical activity. If you are not already physically active, start small and work up to thirty minutes or more of moderate physical activity most days of the week.

Eat a healthy diet: Emphasize fruits, vegetables, whole grains, and fat-free or low-fat milk and milk products; include lean meats, poultry, fish, beans, eggs, and nuts; and eat foods low in saturated fats, trans fats, cholesterol, salt (sodium), and added sugars.

Stay at a healthy weight: Balance calories from foods and beverages with calories you burn off by your activities. To prevent gradual weight gain over time, make small decreases in food and beverage calories and increase physical activity.

Drink alcohol only in moderation: If you drink alcohol, have no more than two drinks a day. (A standard drink is one 12-ounce bottle of beer or wine cooler, one 5-ounce glass of wine, or 1.5 ounces of 80-proof distilled spirits.)

Should You Take Medicines to Prevent Disease?

Aspirin

Ask your doctor about taking aspirin to prevent heart disease if any of the following are true:

- You are older than forty-five
- You are younger than forty-five and:
  - have high blood pressure;
  - have high cholesterol;
  - have diabetes;
  - smoke.

Immunizations

Stay up-to-date with your immunizations:

- Have a flu shot every year starting at age fifty. If you are younger than fifty, ask your doctor whether you need a flu shot.
- Have a pneumonia shot once after you turn sixty-five. If you are younger, ask your doctor whether you need a pneumonia shot.

Section 4.2

Colorectal Cancer Screening

Reprinted from "Colorectal Cancer: Basic Facts on Screening," U.S. Centers for Disease Control and Prevention, January 2006.

What is Colorectal Cancer?

Colorectal cancer is cancer that occurs in the colon or rectum. Sometimes it is called colon cancer, for short. The colon is the large intestine or large bowel. The rectum is the passageway that connects the colon to the anus.

It's the Second Leading Cancer Killer

Colorectal cancer is the second leading cancer killer in the United States, but it doesn't have to be. If everybody age fifty or older had regular screening tests, at least one-third of deaths from this cancer could be avoided. So if you are fifty or older, start screening now.

Who Gets Colorectal Cancer?

- Both men and women can get colorectal cancer.
- Colorectal cancer is most often found in people fifty and older.
- The risk for getting colorectal cancer increases with age.

Are You at High Risk?

Your risk for colorectal cancer may be higher than average if either of the following are true:

- You or a close relative have had colorectal polyps or colorectal cancer.
- You have inflammatory bowel disease.

People at high risk for colorectal cancer may need earlier or more frequent tests than other people. Talk to your doctor about when you should begin screening and how often you should be tested.

Screening Saves Lives

If you're fifty or older, getting a screening test for colorectal cancer could save your life. Here's how:

- Colorectal cancer usually starts from polyps in the colon or rectum. A polyp is a growth that shouldn't be there.
- Over time, some polyps can turn into cancer.
- Screening tests can find polyps, so they can be removed before they turn into cancer.
- Screening tests can also find colorectal cancer early. When it is found early, the chance of being cured is good.

Colorectal Cancer Can Start With No Symptoms

People who have polyps or colorectal cancer sometimes don't have symptoms, especially at first. This means that someone could have polyps or colorectal cancer and not know it. That is why having a screening test is so important.

What Are the Symptoms?

Some people with colorectal polyps or colorectal cancer do have symptoms. They may include the following:

- Blood in or on your stool (bowel movement).
- Pain, aches, or cramps in your stomach that happen a lot and you don't know why.
- A change in bowel habits, such as having stools that are narrower than usual.
- Losing weight and you don't know why.

If you have any of these symptoms, talk to your doctor. These symptoms may also be caused by something other than cancer. However, the only way to know what is causing them is to see your doctor.

Types of Screening Tests

There are several different screening tests that can be used to find polyps or colorectal cancer. Each one can be used alone. Sometimes they are used in combination with each other. Talk to your doctor about which test or tests are right for you and how often you should be tested.

Fecal occult blood test or stool test: For this test, you receive a test kit from your doctor or health care provider. At home, you put a small piece of stool on a test card. You do this for three bowel movements in a row. Then you return the test cards to the doctor or a lab. The stool samples are checked for blood. This test should be done every year.

Flexible sigmoidoscopy: For this test, the doctor puts a short, thin, flexible, lighted tube into your rectum. The doctor checks for polyps or cancer inside the rectum and lower third of the colon. This test should be done every five years.

Fecal occult blood test plus flexible sigmoidoscopy: Your doctor may ask you to have both tests. Some experts believe that by using both tests, there is a better chance of finding polyps or colorectal cancer.

Colonoscopy: This test is similar to flexible sigmoidoscopy, except the doctor uses a longer, thin, flexible, lighted tube to check for polyps or cancer inside the rectum and the entire colon. During the test, the doctor can find and remove most polyps and some cancers. This test should be done every ten years. Colonoscopy may also be used as a follow-up test if anything unusual is found during one of the other screening tests.

Double contrast barium enema: This test is an x-ray of your colon. You are given an enema with a liquid called barium. Then the doctor takes an x-ray. The barium makes it easy for the doctor to see the outline of your colon on the x-ray to check for polyps or other abnormalities. This test should be done every five years.

Will Insurance or Medicare Pay for Screening Tests?

Many insurance plans and Medicare help pay for colorectal cancer screening tests. Check with your plan to find out which tests are covered for you.

Section 4.3

Prostate Cancer Screening

"Prostate Cancer Screening," is reprinted with permission from www.urologyhealth.org,

Currently, digital rectal examination (DRE) and prostate specific antigen (PSA) are used for prostate cancer detection. The age at which time screening for prostate cancer should begin is not known with certainty. However, most experts agree that healthy men over the age of fifty should consider prostate cancer screening with a DRE and PSA test. Screening should occur earlier, at age forty, in those who are at a higher risk of prostate cancer, such as African-American men or those with a family history of prostate cancer. Men who are concerned about their future risk of prostate cancer should be screened to assess their baseline risk for developing the disease.

Digital rectal exam (DRE): The DRE is performed with the man either bending over, lying on his side, or with his knees drawn up to his chest on the examining table. The physician inserts a gloved finger into the rectum and examines the prostate gland, noting any abnormalities in size, contour, or consistency. DRE is inexpensive, easy to perform, and allows the physician to note other abnormalities such as blood in the stool or rectal masses, which may allow for the early detection of rectal or colon cancer. However, DRE is not the most effective way to detect an early cancer, so it should be combined with a PSA test.

Prostate specific antigen test: The PSA test is usually performed in addition to DRE and increases the likelihood of prostate cancer detection. The test measures the level of PSA, a substance produced only by the prostate, in the bloodstream. The PSA should be less than 1.0 ng/ml The median for men in their forties is 0.7 ng/ml. If the PSA is higher than the age-specific median, the risk of developing prostate cancer and the risk of having an aggressive form of the disease are increased. Accordingly, the patient might be well advised to have more frequent screening to detect a rise in the PSA level over time.

This blood test can be performed in a clinical laboratory, hospital, or physician's office and requires no special preparation on the part of the patient. Ideally, the test should be taken before a digital rectal examination is performed or any catheterization or instrumentation of the urinary tract. Furthermore, because ejaculation can transiently elevate the PSA level for twenty-four to forty-eight hours, men should abstain from sexual activity for two days prior to having a PSA test. A tourniquet or rubber strap is tied around the upper arm to mildly restrict the flow of blood and keep blood in the vein. Then, a needle with a tube-like container attached is inserted into a vein, usually in the bend of the elbow or the top of the hand. After a sufficient sample of blood is obtained, the needle is withdrawn, a bandage is placed on the puncture site, and firm pressure is held until the bleeding stops. The entire test takes less than five minutes and produces only mild discomfort. After, the patient may experience slight bruising at the puncture site.

Very little PSA escapes from a healthy prostate into the bloodstream, but certain prostatic conditions can cause larger amounts of PSA to leak into the blood. One possible cause of a high PSA level is benign (noncancerous) enlargement of the prostate, otherwise known as BPH. Inflammation of the prostate, called prostatitis, is another common cause of PSA elevation, as is recent ejaculation. Prostate cancer is the most serious possible cause of an elevated PSA level. The frequency of PSA testing remains a matter of some debate. The American Urological Association (AUA) encourages men to have annual PSA testing starting at age fifty. The AUA also recommends annual PSA testing for men over the age of forty who are African American or have a family history of the disease (for example, a father or brother who was diagnosed with prostate cancer), or for those who are interested in an early risk assessment. Some experts have suggested that men with an initial normal DRE and PSA level of less than 2.5 ng/ml can have PSA testing performed every two years. However, a disadvantage of infrequent testing is that it limits the ability to detect a rapidly rising PSA level that can signal aggressive prostate cancer. Recently, several refinements have been made in the PSA blood test in an attempt to determine more accurately who has prostate cancer and who has false-positive PSA elevations caused by other conditions like BPH. These refinements include PSA density, PSA velocity, PSA age-specific reference ranges and use of free-to-total PSA ratios. Such refinements may increase the ability to detect cancer and these should be discussed with your physician.

Currently, it is recommended that both a DRE and PSA test be used for the early detection of prostate cancer. It is important to realize that in most cases an abnormality in either test is not due to cancer but to benign conditions, the most common being BPH or prostatitis. For instance, it has been shown that only 18 to 30 percent of men with serum PSA values between 4 and 10 ng/ml have prostate cancer. This number rises to approximately 42 to 70 percent for those men whose PSA values exceeding 10 ng/ml.

Section 4.4

New Research Questions Benefit of Annual Prostate Cancer Screening

Excerpted from "U.S. Cancer Screening Trial Shows No Early Mortality Benefit from Annual Prostate Cancer Screening," National Cancer Institute, March 18, 2009.

Six annual screenings for prostate cancer led to more diagnoses of the disease, but no fewer prostate cancer deaths, according to a major new report from the Prostate, Lung, Colorectal, and Ovarian (PLCO) Cancer Screening Trial, a seventeen-year project of the National Cancer Institute (NCI), part of the National Institutes of Health. The PLCO was designed to provide answers about the effectiveness of prostate cancer screening.

"What this report tells us is that there may be some men who are diagnosed with prostate cancer and have the side-effects of treatment, such as impotence and incontinence, with little chance of benefit," said John E. Niederhuber, M.D., director of the NCI. "Clearly, we need a better way of detecting prostate cancer at its earliest stages and as importantly, a method of determining which tumors will progress. Many of the molecular studies we're currently sponsoring will hopefully yield new, better ways of definitively classifying which men need treatment and which can consider watchful waiting. Until we have developed and verified a new test's benefits and harms, as we have done with the PLCO, regular visits to your doctor to monitor your health are still strongly recommended."

Results appeared online March 18, 2009, in the *New England Journal of Medicine*, to coincide with presentation of the data at the European Association of Urology meeting in Stockholm, Sweden. The print version of the results appeared in the March 26, 2009, issue.

NCI does not have a recommendation about prostate cancer screening. The U.S. Preventive Services Task Force, whose recommendations are considered the gold standard for clinical preventive services, recently concluded that there is insufficient evidence to assess the balance of benefits and harms of prostate cancer screening in men younger than age seventy-five and recommended against prostate cancer screening in men age seventy-five and older.

There were 76,693 men in the PLCO trial that was conducted at ten centers around the United States. Of the men in the trial, 38,343 were randomly assigned to screening with annual prostate-specific antigen (PSA) tests for six rounds and digital rectal exams (DRE) for four rounds. The other 38,350 men were randomly assigned to usual care, but received no recommendations for or against annual prostate cancer screening.

Of those men who were screened annually, 85 percent had PSA tests and 86 percent had DREs. Men in the usual-care arm sometimes had these tests as well, due to the growing public acceptance of such screening. Screening by PSA in this usual-care group increased from 40 percent at the beginning of the study to 52 percent of men by the last screening year, and screening with DRE ranged from 41 percent initially to 46 percent by the last screening year. Men in the screening arm were referred to their usual health care provider for follow-up testing for prostate cancer if their PSA level was greater than 4.0 nanograms per milliliter (ng/mL) or if a DRE found an abnormality.

This report includes data for all participants at seven years after they joined the trial and for 67 percent of participants at ten years after they joined the trial. Other important findings are as follows.

At seven years, 22 percent more prostate cancers were diagnosed in the screening arm. This excess is continuing to be observed in data collected up to ten years (currently a 17 percent excess).

The vast majority of men in both groups who developed prostate cancer were diagnosed with relatively early stage II (out of four stages, of which IV is late stage) disease, and the number of later-stage cases was similar in the two groups. However, using the Gleason scoring system, which assesses tumor aggressiveness, men in the usual-care group had more prostate cancers that fell into the Gleason 8 to 10 range, which marks them as more aggressive. The smaller number of men with prostate cancer with a Gleason score of 8 to 10 in the intervention group may eventually lead to a mortality difference between men in the two groups but data analyzed so far have not shown such a difference.

Men in both groups who were diagnosed with prostate cancer at the same stage received similar treatments for their disease. This reflects the PLCO study design policy of not mandating specific therapies.

At seven years, fifty deaths were attributable to prostate cancer in the screening group and forty-four deaths were attributable in the usual-care group. Through year ten, there were ninety-two prostate cancer deaths in the screening group and eighty-two in the usual-care group. The difference between the numbers of deaths in the two groups was not statistically significant. Thus there was no detectable mortality benefit for screening vs. usual-care.

Given the uncertainties about the mortality benefits of PSA testing, NCI has been pursuing many avenues to find new ways of screening for prostate cancer, including several sets of biomarkers that are being validated in its Early Detection Research Network (EDRN), some using specimens from PLCO's biorepository of tissue and blood. Some examples of the marker tests include using microstrands of RNA to detect disease, examining changes in genes such as GSTP1, and imaging of proteins in prostate cancer tissue.

"NCI wants to understand why some prostate cancers are lethal even when found early by annual screening, and what approaches can be used to identify these more aggressive cancers when they can be effectively treated," said Christine Berg, M.D., NCI leader of the PLCO trial and senior author of the study. "The PLCO biorepository is an invaluable resource for such research, with nearly three million biological samples collected from our participants. Our hope is that through all aspects of the PLCO, we will gather the information that tells us whom to treat aggressively and whom to avoid overtreating."

Another report in this same online publication of the *NEJM* [*New England Journal of Medicine*] is from the large European Randomized Study of Screening for Prostate Cancer (ERSPC), which shows a 20 percent reduction in the rate of death from prostate cancer but with a high risk of overdiagnosis. In the ERSPC, unlike the PLCO trial, men were referred for follow-up testing if their PSA level was 3.0 ng/mL or higher and were also screened, on average, every four years as opposed to annually in the PLCO.

"Approaches such as lowering the threshold for what is considered an abnormal PSA level to 3.0 ng/mL will diagnose more cases, but it is not at all clear that it will identify the prostate cancers that are more likely to lead to a man's death," said Berg.

The PLCO data are being made public now because the study's Data and Safety Monitoring Board (DSMB), an independent review committee that meets every six months saw a continuing lack of evidence that screening reduces death due to prostate cancer as well as the suggestion that screening may cause men to be treated unnecessarily. The DSMB also supports continued follow-up of all participants so that every participant is tracked for at least thirteen years from entry onto the trial.

The PLCO is a large-scale clinical trial, sponsored and run by NCI's Division of Cancer Prevention, begun in 1992 to determine whether certain cancer screening tests can help reduce deaths from prostate, lung, colorectal and ovarian cancer. The underlying rationale for the trial is that screening for cancer may enable doctors to discover and treat the disease earlier.

Nearly 155,000 women and men between the ages of fifty-five and seventy-four have joined the PLCO trial. At entry, participants were assigned at random to one of two study groups: One group received routine health care from their health providers. The other received a series of exams to screen for prostate, lung, colorectal, and ovarian cancers. Screening of participants ended in late 2006. Follow-up of participants is anticipated to continue for several more years.

Section 4.5

Adult Immunization Questions and Answers

Excerpted from "Adult Immunization Questions and Answers," © 2008 National Foundation for Infectious Diseases (www.nfid.org). Reprinted with permission.

Are there vaccines that protect against communicable diseases for adults?

Yes! Vaccinations are readily available for such common adult illnesses as influenza (flu), pneumococcal disease, herpes zoster (shingles), human papillomavirus (HPV), pertussis (whooping cough), hepatitis A, and hepatitis B. Vaccinations against less common diseases such as measles, mumps, rubella (German measles), tetanus (lockjaw), diphtheria, and varicella (chickenpox) are also needed by some adults. The Centers for Disease Control and Prevention's (CDC) recommendations clearly identify people who are at risk for these diseases and who should be immunized to prevent these diseases and their complications. Consult your healthcare provider or local health department regarding your own immunization status as well as current immunization recommendations.

Which vaccinations do adults need?

All adults require tetanus and diphtheria (Td) immunizations at ten-year intervals throughout their lives. Adults who deferred Td boosters during 2001 and early 2002 because of vaccine shortages should get back on track—the supply problems have been resolved. Additionally, adults younger than sixty-five years of age should substitute a tetanus, diphtheria, acellular pertussis (Tdap) vaccination for one Td booster.

Adults born after 1956 who are not immune to measles, mumps, or rubella should be immunized.

Women twenty-six years of age or younger should be immunized against human papillomavirus (HPV), the virus that causes about 70 percent of all cervical cancer cases in the United States.

All adults sixty-five years of age or older, as well as persons two to sixty-four years of age who have diabetes or chronic heart, lung, liver, or kidney disorders need protection against pneumococcal disease, and should consult their healthcare providers regarding this vaccine.

Influenza vaccination is recommended for all adults fifty years of age or older, women who will be pregnant during influenza season, and residents of long-term care facilities, as well as for all children six months through eighteen years of age, and persons who have certain chronic medical conditions. Other individuals who should seek annual influenza immunization include healthcare workers and those who live with or provide care for high-risk persons, including those who live with or who provide care for infants younger than six months of age.

Hepatitis B vaccine is recommended for adults in certain high-risk groups, such as healthcare workers and public safety workers exposed to blood on the job; household and sex contacts of persons with chronic hepatitis B virus (HBV) infection; sexually active people who are not in long-term, mutually monogamous relationships; people seeking evaluation or treatment for sexually transmitted disease (STD); men who have sex with men; injection drug users; travelers to countries where HBV infection is common; people with end-stage renal disease; and human immunodeficiency virus (HIV)–infected persons. Hepatitis B vaccine is also recommended for anyone seeking protection from HBV infection. To increase vaccination rates among people at highest risk for HBV infection, hepatitis B vaccine is recommended for all adults in the following settings: STD treatment facilities, HIV testing and treatment facilities, facilities providing drug-abuse treatment and prevention services, healthcare settings targeting services to injection-drug users or men who have sex with men, correctional facilities, end-stage renal disease programs and facilities for chronic hemodialysis patients, and institutions and nonresidential daycare facilities for persons with developmental disabilities.

Hepatitis A vaccine is recommended for adults in certain high-risk groups, including travelers to countries where hepatitis A is common, people with chronic liver disease, people who have blood clotting-factor disorders such as hemophilia, men who have sex with men, and users of injection and non-injection illegal drugs.

Varicella vaccine is recommended for all adults who have not had chickenpox and have not been immunized previously against chickenpox, including teachers of young children and daycare workers, residents and staff in institutional settings, military personnel, nonpregnant women of childbearing age, international travelers, healthcare workers, and family members of immunocompromised persons.

Meningococcal vaccination is recommended for adults (not previously immunized with the meningococcal conjugate vaccine) with asplenia or terminal complement deficiencies, who will be first-year college students living in dormitories, who are military recruits or certain laboratory workers, or who will be traveling to or living in countries in which meningococcal disease is common. The vaccine is also recommended for administration to all adolescents eleven to eighteen years of age.

Adults sixty years of age and older should receive a single dose of zoster vaccine whether or not they report a prior episode of herpes zoster (shingles). Persons with chronic medical conditions may be vaccinated unless a contraindication or precaution exists for their condition.

Where can I obtain my vaccinations?

Vaccinations should be available from family doctors and internists. Additionally, your city or county health department or local hospital may hold clinics to administer influenza, pneumococcal, hepatitis A, and hepatitis B vaccines. Many pharmacies offer these and other immunizations. Clinics may also be available in shopping malls, grocery stores, senior centers, and other community settings.

How often do I need to be immunized?

Immunizations for pneumococcal disease (except for patients at particular risk for pneumococcal complications), measles, mumps, and rubella are usually administered once, and offer protection for life. A single pneumococcal revaccination is recommended for persons who were vaccinated prior to age sixty-five. Some persons born after 1956 may require a second measles and mumps vaccination. Women twenty-six years of age and younger should receive three doses of the HPV vaccine to prevent cervical cancer. Influenza vaccine must be administered yearly because the strains in the vaccine are updated nearly every year and because protection from the vaccine does not last from year to year. Additional booster doses of tetanus and diphtheria vaccines (usually given as a combination Td vaccine) are required every ten years to maintain immunity against these diseases. One of these booster doses should be the tetanus, diphtheria, acellular pertussis (Tdap) vaccine, for adults younger than sixty-five years of age. Two doses of hepatitis A are needed six to twelve months apart to ensure long-term protection. Hepatitis B vaccine is usually administered in three doses given over a six-month period. Two doses of chickenpox vaccine are recommended for people thirteen years old or older who have not had the disease or been immunized. One dose of zoster vaccine is recommended for persons sixty years of age and older.

Are there side effects to these vaccines?

Vaccines are among the safest medical products available. Some common side effects are a sore arm or low-grade fever. As with any medical product, there are very small risks that serious problems could occur after getting a vaccine. However, the potential risks associated with the diseases these vaccines prevent are much greater than the potential risks associated with the vaccines themselves.

What vaccines do I need if I'm traveling abroad?

Contact your healthcare provider or the public health department as early as possible to check on the vaccinations you may need. Vaccines against certain diseases such as hepatitis A, hepatitis B, yellow fever, and typhoid fever are recommended for different countries. The time required to receive all vaccinations will depend on whether you need one dose or a series of doses. A variety of books are available from libraries and bookstores providing information on specific vaccines required by different countries as well as general health measures for travelers. Up-to-date information on immunization recommendations for international travelers is available from the Centers for Disease Control and Prevention.

Section 4.6

Facts about the Seasonal Flu Vaccine

Reprinted from "Key Facts about Seasonal Flu Vaccine," U.S. Centers for Disease Control and Prevention, July 16, 2008.

The single best way to protect against the flu is to get vaccinated each year.

There are two types of vaccines:

- **The "flu shot":** An inactivated vaccine (containing killed virus) that is given with a needle, usually in the arm. The flu shot is approved for use in people older than six months, including healthy people and people with chronic medical conditions.
- **The nasal-spray flu vaccine:** A vaccine made with live, weakened flu viruses that do not cause the flu (sometimes called LAIV for "live attenuated influenza vaccine" or FluMist®). LAIV (FluMist®) is approved for use in healthy people two to forty-nine years of age who are not pregnant.

Each vaccine contains three influenza viruses—one A (H3N2) virus, one A (H1N1) virus, and one B virus. The viruses in the vaccine change each year based on international surveillance and scientists' estimations about which types and strains of viruses will circulate in a given year.

About two weeks after vaccination, antibodies that provide protection against influenza virus infection develop in the body.

When to Get Vaccinated

Yearly flu vaccination should begin in September or as soon as vaccine is available and continue throughout the influenza season, into December, January, and beyond. This is because the timing and duration of influenza seasons vary. While influenza outbreaks can happen as early as October, most of the time influenza activity peaks in January or later.

Who Should Get Vaccinated

In general, anyone who wants to reduce their chances of getting the flu can get vaccinated. However, it is recommended by the Advisory Committee on Immunization Practices (ACIP) that certain people should get vaccinated each year. They are either people who are at high risk of having serious flu complications or people who live with or care for those at high risk for serious complications. During flu seasons when vaccine supplies are limited or delayed, ACIP makes recommendations regarding priority groups for vaccination.

People who should get vaccinated each year are as follows:

- Children aged six months up to their nineteenth birthday
- Pregnant women
- People fifty years of age and older
- People of any age with certain chronic medical conditions
- People who live in nursing homes and other long-term care facilities
- People who live with or care for those at high risk for complications from flu, including health care workers, household contacts of persons at high risk for complications from the flu, or household contacts and out of home caregivers of children less than six months of age (these children are too young to be vaccinated)

Use of the Nasal Spray Flu Vaccine

It should be noted that vaccination with the nasal-spray flu vaccine is always an option for healthy people two to forty-nine years of age who are not pregnant.

Who Should Not Be Vaccinated

There are some people who should not be vaccinated without first consulting a physician. These include the following:

- People who have a severe allergy to chicken eggs
- People who have had a severe reaction to an influenza vaccination

- People who developed Guillain-Barré syndrome (GBS) within six weeks of getting an influenza vaccine
- Children less than six months of age (influenza vaccine is not approved for this age group)
- People who have a moderate-to-severe illness with a fever (they should wait until they recover to get vaccinated)

Vaccine Effectiveness

The ability of flu vaccine to protect a person depends on the age and health status of the person getting the vaccine, and the similarity or "match" between the virus strains in the vaccine and those in circulation. Testing has shown that both the flu shot and the nasal-spray vaccine are effective at preventing the flu.

Vaccine Side Effects (What to Expect)

Different side effects can be associated with the flu shot and LAIV.

The Flu Shot

The viruses in the flu shot are killed (inactivated), so you cannot get the flu from a flu shot. Some minor side effects that could occur are as follows:

- Soreness, redness, or swelling where the shot was given
- Fever (low grade)
- Aches

If these problems occur, they begin soon after the shot and usually last one to two days. Almost all people who receive influenza vaccine have no serious problems from it. However, on rare occasions, flu vaccination can cause serious problems, such as severe allergic reactions. As of July 1, 2005, people who think that they have been injured by the flu shot can file a claim for compensation from the National Vaccine Injury Compensation Program (VICP).

LAIV (FluMist®)

The viruses in the nasal-spray vaccine are weakened and do not cause severe symptoms often associated with influenza illness. (In clinical studies, transmission of vaccine viruses to close contacts has occurred only rarely.)

In children, side effects from LAIV (FluMist®) can include the following:

- Runny nose
- Wheezing
- Headache
- Vomiting
- Muscle aches
- Fever

In adults, side effects from LAIV (FluMist®) can include the following:

- Runny nose
- Headache
- Sore throat
- Cough

Chapter 5

Self-Examinations Can Lead to Early Cancer Detection

Chapter Contents

Section 5.1

Skin Cancer Self-Examination

Reprinted from "Self-Examination: How to Spot Skin Cancer," "Warning Signs: The ABCDEs of Melanoma," and "The Ugly Duckling Sign: An Early Melanoma Recognition Tool," © 2008 Skin Cancer Foundation (www.skincancer.org). Reprinted with permission.

Self-Examination

Coupled with a yearly skin exam by a doctor, self-examination of your skin once a month is the best way to detect the early warning signs of basal cell carcinoma, squamous cell carcinoma, and melanoma, the three main types of skin cancer. Look for a new growth or any skin change.

What you'll need: a bright light; a full-length mirror; a hand mirror; two chairs or stools; a blow dryer.

Examine head and face, using one or both mirrors. Use blow dryer to inspect scalp.

Check hands, including nails. In full-length mirror, examine elbows, arms, underarms.

Focus on neck, chest, torso. Women: Check under breasts.

With back to the mirror, use hand mirror to inspect back of neck, shoulders, upper arms, back, buttocks, legs.

Sitting down, check legs and feet, including soles, heels, and nails. Use hand mirror to examine genitals.

Melanoma, the deadliest form of skin cancer, is especially hard to stop once it has spread (metastasized) to other parts of the body. But it can be readily treated in its earliest stages.

Warning Signs: The ABCDEs of Melanoma

Moles, brown spots, and growths on the skin are usually harmless—but not always. Anyone who has more than one hundred moles is at greater risk for melanoma. The first signs can appear in one or more of these moles. That's why it's so important to get to know your skin very well, so you can recognize any changes in the moles on your body. Look for the ABCDEs of melanoma, and if you see one or more, make an appointment with a dermatologist immediately.

Asymmetry: If you draw a line through the mole, the two halves will not match, meaning it is asymmetrical, a warning sign for melanoma.

Border: The borders of an early melanoma tend to be uneven. The edges may be scalloped or notched.

Color: Having a variety of colors is another warning signal. A number of different shades of brown, tan, or black could appear. A melanoma may also become red, white, or blue.

Diameter: Melanomas usually are larger in diameter than the size of the eraser on your pencil (1/4 inch or 6 mm), but they may sometimes be smaller when first detected.

Evolving: Any change—in size, shape, color, elevation, or another trait, or any new symptom such as bleeding, itching, or crusting—points to danger.

Prompt action is your best protection. Common moles and melanomas do not look alike.

Table 5.1. Characteristics of Benign and Malignant Skin Growths

Benign	Malignant
Symmetrical	Asymmetrical
Borders are even	Borders are uneven
One shade	Two or more shades
Smaller than 1/4 inch	Larger than 1/4 inch

The Ugly Duckling Sign: An Early Melanoma Recognition Tool

A recently developed early detection tool can improve early diagnosis critical to the successful treatment of melanoma.

For many years, the early warning signs of melanoma have been identified by the acronym "ABCDE" (A stands for asymmetry, B stands for border, C for color, D for diameter, and E for evolving or changing was recently added.). While the ABCDE rule helps detect many melanomas, there are a group of melanomas that do not manifest the ABCDE features. Recently, several melanoma specialists developed a new method of sight detection for skin lesions which could be melanoma.

This new method of sight detection for skin lesions is based on the concept that these melanomas look different—i.e., "the ugly duckling"—compared to surrounding moles. Thus, during skin self examination, patients and physicians should be looking for lesions that manifest the ABCDEs *and* for lesions that look different compared to surrounding moles.

As reported in the December 2007 issue of *The Melanoma Letter*, a publication of the Skin Cancer Foundation, an approach combining the ABCDEs and the "Ugly Duckling" technique should improve the chances of early detection of all types of melanoma. In the article "The 'Ugly Duckling' Sign: An Early Melanoma Recognition Tool For Clinicians and the Public" by Dr. Alon Scope and Dr. Ashfaq A. Marghoob of Memorial Sloan Kettering Cancer Center (New York, N.Y.), the premise of the ugly duckling sign is that the patient's "normal" moles resemble each other, like siblings.

The doctors suggest thinking of "the ugly duckling" mole, a.k.a. "the outlier," as the lesion that, at a given moment in time, looks or feels different than the patient's other moles, or that over time, changes differently than the patient's other moles. The "ugly duckling" methodology may be especially useful in the detection of nodular melanoma, a dangerous type of melanoma, which notoriously lacks the classic ABCDE signs.

Section 5.2

Testicular Self-Examination

The testicular self-examination (TSE) is an easy way for guys to check their own testicles to make sure there aren't any unusual lumps or bumps—which can be the first sign of testicular cancer.

Although testicular cancer is rare in teenage guys, overall it is the most common cancer in males between the ages of fifteen and thirty-five. It's important to try to do a TSE every month so you can become familiar with the normal size and shape of your testicles, making it easier to tell if something feels different or abnormal in the future.

Here's what to do:

- It's best to do a TSE during or right after a hot shower or bath. The scrotum (skin that covers the testicles) is most relaxed then, which makes it easier to examine the testicles.
- Examine one testicle at a time. Use both hands to gently roll each testicle (with slight pressure) between your fingers. Place your thumbs over the top of your testicle, with the index and middle fingers of each hand behind the testicle, and then roll it between your fingers.
- You should be able to feel the epididymis (the sperm-carrying tube), which feels soft, rope-like, and slightly tender to pressure, and is located at the top of the back part of each testicle. This is a normal lump.
- Remember that one testicle (usually the right one) is slightly larger than the other for most guys—this is also normal.
- When examining each testicle, feel for any lumps or bumps along the front or sides. Lumps may be as small as a piece of rice or a pea.

- If you notice any swelling, lumps, or changes in the size or color of a testicle, or if you have any pain or achy areas in your groin, let your doctor know right away.

Lumps or swelling may not be cancer, but they should be checked by your doctor as soon as possible. Testicular cancer is almost always curable if it is caught and treated early.

Chapter 6

Nutrition and Wellness

Chapter Contents

Section 6.1

Dietary Changes for a Healthier You

Reprinted from "Finding Your Way to a Healthier You," U.S. Department of Agriculture, April 5, 2005.

Feel Better Today, Stay Healthy for Tomorrow

The food and physical activity choices you make every day affect your health—how you feel today, tomorrow, and in the future. The science-based advice of the *Dietary Guidelines for Americans, 2005* highlights how make smart choices from every food group, find your balance between food and physical activity, and get the most nutrition out of your calories.

You may be eating plenty of food, but not eating the right foods that give your body the nutrients you need to be healthy. You may not be getting enough physical activity to stay fit and burn those extra calories. This chapter is a starting point for finding your way to a healthier you.

Eating right and being physically active aren't just a "diet" or a "program"—they are keys to a healthy lifestyle. With healthful habits, you may reduce your risk of many chronic diseases such as heart disease, diabetes, osteoporosis, and certain cancers, and increase your chances for a longer life.

The sooner you start, the better for you, your family, and your future.

Make Smart Choices from Every Food Group

The best way to give your body the balanced nutrition it needs is by eating a variety of nutrient-packed foods every day. Just be sure to stay within your daily calorie needs.

A healthy eating plan is one that does the following:

- Emphasizes fruits, vegetables, whole grains, and fat-free or low-fat milk and milk products
- Includes lean meats, poultry, fish, beans, eggs, and nuts

- Is low in saturated fats, trans fats, cholesterol, salt (sodium), and added sugars.

Don't Give in When You Eat Out and Are on the Go

It's important to make smart food choices and watch portion sizes wherever you are—at the grocery store, at work, in your favorite restaurant, or running errands. Try these tips:

- At the store, plan ahead by buying a variety of nutrient-rich foods for meals and snacks throughout the week.
- When grabbing lunch, have a sandwich on whole-grain bread and choose low-fat/fat-free milk, water, or other drinks without added sugars.
- In a restaurant, opt for steamed, grilled, or broiled dishes instead of those that are fried or sautéed.
- On a long commute or shopping trip, pack some fresh fruit, cut-up vegetables, string cheese sticks, or a handful of unsalted nuts—to help you avoid impulsive, less healthful snack choices.

Mix Up Your Choices within Each Food Group

Focus on fruits: Eat a variety of fruits—whether fresh, frozen, canned, or dried—rather than fruit juice for most of your fruit choices. For a two-thousand-calorie diet, you will need two cups of fruit each day (for example, one small banana, one large orange, and 1/4 cup of dried apricots or peaches).

Vary your veggies: Eat more dark green veggies, such as broccoli, kale, and other dark leafy greens; orange veggies, such as carrots, sweet potatoes, pumpkin, and winter squash; and beans and peas, such as pinto beans, kidney beans, black beans, garbanzo beans, split peas, and lentils.

Get your calcium-rich foods: Get three cups of low-fat or fat-free milk—or an equivalent amount of low-fat yogurt and/or low-fat cheese (1½ ounces of cheese equals one cup of milk)—every day. For kids aged two to eight, it's two cups of milk. If you don't or can't consume milk, choose lactose-free milk products or calcium-fortified foods and beverages.

Make half your grains whole: Eat at least 3 ounces of whole-grain cereals, breads, crackers, rice, or pasta every day. One ounce is about 1 slice of bread, 1 cup of breakfast cereal, or ½ cup of cooked rice or pasta. Look to see that grains such as wheat, rice, oats, or corn are referred to as "whole" in the list of ingredients.

Go lean with protein: Choose lean meats and poultry. Bake it, broil it, or grill it. And vary your protein choices—with more fish, beans, peas, nuts, and seeds.

Know the limits on fats, salt, and sugars: Read the Nutrition Facts label on foods. Look for foods low in saturated fats and trans fats. Choose and prepare foods and beverages with little salt (sodium) or added sugars (caloric sweeteners).

Find Your Balance between Food and Physical Activity

Becoming a healthier you isn't just about eating healthy—it's also about physical activity. Regular physical activity is important for your overall health and fitness. It also helps you control body weight by balancing the calories you take in as food with the calories you expend each day. Here are some tips:

- Be physically active for at least thirty minutes most days of the week.
- Increasing the intensity or the amount of time that you are physically active can have even greater health benefits and may be needed to control body weight. About sixty minutes a day may be needed to prevent weight gain.
- Children and teenagers should be physically active for sixty minutes every day, or most every day.

Consider this: If you eat one hundred more food calories a day than you burn, you'll gain about one pound in a month. That's about ten pounds in a year. The bottom line is that to lose weight, it's important to reduce calories and increase physical activity.

Get the Most Nutrition out of Your Calories

There is a right number of calories for you to eat each day. This number depends on your age, activity level, and whether you're trying to gain, maintain, or lose weight. You could use up the entire amount on a few high-calorie items, but chances are you won't get the full range of vitamins and nutrients your body needs to be healthy.

Choose the most nutritionally rich foods you can from each food group each day—those packed with vitamins, minerals, fiber, and other nutrients but lower in calories. Pick foods like fruits, vegetables, whole grains, and fat-free or low-fat milk and milk products more often.

Nutrition: Know the Facts, Use the Label

Most packaged foods have a Nutrition Facts label. For a healthier you, use this tool to make smart food choices quickly and easily. Try these tips:

- **Keep these low:** saturated fats, trans fats, cholesterol, and sodium.
- **Get enough of these:** potassium, fiber, vitamins A and C, calcium, and iron.
- **Use the % Daily Value (DV) column when possible:** 5 percent DV or less is low, 20 percent DV or more is high.

Check servings and calories: Look at the serving size and how many servings you are actually consuming. If you double the servings you eat, you double the calories and nutrients, including the % DVs.

Make your calories count: Look at the calories on the label and compare them with what nutrients you are also getting to decide whether the food is worth eating. When one serving of a single food item has more than 400 calories per serving, it is high in calories.

Don't sugarcoat it: Since sugars contribute calories with few, if any, nutrients, look for foods and beverages low in added sugars. Read the ingredient list and make sure that added sugars are not one of the first few ingredients. Some names for added sugars (caloric sweeteners) include sucrose, glucose, high fructose corn syrup, corn syrup, maple syrup, and fructose.

Know your fats: Look for foods low in saturated fats, trans fats, and cholesterol to help reduce the risk of heart disease (5% DV or less is low, 20% DV or more is high). Most of the fats you eat should be polyunsaturated and monounsaturated fats. Keep total fat intake between 20 percent and 35 percent of calories.

Reduce sodium (salt), increase potassium: Research shows that eating less than 2,300 milligrams of sodium (about 1 tsp of salt) per day may reduce the risk of high blood pressure. Most of the sodium people eat comes from processed foods, not from the saltshaker. Also look for foods high in potassium, which counteracts some of sodium's effects on blood pressure.

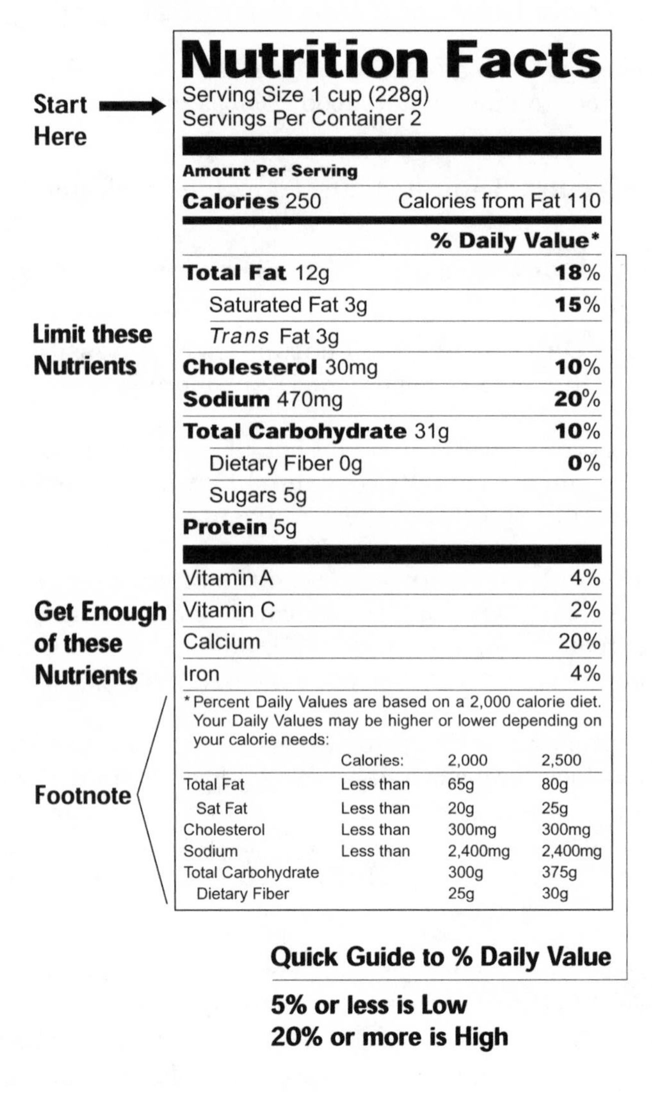

Figure 6.1. Nutrition Facts Label

Play It Safe with Food

Know how to prepare, handle, and store food safely to keep you and your family safe:

- Clean hands, food-contact surfaces, fruits, and vegetables. To avoid spreading bacteria to other foods, meat and poultry should not be washed or rinsed.
- Separate raw, cooked, and ready-to-eat foods while shopping, preparing, or storing.
- Cook meat, poultry, and fish to safe internal temperatures to kill microorganisms.
- Chill perishable foods promptly and thaw foods properly.

Table 6.1. Safe Cooking and Holding Temperatures for Foods

180° F	Whole poultry
170° F	Poultry breasts
165° F	Stuffing, ground poultry, reheat leftovers
160° F	Meats (medium), egg dishes, pork, and ground meats
145° F	Beef steaks, roasts, veal, lamb (medium rare)
140° F	Hold hot foods
41°–139° F	DANGER ZONE
40° F	Refrigerator temperatures
0° F	Freezer temperatures

About Alcohol

If you choose to drink alcohol, do so in moderation. Moderate drinking means up to one drink a day for women and up to two drinks for men. Twelve ounces of regular beer, 5 ounces of wine, or 1.5 ounces of 80-proof distilled spirits count as a drink for purposes of explaining moderation. Remember that alcoholic beverages have calories but are low in nutritional value.

Generally, anything more than moderate drinking can be harmful to your health. Some people, or people in certain situations, shouldn't drink at all. If you have questions or concerns, talk to your doctor or healthcare provider.

Section 6.2

Diet and Disease

Reprinted from "Diet and Disease,"

There are nutritional and dietary elements that have proven relationships to certain diseases or conditions. For additional information on U.S. Food and Drug Administration (FDA)–approved health claims, refer to nutrition labeling.

Calcium and Osteoporosis

Calcium is one of the most important minerals for human life. The body uses it to form and maintain healthy bones and teeth. Calcium also plays a vital role in nerve conduction, muscle contraction, and blood clotting.

Osteoporosis is a disease in which the calcium content of bones is very low. In this disease, calcium and phosphorus, which are normally present in the bones, become reabsorbed back into the body. This process results in brittle, fragile bones that are easily broken.

Getting enough calcium in the diet throughout childhood and puberty is one key to preventing osteoporosis. A person who does not get enough calcium growing up will not have sturdy bones. An older person who consumes a low-calcium diet is also at great risk for osteoporosis.

The recommended dietary allowances (RDA) for calcium are based on age, gender, and hormonal factors. Many foods, such as some vegetables, contain calcium. However, milk and dairy products are some of the best food sources. Calcium may also be obtained by taking supplements.

Fiber and Cancer

Dietary fiber is found in plant foods, where it occurs in two forms: soluble and insoluble. Soluble fiber attracts water and turns to gel during digestion. This process slows digestion and the rate of nutrient absorption from the stomach and intestine.

Soluble fiber is found in oat bran, barley, nuts, seeds, dried beans and legumes, lentils, peas, and some fruits and vegetables. Insoluble fiber also adds bulk (fiber) to the stool. It is found in wheat bran, vegetables, and whole grains.

A diet high in fiber is thought to reduce the risk of cancers of the rectum and colon.

Fruits, Vegetables, and Cancer

Eating more fruits and vegetables helps provide a good supply of fiber, vitamin A, vitamin C, beta carotene and other carotenoids, and valuable substances called phytochemicals. Studies have shown that a diet high in these nutrients and fiber can reduce the risk of developing cancers of the stomach, colon, rectum, esophagus, larynx, and lung.

Vitamin C and beta carotene, which forms vitamin A, are antioxidants. As such, they protect body cells from oxidation, a process that can lead to cell damage and may play a role in cancer.

In addition to nutrients that are needed for normal metabolism, plant foods also contain phytochemicals, plant chemicals that may affect human health. There are hundreds of phytochemicals, and their exact role in promoting health is still uncertain. However, a growing body of evidence indicates that phytochemicals may help protect against cancer.

To get these benefits, eat more fruits and vegetables that contain vitamins A and C and beta carotene. These include dark-green leafy vegetables such as spinach, kale, collards, and turnip greens. Citrus fruits, such as oranges, grapefruit, and tangerines, are also high in antioxidants. Other red, yellow, and orange fruits and vegetables or their juices are also healthful choices. Note: Juicing removes the fiber.

Fiber and Coronary Heart Disease

Some fiber, especially soluble fiber, binds to lipids such as cholesterol. The fiber then carries the lipids out of the body through the stool. This lowers the concentration of lipids in the blood and may reduce the risk of coronary heart disease.

Fat and Cancer

A diet high in fat has been shown to increase the risk of cancers of the breast, colon, and prostate. A high-fat diet does not necessarily cause cancer. Rather, it may promote the development of cancer in people who are exposed to cancer-causing agents.

A diet high in fat may promote cancer by causing the body to secrete more of certain hormones that create a favorable environment for certain types of cancer. Breast cancer is one of these hormone-influenced cancers. High-fat diets also may change the characteristics of the cells to make them more vulnerable to cancer-causing agents.

To reduce fat in the diet, choose lean cuts of beef, lamb, and pork as well as skinless poultry and fish. Baking, broiling, poaching, and steaming are recommended cooking methods. Choose skim or low-fat milk and dairy products, as well as low-fat salad dressings.

Saturated Fat, Cholesterol, and Coronary Heart Disease

Eating too much saturated fat is one of the major risk factors for heart disease. A diet high in saturated fat causes cholesterol, a soft, waxy substance, to build up in the arteries. Eventually, the arteries harden and narrow. The result is an increased pressure in the arteries as well as strain on the heart to maintain adequate blood flow throughout the body.

Because of its high calorie content, too much dietary fat also increases the risk of heart disease in that it increases the likelihood that a person will become obese. Obesity is another risk factor for heart disease.

Sodium and Hypertension

Sodium is a mineral that helps the body regulate blood pressure. Sodium is also commonly known as salt. It also plays a role in the proper functioning of cell membranes, muscles, and nerves. Sodium concentration in the body is mainly controlled by the kidneys, adrenal glands, and the pituitary gland in the brain.

The balance between dietary intake and kidney excretion through urine determines the amount of sodium in the body. Only a small amount of sodium is lost through the stool or sweat. The amount of sodium in urine is controlled by the steroid hormone aldosterone. Water and sodium are also related. Retention of more sodium is followed by retention of more fluid, and vice versa.

Sodium-sensitive individuals may experience high blood pressure from too much sodium in the diet. The American Heart Association has developed specific guidelines for sodium intake. Dietary changes may be helpful. Sodium intake may have little effect in persons without high blood pressure, but it may have a profound effect in sodium-sensitive individuals. Blood pressure is often controlled by diuretics that cause sodium excretion in the urine.

Alcohol

Alcohol use increases the risk of liver cancer. When combined with smoking, alcohol intake also increases the risk of cancers of the mouth, throat, larynx, and esophagus. In addition, alcohol intake is associated with an increased risk of breast cancer in women.

Alcohol is processed by the liver into energy for the body. Continued and excessive use of alcohol can damage the liver in various ways, including the development of a fatty liver. A fatty liver can lead to cirrhosis of the liver.

Alcohol can damage the lining of the small intestine and stomach, where most nutrients are digested. As a result, alcohol can impair the absorption of essential nutrients. Alcohol also increases the body's need for some nutrients, and interferes with the absorption and storage of other nutrients.

Continued and excessive use of alcohol can result in an increase in blood pressure. Chronic heavy drinking also can cause damage to the heart muscle (cardiomyopathy). In addition, stroke is associated with both chronic heavy drinking and binge drinking.

If you choose to drink alcohol, do so in moderation—no more than two drinks per day for a man, one per day for a woman.

Nitrates and Cancer

Countries in which people eat a lot of salt-cured, smoked, and nitrite-cured foods have a high rate of cancer of the stomach and esophagus. Examples of such foods include bacon, ham, hot dogs, and salt-cured fish.

Eat salted, smoked, or cured foods only on occasion.

Chapter 7

Managing Your Weight: Avoiding Overweight and Obesity

What Are Overweight and Obesity?

The terms "overweight" and "obesity" refer to a person's overall body weight and where the extra weight comes from. Overweight is having extra body weight from muscle, bone, fat, and/or water. Obesity is having a high amount of extra body fat. The most useful measure of overweight and obesity is the body mass index (BMI). BMI is based on height and weight and is used for adults, children, and teens.

Millions of Americans and people worldwide are overweight or obese. Being overweight or obese puts you at risk for many diseases and conditions. The more body fat that you carry around and the more you weigh, the more likely you are to develop heart disease, high blood pressure, type 2 diabetes, gallstones, breathing problems, and certain cancers.

A person's weight is a result of many factors. These factors include environment, family history and genetics, metabolism (the way your body changes food and oxygen into energy), behavior or habits, and other factors.

Certain things, like family history, can't be changed. However, other things—like a person's lifestyle habits—can be changed. You can help prevent or treat overweight and obesity if you do the following things:

- Follow a healthful diet, while keeping your calorie needs in mind

---

Excerpted from "Overweight and Obesity," National Heart Lung and Blood Institute, National Institutes of Health, May 2008.

- Be physically active
- Limit the time you spend being physically inactive

Weight loss medicines and surgery also are options for some people who need to lose weight if lifestyle changes don't work.

Outlook

Reaching and staying at a healthy weight is a long-term challenge for people who are overweight or obese. But it also can be a chance to lower your risk of other serious health problems. With the right treatment and motivation, it's possible to lose weight and lower your long-term disease risk.

What Causes Overweight and Obesity?

Energy Balance

For most people, overweight and obesity are caused by not having energy balance. Weight is balanced by the amount of energy or calories you get from food and drinks (this is called energy IN) equaling the energy your body uses for things like breathing, digesting, and being physically active (this is called energy OUT).

Energy balance means that your energy IN equals your energy OUT. To maintain a healthy weight, your energy IN and OUT don't have to balance exactly every day. It's the balance over time that helps you maintain a healthy weight:

- The same amount of energy IN and energy OUT over time = weight stays the same
- More IN than OUT over time = weight gain
- More OUT than IN over time = weight loss

Overweight and obesity happen over time when you take in more calories than you use.

Other Causes

Physical inactivity: Many Americans aren't very physically active. There are many reasons for this. One reason is that many people spend hours in front of TVs and computers doing work, schoolwork, and leisure activities. In fact, more than two hours a day of regular TV viewing time has been linked to overweight and obesity.

Other reasons for not being active include: relying on cars instead of walking to places, fewer physical demands at work or at home because modern technology and conveniences reduce the need to burn calories, and lack of physical education classes in schools for children.

People who are inactive are more likely to gain weight because they don't burn up the calories that they take in from food and drinks. An inactive lifestyle also raises your risk for heart disease, high blood pressure, diabetes, colon cancer, and other health problems.

Environment: Our environment doesn't always help with healthy lifestyle habits; in fact, it encourages obesity. Some reasons are as follows:

- *Lack of neighborhood sidewalks and safe places for recreation:* Not having area parks, trails, sidewalks, and affordable gyms makes it hard for people to be physically active.
- *Work schedules:* People often say that they don't have time to be physically active, given the long hours at work and the time spent commuting back and forth to work.
- *Oversized food portions:* Americans are surrounded by huge food portions in restaurants, fast food places, gas stations, movie theaters, supermarkets, and even home. Some of these meals and snacks can feed two or more people. Eating large portions means too much energy IN. Over time, this will cause weight gain if it isn't balanced with physical activity.
- *Lack of access to healthy foods:* Some people don't live in neighborhoods that have supermarkets that sell healthy foods such as fresh fruits and vegetables. Or if they do, these items are often too costly.
- *Food advertising:* Americans are surrounded by ads from food companies. Often children are the targets of advertising for high-calorie, high-fat snacks and sugary drinks. The goal of these ads is to sway people to buy these high-calorie foods, and often they do.

Genes and family history: Studies of identical twins who have been raised apart show that genes have a strong influence on one's weight. Overweight and obesity tend to run in families. Your chances of being overweight are greater if one or both of your parents are overweight or obese. Your genes also may affect the amount of fat you store in your body and where on your body you carry the extra fat.

Because families also share food and physical activity habits, there is a link between genes and the environment. Children adopt the habits of their parents. So, a child with overweight parents who eat high-calorie foods and are inactive will likely become overweight like the parents. On the other hand, if a family adopts healthful food and physical activity habits, the child's chance of being overweight or obese is reduced.

Health conditions: Sometimes hormone problems cause overweight and obesity. These problems include the following:

- *Underactive thyroid (also called hypothyroidism):* This is a condition in which the thyroid gland doesn't make enough thyroid hormone. Lack of thyroid hormone will slow down your metabolism and cause weight gain. You'll also feel tired and weak.
- *Cushing syndrome:* This is a condition in which the body's adrenal glands make too much of the hormone cortisol. Cushing syndrome also can happen when people take high levels of medicines such as prednisone for long periods of time. People with Cushing syndrome gain weight and have upper-body obesity, a rounded face, fat around the neck, and thin arms and legs.
- *Polycystic ovarian syndrome (PCOS):* This is a condition that affects about 5 to 10 percent of women of childbearing age. Women with PCOS often are obese, have excess hair growth, and have reproductive and other health problems due to high levels of hormones called androgens.

Medicines: Certain medicines, such as corticosteroids (for example, prednisone), antidepressants (for example, Elavil®), and medicines for seizures (for example, Neurontin®), may cause you to gain weight. These medicines can slow the rate at which your body burns calories, increase your appetite, or cause your body to hold on to extra water—all of which can lead to weight gain.

Emotional factors: Some people eat more than usual when they are bored, angry, or stressed. Over time, overeating will lead to weight gain and may cause overweight or obesity.

Smoking: Some people gain weight when they stop smoking. One reason is that food often tastes and smells better. Another reason is because nicotine raises the rate at which your body burns calories, so you burn fewer calories when you stop smoking. However, smoking is a serious health risk, and quitting is more important than possible weight gain.

Age: As you get older, you tend to lose muscle, especially if you're less active. Muscle loss can slow down the rate at which your body burns calories. If you don't reduce your calorie intake as you get older, you may gain weight. Midlife weight gain in women is mainly due to aging and lifestyle, but menopause also plays a role. Many women gain around five pounds during menopause and have more fat around the waist than they did before.

Pregnancy: During pregnancy, women gain weight so that the baby gets proper nourishment and develops normally. After giving birth, some women find it hard to lose the weight. This may lead to overweight or obesity, especially after a few pregnancies.

Lack of sleep: Studies find that the less people sleep, the more likely they are to be overweight or obese. People who report sleeping five hours a night, for example, are much more likely to become obese compared to people who sleep seven to eight hours a night.

People who sleep fewer hours also seem to prefer eating foods that are higher in calories and carbohydrates, which can lead to overeating, weight gain, and obesity over time. Hormones that are released during sleep control appetite and the body's use of energy. For example, insulin controls the rise and fall of blood sugar levels during sleep. People who don't get enough sleep have insulin and blood sugar levels that are similar to those in people who are likely to have diabetes.

Also, people who don't get enough sleep on a regular basis seem to have high levels of a hormone called ghrelin (which causes hunger) and low levels of a hormone called leptin (which normally helps to curb hunger).

What Are the Health Risks of Overweight and Obesity?

Being overweight or obese isn't a cosmetic problem. It greatly raises the risk in adults for many diseases and conditions.

Heart disease: This condition occurs when a fatty material called plaque builds up on the inside walls of the coronary arteries (the arteries that supply blood and oxygen to your heart). Plaque narrows the coronary arteries, which reduces blood flow to your heart. Your chances for having heart disease and a heart attack get higher as your body mass index (BMI) increases. Obesity also can lead to congestive heart failure, a serious condition in which the heart can't pump enough blood to meet your body's needs.

High blood pressure (hypertension): This condition occurs when the force of the blood pushing against the walls of the arteries is too high. Your chances for having high blood pressure are greater if you're overweight or obese.

Stroke: Being overweight or obese can lead to a buildup of fatty deposits in your arteries that form a blood clot. If the clot is close to your brain, it can block the flow of blood and oxygen and cause a stroke. The risk of having a stroke rises as BMI increases.

Type 2 diabetes: This is a disease in which blood sugar (glucose) levels are too high. Normally, the body makes insulin to move the blood sugar into cells where it's used. In type 2 diabetes, the cells don't respond enough to the insulin that's made. Diabetes is a leading cause of early death, heart disease, stroke, kidney disease, and blindness. More than 80 percent of people with type 2 diabetes are overweight.

Abnormal blood fats: If you're overweight or obese, you have a greater chance of having abnormal levels of blood fats. These include high amounts of triglycerides and low-density lipoprotein (LDL) cholesterol (a fat-like substance often called "bad" cholesterol), and low amounts of high-density lipoprotein (HDL) cholesterol (often called "good" cholesterol). Abnormal levels of these blood fats are a risk for heart disease.

Metabolic syndrome: This is the name for a group of risk factors linked to overweight and obesity that raise your chance for heart disease and other health problems such as diabetes and stroke. A person can develop any one of these risk factors by itself, but they tend to occur together. Metabolic syndrome occurs when a person has at least three of these heart disease risk factors:

- A large waistline. This is also called abdominal obesity or "having an apple shape." Having extra fat in the waist area is a greater risk factor for heart disease than having extra fat in other parts of the body, such as on the hips.

- Abnormal blood fat levels, including high triglycerides and low HDL cholesterol.
- Higher than normal blood pressure.
- Higher than normal fasting blood sugar levels.

Cancer: Being overweight or obese raises the risk for colon, breast, endometrial, and gallbladder cancers.

Osteoarthritis: This is a common joint problem of the knees, hips, and lower back. It occurs when the tissue that protects the joints wears away. Extra weight can put more pressure and wear on joints, causing pain.

Sleep apnea: This condition causes a person to stop breathing for short periods during sleep. A person with sleep apnea may have more fat stored around the neck. This can make the breathing airway smaller so that it's hard to breathe.

Reproductive problems: Obesity can cause menstrual irregularity and infertility in women.

Gallstones: These are hard pieces of stone-like material that form in the gallbladder. They're mostly made of cholesterol and can cause abdominal or back pain. People who are overweight or obese have a greater chance of having gallstones. Also, being overweight may result in an enlarged gallbladder that may not work properly.

How Are Overweight and Obesity Diagnosed?

Body Mass Index

The most common way to find out whether you're overweight or obese is to figure out your body mass index (BMI). BMI is an estimate of body fat and a good gauge of your risk for diseases that occur with more body fat. The higher your BMI, the higher your risk of disease. BMI is calculated from your height and weight. You can use Table 7.1 to figure out your BMI.

Use this table to learn your BMI. First, find your height on the far left column. Next, move across the row to find your weight. Once you've found your weight, move to the very top of that column. This number is your BMI.

Table 7.1. Body Mass Index for Adults

Height	21	22	23	24	25	26	27	28	29	30	31
4'10"	100	105	110	115	119	124	129	134	138	143	148
5'0"	107	112	118	123	128	133	138	143	148	153	158
5'1"	111	116	122	127	132	137	143	148	153	158	164
5'3"	118	124	130	135	141	146	152	158	163	169	175
5'5"	126	132	138	144	150	156	162	168	174	180	186
5'7"	134	140	146	153	159	166	172	178	185	191	198
5'9"	142	149	155	162	169	176	182	189	196	203	209
5'11"	150	157	165	172	179	186	193	200	208	215	222
6'1"	159	166	174	182	189	197	204	212	219	227	235
6'3"	168	176	184	192	200	208	216	224	232	240	248

Note: Weight is measured with underwear but no shoes.

Table 7.2. What Does Body Mass Index Mean?

BMI	
18.5–24.9	Normal weight
25.0–29.9	Overweight
30.0–39.9	Obese
40.0 and above	Extreme obesity

Although BMI can be used for most men and women, it does have some limits:

- It may overestimate body fat in athletes and others who have a muscular build.
- It may underestimate body fat in older persons and others who have lost muscle.

Waist Circumference

Health care professionals also may take your waist measurement. This helps to screen for the possible health risks that come with overweight and obesity in adults. If you have abdominal obesity and most of your fat is around your waist rather than at your hips, you're at higher risk for heart disease and type 2 diabetes. This risk goes up with a waist size that is greater than thirty-five inches for women or greater than forty inches for men.

You, too, may want to measure your waist size. To do so correctly, stand and place a tape measure around your middle, just above your hipbones. Measure your waist just after you breathe out.

How Are Overweight and Obesity Treated?

Successful treatments for weight loss include setting goals and making lifestyle changes such as eating fewer calories and being more physically active. Drug therapy and weight loss surgery are also options for some people if lifestyle changes don't work.

Set Realistic ("Do-able") Goals

Setting the right weight loss goals is an important first step to losing and maintaining weight:

- Lose just 5 to 10 percent of your current weight over six months. This will lower your risk for heart disease and other conditions.
- The best way to lose weight is slowly. A weight loss of one to two pounds a week is do-able, safe, and will help you keep off the weight. It also will give you the time to make new, healthy lifestyle changes.
- If you've lost 10 percent of your body weight, have kept it off for six months, and are still overweight or obese, you may want to consider further weight loss.

Lifestyle Changes

For long-term weight loss success, it's important for you and your family to make lifestyle changes:

- Focus on energy IN (calories from food and drinks) and energy OUT (physical activity).
- Follow a healthy eating plan.
- Learn how to adopt more healthful lifestyle habits.

Over time, these changes will become part of your everyday life.

Calories

Cutting back on calories (energy IN) will help you lose weight. To lose one to two pounds a week, adults should cut back their calorie intake by 500 to 1,000 calories a day:

- In general, 1,000 to 1,200 calories a day will help most women lose weight safely.
- In general, 1,200 to 1,600 calories a day will help most men lose weight safely. This calorie range is also suitable for women who weigh 165 pounds or more or who exercise routinely.

These calorie levels are a guide and may need to be adjusted. If you eat 1,600 calories a day but don't lose weight, then you may want to cut back to 1,200 calories. If you're hungry on either diet, then you may want to boost your calories by 100 to 200 a day. Very-low-calorie diets of less than 800 calories a day shouldn't be used unless your doctor is monitoring you.

Healthy Eating Plan

A healthy eating plan gives your body the nutrients it needs every day. It has enough calories for good health, but not so many that you gain weight.

A healthy eating plan also will lower your risk for heart disease and other conditions. A plan low in total, saturated, and trans fat; cholesterol; and sodium (salt) will help to lower your risk for heart disease. Cutting down on fats and added sugars also can help you eat fewer calories and lose weight. Healthful foods include the following:

- Fat-free and low-fat milk and milk products such as low-fat yogurt, cheese, and milk.
- Lean meat, fish, poultry, cooked beans, and peas.
- Whole-grain foods such as whole wheat bread, oatmeal, and brown rice. Other grain foods like pasta, cereal, bagels, bread, tortillas, couscous, and crackers.
- Fruits, which can be canned (in juice or water), fresh, frozen, or dried.
- Vegetables, which can be canned (without salt), fresh, frozen, or dried.

Canola or olive oils and soft margarines made from these oils are heart healthy. They should be used in small amounts because they're high in calories. Unsalted nuts, like walnuts and almonds, also can be built into a healthful diet as long as you watch the amount you eat, because nuts are high in calories.

Foods to limit: Foods that are high in saturated and trans fats and cholesterol raise blood cholesterol levels and also may be high in calories. These fats raise the risk of heart disease, so they should be limited.

Saturated fat is found mainly in the following:

- Fatty cuts of meat such as ground beef, sausage, and processed meats such as bologna, hot dogs, and deli meats
- Poultry with the skin
- High-fat milk and milk products like whole-milk cheeses, whole milk, cream, butter, and ice cream
- Lard, coconut, and palm oils found in many processed foods

Trans fat is found mainly in the following:

- Foods with partially hydrogenated oils such as many hard margarines and shortening
- Baked products and snack foods such as crackers, cookies, doughnuts, and breads
- Food fried in hydrogenated shortening such as French fries and chicken

Cholesterol is found mainly in the following:

- Egg yolks
- Organ meats such as liver
- Shrimp
- Whole milk or whole-milk products, including butter, cream, and cheese

Limiting foods and drinks with added sugars, like high-fructose corn syrup, is important. Added sugars will give you extra calories without nutrients like vitamins and minerals. Added sugars are found in many desserts, canned fruit packed in syrup, fruit drinks, and nondiet drinks. Check the nutrition label on food packages for added sugars like high-fructose corn syrup. Drinks with alcohol also will add calories, so it's a good idea to watch alcohol intake.

Portion size: A portion is the amount of food that you choose to eat for a meal or snack. It's different from a serving, which is a measured amount of food and is noted on the nutrition label on food packages.

Anyone who has eaten out lately is likely to notice how big the portions are. In fact, they're oversized. These ever-larger portions have changed what we think of as normal.

Cutting back on portion size is a good way to help you eat fewer calories and balance your energy IN.

Food weight: Studies have shown that we all tend to eat a constant "weight" of food. Ounce for ounce, our food intake is fairly constant. Knowing this, you can lose weight if you eat foods that are lower in calories and fat for a given measure of food. For example, replacing a full-fat food product that weighs two ounces with one that's the same weight but lower in fat helps you cut back on calories. Another helpful practice is to eat foods that contain a lot of water, like vegetables, fruits, and soups.

Physical Activity

Staying active and eating fewer calories will help you lose weight and keep the weight off over time. Physical activity also will benefit you in other ways. It will do the following:

- Lower the risk of heart disease, diabetes, and cancers (such as breast, uterus, and colon)
- Strengthen your lungs and help them to work better
- Strengthen your muscles and keep your joints in good condition
- Slow bone loss
- Give you more energy
- Help you to relax and cope better with stress
- Allow you to fall asleep more quickly and sleep more soundly
- Give you an enjoyable way to share time with friends and family

In general, adults should follow these guidelines in relation to physical activity:

- For overall health and to lower the risk of disease, aim for at least thirty minutes of moderate-intensity physical activity most days of the week.
- To help manage body weight and prevent gradual weight gain, aim for sixty minutes of moderate-to-vigorous-intensity physical activity most days of the week.
- To maintain weight loss, aim for at least sixty to ninety minutes of daily moderate-intensity physical activity.

Many people lead inactive lives and may not be motivated to do more physical activity. Some people may need help and supervision when they start a physical activity program to avoid injury.

If you're obese, or if you haven't been active in the past, start physical activity slowly and build up the intensity a little at a time. When starting out, one way to be active is to do more "everyday" activities such as taking the stairs instead of the elevator and doing household chores and yard work. The next step is to start walking, biking, or swimming at a slow pace, and then build up the amount of time you exercise or the intensity level of the activity.

To lose weight and gain better health, it's important to get moderate-intensity physical activity. Choose activities that you enjoy and that fit into your daily life. A daily, brisk walk is an easy way to be more active and improve your health. Use a pedometer to count your daily steps and keep track of how much you're walking. Try to increase the number of steps you take each day.

Other examples of moderate-intensity physical activity include dancing, bicycling, gardening, and swimming. For greater health benefits, try to step up your level of activity or the length of time you're active. For example, start walking for ten to fifteen minutes three times a week, and then build up to brisk walking for sixty minutes, five days a week. You also can break up the amount of time that you're physically active into shorter amounts, such as fifteen minutes at a time.

Behavioral Changes

Changing your behaviors or habits around food and physical activity is important for losing weight. The first step is to understand the things that lead you to overeat or have an inactive lifestyle. The next step is to change these habits.

The list below gives you some simple tips to help build healthier habits.

Change your surroundings: You may be more likely to overeat when watching TV, when treats are available in the office break room, or when you're with a certain friend. You also may not be motivated to take the exercise class you signed up for. But you can change these habits. Here are some things you can do:

- Instead of watching TV, dance to music in your living room or go for a walk.
- Leave the office break room right after you get a cup of coffee.
- Bring a change of clothes to work. Head straight to the exercise class on the way home from work.
- Put a note on your calendar to remind yourself to take a walk or go to your activity class.

Keep a record: A record of your food intake and the amount of physical activity that you do each day will help to inspire you. You also can keep track of your weight. For example, when the record shows that you've been meeting your goal to be more active, you'll want to keep it up. A record is also an easy way to track how you're doing, especially if you're working with a registered dietitian or nutritionist.

Seek support: Ask for help or encouragement from your friends, family, and health care provider. You can get support in person, through e-mail, or by talking on the phone. You also can join a support group.

Reward success: Reward your success for meeting your weight loss goals or other achievements with something you would like to do, not with food. Choose rewards that you'll enjoy, such as a movie, a music CD, an afternoon off from work, a massage, or personal time.

Weight Loss Medicines

Weight loss medicines approved by the Food and Drug Administration (FDA) may be an option for some people. If you're not successful at losing one pound a week after six months of using lifestyle changes, medicines may help. These medicines should be used only as part of a program that includes diet, physical activity, and behavioral changes.

Weight loss medicines may be suitable for adults who are obese (a BMI of 30 or greater). People who have BMIs of 27 or greater and a risk for heart disease and other health conditions also may benefit from medicines.

The FDA has approved two prescription weight loss medicines for long-term use: sibutramine (Meridia®) and orlistat (Xenical®). These medicines cause a weight loss between four and twenty-two pounds, although some people lose more weight. Most of the weight loss occurs within the first six months of taking the medicine.

Sibutramine (Meridia): This medicine sends signals to your brain to curb your appetite. Sibutramine raises blood pressure and pulse. You shouldn't take it if you have high blood pressure or a history of heart disease or stroke.

Orlistat (Xenical): This medicine reduces the absorption of fats, fat calories, and vitamins A, D, E, and K by the body. Orlistat can result in mild side effects such as oily and loose stools.

The FDA also has approved Alli®, an over-the-counter weight loss aid for adults. Alli is the lower-dose form of orlistat. It's meant to be used along with a reduced-calorie, low-fat diet and physical activity. In studies, most people taking Alli lost five to ten pounds over six months.

Like orlistat, Alli reduces the absorption of fats, fat calories, and vitamins A, D, E, and K to promote weight loss. It also has similar side effects to orlistat. If you're taking orlistat or Alli, you should take a multivitamin at bedtime due to the possible loss of some vitamins. You also should talk to your doctor before starting Alli if you're taking blood-thinning medicines or being treated for diabetes or thyroid disease.

Combined with healthy eating and physical activity, these medicines can help people lose weight. If you think you would benefit from the prescription medicines sibutramine or orlistat, talk to your doctor. People taking these medicines need regular checkups with their doctors, especially in the first year after starting the medicine. During checkups, your doctor will check your weight, blood pressure, and pulse and order laboratory tests. He or she also will discuss any medicine side effects and answer your questions.

Over-the-Counter Products

Over-the-counter (OTC) products often claim that a person taking them will lose weight. The FDA doesn't regulate these products because they're considered dietary supplements, not medicines. However, many of these products have serious side effects and aren't generally recommended. A few OTC products include the following:

- **Ephedra (also called Ma-huang):** Ephedra comes from plants and has been sold as a dietary supplement. The active ingredient in the plant is called ephedrine. Ephedra can cause short-term weight loss. It also has serious side effects. It causes high blood pressure and stresses the heart. In fact, because ephedra poses a serious health risk, the FDA has advised people to stop using dietary supplements that contain it.
- **Chromium:** This is a mineral that's sold as a dietary supplement to reduce body fat. While studies haven't found any weight loss benefit from chromium, there are few serious side effects from taking it.
- **Diuretics and herbal laxatives:** These products cause you to lose water weight, not fat. They also can lower your body's potassium levels, which may cause heart and muscle problems.
- **Hoodia:** Hoodia is a cactus that is native to Africa. It's sold in pill form as an appetite suppressant. However, there is no firm evidence that hoodia works. No large-scale research has been done on humans to show whether hoodia is effective or safe.

Weight Loss Surgery

Weight loss surgery may be an option for people with extreme obesity (BMI of 40 or greater) when other treatments have failed. It's also an option for people with a BMI of 35 or greater who have life-threatening conditions such as the following:

- Severe sleep apnea (a condition in which your breathing stops or gets very shallow while you're sleeping)
- Obesity-related cardiomyopathy (diseases of the heart muscle)
- Severe type 2 diabetes

There are two common weight loss surgeries:

- **Banded gastroplasty:** For this surgery, a band or staples are used to create a small pouch at the top of your stomach. This surgery limits the amount of food and liquids the stomach can hold.
- **Roux-en-Y gastric bypass:** For this surgery, a small stomach pouch is created with a bypass around part of the small intestine where most of the calories you eat are absorbed. This surgery limits food intake and reduces the calories your body absorbs.

Weight loss surgery can improve your health and weight. However, the surgery can be risky depending on your overall health. There are few long-term side effects with gastroplasty; however, you must limit your food intake dramatically. Roux-en-Y gastric bypass has more side effects. These include nausea, bloating, diarrhea, and faintness (which are all part of a condition called dumping syndrome). After Roux-en-Y gastric bypass, multivitamins and minerals may be needed to prevent nutrient deficiencies.

Lifelong medical follow-up is needed after both surgeries. A monitoring program both before and after surgery also is advised to help you with diet, physical activity, and coping skills.

If you think you would benefit from weight loss surgery, talk to your doctor. Ask whether you're a candidate for the surgery and discuss the risks, benefits, and what to expect.

Weight Loss Maintenance

Maintaining your weight loss over time can be a challenge. For adults, weight loss is a success if you lose at least 10 percent of your initial weight and you don't regain more than six or seven pounds in two years. You also must keep a lower waist circumference—at least two inches lower than your waist circumference before you lost weight.

After six months of keeping off the weight, you can think about losing more if the following are true:

- You've already lost 5 to 10 percent of your body weight
- You're still overweight or obese

The key to further weight loss or to maintain your weight loss is to continue with lifestyle changes. Adopt these changes as a new way of life. However, if you want to lose more weight, you may need to eat fewer calories and increase your activity level. For example, if you eat 1,600 calories a day but don't lose weight, you may want to cut back to 1,200 calories.

Adults should aim for sixty to ninety minutes of daily moderate-intensity physical activity.

How Can Overweight and Obesity Be Prevented?

Staying at a healthy weight and preventing overweight and obesity can be achieved through living a healthy lifestyle. Because lifetime habits begin in childhood, it's important for parents and families to create habits that encourage healthy food choices and physical activity early in life.

Chapter 8

Physical Activity: Key to a Healthy Lifestyle

Physical Activity and Health

The Benefits of Physical Activity

Regular physical activity is one of the most important things you can do for your health. It can help:

- control your weight;
- reduce your risk of cardiovascular disease;
- reduce your risk for type 2 diabetes and metabolic syndrome;
- reduce your risk of some cancers;
- strengthen your bones and muscles;
- improve your mental health and mood;
- improve your ability to do daily activities and prevent falls, if you're an older adult;
- increase your chances of living longer.

If you're not sure about becoming active or boosting your level of physical activity because you're afraid of getting hurt, the good news

---

Excerpted from the following documents from the Centers for Disease Control and Prevention: "Physical Activity and Health," December 3, 2008; "How Much Physical Activity Do Adults Need?" December 17, 2008; and "Adding Physical Activity to Your Life," January 15, 2009.

is that moderate-intensity aerobic activity, like brisk walking, is generally safe for most people.

Start slowly. Cardiac events, such as a heart attack, are rare during physical activity. But the risk does go up when you suddenly become much more active than usual. For example, you can put yourself at risk if you don't usually get much physical activity and then all of a sudden do vigorous-intensity aerobic activity, like shoveling snow. That's why it's important to start slowly and gradually increase your level of activity.

If you have a chronic health condition such as arthritis, diabetes, or heart disease, talk with your doctor to find out if your condition limits, in any way, your ability to be active. Then, work with your doctor to come up with a physical activity plan that matches your abilities. If your condition stops you from meeting the minimum guidelines, try to do as much as you can. What's important is that you avoid being inactive. Even sixty minutes a week of moderate-intensity aerobic activity is good for you.

The bottom line is, the health benefits of physical activity far outweigh the risks of getting hurt.

Control Your Weight

Looking to get to or stay at a healthy weight? Both diet and physical activity play a critical role in controlling your weight. You gain weight when the calories you burn, including those burned during physical activity, are less than the calories you eat or drink. When it comes to weight management, people vary greatly in how much physical activity they need. You may need to be more active than others to achieve or maintain a healthy weight.

To maintain your weight: Work your way up to 150 minutes of moderate-intensity aerobic activity, 75 minutes of vigorous-intensity aerobic activity, or an equivalent mix of the two each week. Strong scientific evidence shows that physical activity can help you maintain your weight over time. However, the exact amount of physical activity needed to do this is not clear since it varies greatly from person to person. It's possible that you may need to do more than the equivalent of 150 minutes of moderate-intensity activity a week to maintain your weight.

To lose weight and keep it off: You will need a high amount of physical activity unless you also adjust your diet and reduce the number of calories you're eating and drinking. Getting to and staying at a healthy weight requires both regular physical activity and a healthy eating plan.

Reduce Your Risk of Cardiovascular Disease

Heart disease and stroke are two of the leading causes of death in the United States. But following the guidelines and getting at least 150 minutes a week (2 hours and 30 minutes) of moderate-intensity aerobic activity can put you at a lower risk for these diseases. You can reduce your risk even further with more physical activity. Regular physical activity can also lower your blood pressure and improve your cholesterol levels.

Reduce your Risk of Type 2 Diabetes and Metabolic Syndrome

Regular physical activity can reduce your risk of developing type 2 diabetes and metabolic syndrome. Metabolic syndrome is a condition in which you have some combination of too much fat around the waist, high blood pressure, low high-density lipoprotein (HDL) cholesterol, high triglycerides, or high blood sugar. Research shows that lower rates of these conditions are seen with 120 to 150 minutes (2 hours to 2 hours and 30 minutes) a week of at least moderate-intensity aerobic activity. And the more physical activity you do, the lower your risk will be.

Already have type 2 diabetes? Regular physical activity can help control your blood glucose levels.

Reduce Your Risk of Some Cancers

Being physically active lowers your risk for two types of cancer: colon and breast. Research shows that the following is true:

- Physically active people have a lower risk of colon cancer than do people who are not active.
- Physically active women have a lower risk of breast cancer than do people who are not active.

Improve your quality of life: If you are a cancer survivor, research shows that getting regular physical activity not only helps give you a better quality of life, but also improves your physical fitness.

Strengthen Your Bones and Muscles

As you age, it's important to protect your bones, joints, and muscles. Not only do they support your body and help you move, but keeping bones, joints, and muscles healthy can help ensure that you're able to do your daily activities and be physically active. Research shows that doing aerobic, muscle-strengthening, and bone-strengthening physical activity of at least a moderately intense level can slow the loss of bone density that comes with age.

Hip fracture is a serious health condition that can have life-changing negative effects, especially if you're an older adult. But research shows that people who do 120 to 300 minutes of at least moderate-intensity aerobic activity each week have a lower risk of hip fracture.

Regular physical activity helps with arthritis and other conditions affecting the joints. If you have arthritis, research shows that doing 130 to 150 (2 hours and 10 minutes to 2 hours and 30 minutes) a week of moderate-intensity, low-impact aerobic activity can not only improve your ability to manage pain and do everyday tasks, but it can also make your quality of life better.

Build strong, healthy muscles. Muscle-strengthening activities can help you increase or maintain your muscle mass and strength. Slowly increasing the amount of weight and number of repetitions you do will give you even more benefits, no matter your age.

Improve Your Mental Health and Mood

Regular physical activity can help keep your thinking, learning, and judgment skills sharp as you age. It can also reduce your risk of depression and may help you sleep better.

Improve Your Ability to Do Daily Activities and Prevent Falls

A functional limitation is a loss of the ability to do everyday activities such as climbing stairs, grocery shopping, or playing with your grandchildren.

How does this relate to physical activity? If you're a physically active middle-aged or older adult, you have a lower risk of functional limitations than people who are inactive.

Already have trouble doing some of your everyday activities? Aerobic and muscle-strengthening activities can help improve your ability to do these types of tasks.

Are you an older adult who is at risk for falls? Research shows that doing balance and muscle-strengthening activities each week along with moderate-intensity aerobic activity, like brisk walking, can help reduce your risk of falling.

Increase Your Chances of Living Longer

Science shows that physical activity can reduce your risk of dying early from the leading causes of death, like heart disease and some cancers. This is remarkable in two ways:

- Only a few lifestyle choices have as large an impact on your health as physical activity. People who are physically active for about seven hours a week have a 40 percent lower risk of dying early than those who are active for less than 30 minutes a week.
- You don't have to do high amounts of activity or vigorous-intensity activity to reduce your risk of premature death. You can put yourself at lower risk of dying early by doing at least 150 minutes a week of moderate-intensity aerobic activity.

How Much Physical Activity Do Adults Need?

Physical activity is anything that gets your body moving. According to the 2008 Physical Activity Guidelines for Americans, you need to do two types of physical activity each week to improve your health—aerobic and muscle-strengthening.

For Important Health Benefits

Adults need at least:

- Two hours and 30 minutes (150 minutes) of moderate-intensity aerobic activity (i.e., brisk walking) every week and muscle-strengthening activities on two or more days a week that work all major muscle groups (legs, hips, back, abdomen, chest, shoulders, and arms); or
- One hour and 15 minutes (75 minutes) of vigorous-intensity aerobic activity (i.e., jogging or running) every week and muscle-strengthening activities on two or more days a week that work all major muscle groups (legs, hips, back, abdomen, chest, shoulders, and arms); or
- An equivalent mix of moderate- and vigorous-intensity aerobic activity and muscle-strengthening activities on two or more days

a week that work all major muscle groups (legs, hips, back, abdomen, chest, shoulders, and arms).

Ten minutes at a time is fine: We know 150 minutes each week sounds like a lot of time, but you don't have to do it all at once. Not only is it best to spread your activity out during the week, but you can break it up into smaller chunks of time during the day, as long as you're doing your activity at a moderate or vigorous effort for at least ten minutes at a time.

For Even Greater Health Benefits

Adults should increase their activity to:

- Five hours (300 minutes) each week of moderate-intensity aerobic activity and muscle-strengthening activities on two or more days a week that work all major muscle groups (legs, hips, back, abdomen, chest, shoulders, and arms); or
- Two hours and 30 minutes (150 minutes) each week of vigorous-intensity aerobic activity and muscle-strengthening activities on two or more days a week that work all major muscle groups (legs, hips, back, abdomen, chest, shoulders, and arms); or
- An equivalent mix of moderate- and vigorous-intensity aerobic activity and muscle-strengthening activities on two or more days a week that work all major muscle groups (legs, hips, back, abdomen, chest, shoulders, and arms).

More time equals more health benefits: If you go beyond 300 minutes a week of moderate-intensity activity, or 150 minutes a week of vigorous-intensity activity, you'll gain even more health benefits.

Aerobic Activity—What Counts?

Aerobic activity or "cardio" gets you breathing harder and your heart beating faster. From pushing a lawn mower, to taking a dance class, to biking to the store—all types of activities count, as long as you're doing them at a moderate or vigorous intensity for at least ten minutes at a time.

Intensity is how hard your body is working during aerobic activity.

How do you know if you're doing light-, moderate-, or vigorous-intensity aerobic activities? For most people, light daily activities such as shopping, cooking, or doing the laundry don't count toward the guidelines. Why? Your body isn't working hard enough to get your heart rate up.

Moderate-intensity aerobic activity means you're working hard enough to raise your heart rate and break a sweat. One way to tell is that you'll be able to talk, but not sing the words to your favorite song. Here are some examples of activities that require moderate effort:

- Walking fast
- Doing water aerobics
- Riding a bike on level ground or with few hills
- Playing doubles tennis
- Pushing a lawn mower

Vigorous-intensity aerobic activity means you're breathing hard and fast, and your heart rate has gone up quite a bit. If you're working at this level, you won't be able to say more than a few words without pausing for a breath. Here are some examples of activities that require vigorous effort:

- Jogging or running
- Swimming laps
- Riding a bike fast or on hills
- Playing singles tennis
- Playing basketball

You can do moderate- or vigorous-intensity aerobic activity, or a mix of the two each week. A rule of thumb is that one minute of vigorous-intensity activity is about the same as two minutes of moderate-intensity activity.

Muscle-Strengthening Activities—What Counts?

Besides aerobic activity, you need to do things to strengthen your muscles at least two days a week. These activities should work all the major muscle groups of your body (legs, hips, back, chest, abdomen, shoulders, and arms).

To gain health benefits, muscle-strengthening activities need to be done to the point where it's hard for you to do another repetition without help. A repetition is one complete movement of an activity, like lifting a weight or doing a sit-up. Try to do eight to twelve repetitions per activity that count as one set. Try to do at least one set of muscle-strengthening activities, but to gain even more benefits, do two or three sets.

There are many ways you can strengthen your muscles, whether it's at home or the gym. You may want to try the following:

- Lifting weights
- Working with resistance bands
- Doing exercises that use your body weight for resistance (i.e., push-ups, sit-ups)
- Heavy gardening (i.e., digging, shoveling)
- Yoga

Chapter 9

How Much Sleep Do We Really Need?

Our Sleep Needs

What the Research Says about Sleep Duration

The first thing experts will tell you about sleep is that there is no "magic number." Not only do different age groups need different amounts of sleep, but sleep needs are also individual. Just like any other characteristics you are born with, the amount of sleep you need to function best may be different for you than for someone who is of the same age and gender. While you may be at your absolute best sleeping seven hours a night, someone else may clearly need nine hours to have a happy, productive life. In fact, a 2005 study confirmed the fact that sleep needs vary across populations, and the study calls for further research to identify traits within genes that may provide a "map" to explain how sleep needs differ among individuals.

Another reason there is "no magic number" for your sleep results from two different factors that researchers are learning about: a person's basal sleep need—the amount of sleep our bodies need on a regular basis for optimal performance—and sleep debt, the accumulated sleep that is lost to poor sleep habits, sickness, awakenings due to environmental factors, or other causes. Two studies suggest that

---

"Our Sleep Needs" is excerpted from "How Much Sleep Do We Really Need?" and the "Sleep Needs over the Life Cycle" table is excerpted from "Let Sleep Work for You," © 2007 National Sleep Foundation (www.sleepfoundation.org). Reprinted with permission.

healthy adults have a basal sleep need of seven to eight hours every night, but where things get complicated is the interaction between the basal need and sleep debt. For instance, you might meet your basal sleep need on any single night or a few nights in a row, but still have an unresolved sleep debt that may make you feel more sleepy and less alert at times, particularly in conjunction with circadian dips, those times in the twenty-four-hour cycle when we are biologically programmed to be more sleepy and less alert, such as overnight hours and mid-afternoon. You may feel overwhelmingly sleepy quite suddenly at these times, shortly before bedtime, or feel sleepy upon awakening. The good news is that some research suggests that the accumulated sleep debt can be worked down or "paid off."

Though scientists are still learning about the concept of basal sleep need, one thing sleep research certainly has shown is that sleeping too little can not only inhibit your productivity and ability to remember and consolidate information, but lack of sleep can also lead to serious health consequences and jeopardize your safety and the safety of individuals around you.

For example, short sleep duration is linked with:

- increased risk of motor vehicle accidents;
- increase in body mass index—a greater likelihood of obesity due to an increased appetite caused by sleep deprivation;
- increased risk of diabetes and heart problems;
- increased risk for psychiatric conditions including depression and substance abuse;
- decreased ability to pay attention, react to signals, or remember new information.

According to researchers Michael H. Bonnet and Donna L. Arand, "There is strong evidence that sufficient shortening or disturbance of the sleep process compromises mood, performance and alertness and can result in injury or death. In this light, the most common-sense 'do no injury' medical advice would be to avoid sleep deprivation."

On the other hand, some research has found that long sleep durations (nine hours or more) are also associated with increased morbidity (illness, accidents) and mortality (death). Researchers describe this relationship as a "U-shaped" curve, where both sleeping too little and sleeping too much may put you at risk. This research found that variables such as low socioeconomic status and depression were significantly associated with long sleep. Some researchers argue that these other variables might be the cause of the longer sleep: the fact that individuals with low socioeconomic status are more likely to have undiagnosed illnesses because of poor medical care explains the relationship between low socioeconomic status, long sleep, and morbidity/mortality. Researchers caution that there is not a definitive conclusion that getting more than nine hours of sleep per night is consistently linked with health problems and/or mortality in adults, while short sleep has been linked to both these consequences in numerous studies.

"Currently, there is no strong evidence that sleeping too much has detrimental health consequences, or even evidence that our bodies will allow us to sleep much beyond what is required," says Kristen L. Knutson, Ph.D., Department of Health Studies, University of Chicago. "There is laboratory evidence that short sleep durations of four to five hours have negative physiological and neurobehavioral consequences. We need similar laboratory and intervention studies to determine whether long sleep durations (if they can be obtained) result in physiological changes that could lead to disease before we make any recommendations against sleep extension."

But a key question is how much is too much or too little. Researchers Shawn Youngstedt and Daniel Kripke reviewed two surveys of more than one million adults conducted by the American Cancer Society and found that the group of people who slept seven hours had less mortality after six years than those sleeping both more and less. The group of people who slept shorter amounts and those who slept longer than eight hours had an average mortality risk that was greater, but the risk was higher for longer sleepers. Youngstedt and Kripke argue that for those who would normally sleep longer than eight hours, restricting their sleep may actually be healthier for them, just as eating less than one's appetite may be healthier in a more sedentary society.

Though research cannot pinpoint an exact amount of sleep need by people at different ages, Table 9.1 identifies the "rule-of-thumb" amounts most experts have agreed upon. Nevertheless, it's important to pay attention to your own individual needs by assessing how you feel on different amounts of sleep. Are you productive, healthy, and happy on seven hours of sleep? Or does it take you nine hours of quality ZZZs to get you into high gear? Do you have health issues such as being overweight? Are you at risk for any disease? Are you experiencing sleep problems? Do you depend on caffeine to get you through the day? Do you feel sleepy when driving? These are questions that must be asked before you can find the number that works for you.

Table 9.1. Sleep Needs over the Life Cycle

Infants/babies (including naps)	
0 to 2 months	10.5 to 18.5 hours
2 to 12 months	14 to 15 hours
Toddlers/Children (including naps)	
12 to 18 months	13 to 15 hours
18 months to 3 years	12 to 14 hours
3 to 5 years	11 to 13 hours
5 to 12 years	9 to 11 hours
Adolescents	8.5 to 9.5 hours
Adults/Older Persons	7 to 9 hours

Source: "Let Sleep Work for You," © 2007 National Sleep Foundation. Reprinted with permission.

What You Can Do

To begin a new path toward healthier sleep and a healthier lifestyle, begin by assessing your own individual needs and habits. See how you respond to different amounts of sleep. Pay careful attention to your mood, energy, and health after a poor night's sleep versus a good one. Ask yourself, "How often do I get a good night's sleep?" If the answer is "not often", then you may need to consider changing your sleep habits or consulting a physician or sleep specialist.

To pave the way for better sleep, experts recommend that you and your family members follow these sleep tips:

- Establish consistent sleep and wake schedules, even on weekends.
- Create a regular, relaxing bedtime routine such as soaking in a hot bath or listening to soothing music—begin an hour or more before the time you expect to fall asleep.
- Create a sleep-conducive environment that is dark, quiet, comfortable, and cool.
- Sleep on a comfortable mattress and pillows.
- Use your bedroom only for sleep and sex (keep "sleep stealers" out of the bedroom—avoid watching TV, using a computer, or reading in bed).

- Finish eating at least two to three hours before your regular bedtime.
- Exercise regularly during the day or at least a few hours before bedtime.
- Avoid caffeine and alcohol products close to bedtime and give up smoking.

If you or a family member are experiencing symptoms such as sleepiness during the day or when you expect to be awake and alert, snoring, leg cramps or tingling, gasping or difficulty breathing during sleep, prolonged insomnia, or another symptom that is preventing you from sleeping well, you should consult your primary care physician or sleep specialist to determine the underlying cause. You may also try keeping a sleep diary to track your sleep habits over a one- or two-week period and bring the results to your physician.

Most importantly, make sleep a priority. You must schedule sleep like any other daily activity, so put it on your "to-do list" and cross it off every night. But don't make it the thing you do only after everything else is done—stop doing other things so you get the sleep you need.

Chapter 10

Avoiding Risk Factors for Common Health Concerns

Chapter Contents

Section 10.1

Alcohol and Its Effects

Reprinted from "Alcohol: Frequently Asked Questions" and "Excessive Alcohol Use and Risks to Men's Health," Centers for Disease Control and Prevention, August 6, 2008.

Alcohol: Frequently Asked Questions

What Is Alcohol?

Ethyl alcohol, or ethanol, is an intoxicating ingredient found in beer, wine, and liquor. Alcohol is produced by the fermentation of yeast, sugars, and starches.

How Does Alcohol Affect a Person?

Alcohol affects every organ in the body. It is a central nervous system depressant that is rapidly absorbed from the stomach and small intestine into the bloodstream. Alcohol is metabolized in the liver by enzymes; however, the liver can only metabolize a small amount of alcohol at a time, leaving the excess alcohol to circulate throughout the body. The intensity of the effect of alcohol on the body is directly related to the amount consumed.

Why Do Some People React Differently to Alcohol Than Others?

Individual reactions to alcohol vary, and are influenced by many factors, including but not limited to the following:

- Age
- Gender
- Race or ethnicity
- Physical condition (weight, fitness level, etc.)
- Amount of food consumed before drinking
- How quickly the alcohol was consumed

- Use of drugs or prescription medicines
- Family history of alcohol problems

What Is a Standard Drink in the United States?

A standard drink is equal to 13.7 grams (0.6 ounces) of pure alcohol or:

- twelve ounces of beer;
- eight ounces of malt liquor;
- five ounces of wine;
- one and a half ounces, or a "shot," of 80-proof distilled spirits or liquor (e.g., gin, rum, vodka, or whiskey).

Is Beer or Wine Safer to Drink Than Liquor?

No. One 12-ounce beer has about the same amount of alcohol as one 5-ounce glass of wine, or a 1.5-ounce shot of liquor. It is the amount of ethanol consumed that affects a person most, not the type of alcoholic drink.

What Does Moderate Drinking Mean?

There is no one definition of moderate drinking, but generally the term is used to describe a lower risk pattern of drinking. According to the Dietary Guidelines for Americans,[1] drinking in moderation is defined as having no more than one drink per day for women and no more than two drinks per day for men. This definition is referring to the amount consumed on any single day and is not intended as an average over several days.

Is It Safe to Drink Alcohol and Drive?

No, alcohol use slows reaction time and impairs judgment and coordination, which are all skills needed to drive a car safely.[2] The more alcohol consumed, the greater the impairment.

What Does It Mean to Be Above the Legal Limit for Drinking?

The legal limit for drinking is the alcohol level above which an individual is subject to legal penalties (e.g., arrest or loss of a driver's license).

Legal limits are measured using either a blood alcohol test or a breathalyzer.

Legal limits are typically defined by state law, and may vary based on individual characteristics such as age and occupation.

All states in the United States have adopted 0.08 percent (80 mg/dL) as the legal limit for operating a motor vehicle for drivers aged twenty-one years or older. However, drivers under age twenty-one years are not allowed to operate a motor vehicle with any level of alcohol in their system.

Note: Legal limits do not define a level below which it is safe to operate a vehicle or engage in some other activity. Impairment due to alcohol use begins to occur at levels well below the legal limit.

How Do I Know If It's Okay to Drink?

The current *Dietary Guidelines for Americans*[1] recommend that if you choose to drink alcoholic beverages, you do not exceed one drink per day for women and two drinks per day for men. These guidelines also specify that there are some people who should not drink alcoholic beverages at all, including the following:

- Children and adolescents
- Individuals of any age who cannot limit their drinking to low levels
- Women who may become pregnant or who are pregnant
- Individuals who plan to drive, operate machinery, or take part in other activities that require attention, skill, or coordination
- Individuals taking prescription or over-the-counter medications that can interact with alcohol
- Individuals with certain medical conditions
- Persons recovering from alcoholism

What Do You Mean by Heavy Drinking?

For men, heavy drinking is typically defined as consuming an average of more than two drinks per day. For women, heavy drinking is typically defined as consuming an average of more than one drink per day.

What Is Binge Drinking?

According to the National Institute on Alcohol Abuse and Alcoholism, binge drinking is defined as a pattern of alcohol consumption that brings the blood alcohol concentration (BAC) level to 0.08 percent or above. This pattern of drinking usually corresponds to five or more drinks on a single occasion for men or four or more drinks on a single occasion for women, generally within about two hours.[3]

What Is the Difference between Alcoholism and Alcohol Abuse?

Alcoholism or alcohol dependence is a diagnosable disease characterized by several factors, including a strong craving for alcohol, continued use despite harm or personal injury, the inability to limit drinking, physical illness when drinking stops, and the need to increase the amount drunk to feel the effects.[4]

Alcohol abuse is a pattern of drinking that results in harm to one's health, interpersonal relationships, or ability to work. Certain manifestations of alcohol abuse include failure to fulfill responsibilities at work, school, or home; drinking in dangerous situations, such as while driving; legal problems associated with alcohol use; and continued drinking despite problems that are caused or worsened by drinking. Alcohol abuse can lead to alcohol dependence.[4]

What Does It Mean to Get Drunk?

"Getting drunk" or intoxicated is the result of consuming excessive amounts of alcohol. Binge drinking typically results in acute intoxication.

Alcohol intoxication can be detrimental to health for a variety of reasons, including, but not limited to, the following:

- Impaired brain function resulting in poor judgment, reduced reaction time, loss of balance and motor skills, or slurred speech
- Dilation of blood vessels causing a feeling of warmth but resulting in rapid loss of body heat
- Increased risk of certain cancers, stroke, and liver diseases (e.g., cirrhosis), particularly when excessive amounts of alcohol are consumed over extended periods of time
- Damage to a developing fetus if consumed by pregnant women[5]
- Increased risk of motor-vehicle traffic crashes, violence, and other injuries

Coma and death can occur if alcohol is consumed rapidly and in large amounts because of depression of the central nervous system.

How Do I Know If I Have a Drinking Problem?

Drinking is a problem if it causes trouble in your relationships, in school, in social activities, or in how you think and feel. If you are concerned that either you or someone in your family might have a drinking problem, consult your personal health care provider.

What Can I Do If I or Someone I Know Has a Drinking Problem?

Consult your personal health care provider if you feel you or someone you know has a drinking problem. Other resources include the National Drug and Alcohol Treatment Referral Routing Service available at 800-662-HELP. This service can provide you with information about treatment programs in your local community and allow you to speak with someone about alcohol problems.[6]

What Health Problems Are Associated with Excessive Alcohol Use?

Excessive drinking, in the form of either heavy drinking or binge drinking, is associated with numerous health problems, including but not limited to the following:

- Chronic diseases such as liver cirrhosis (damage to liver cells); pancreatitis (inflammation of the pancreas); various cancers, including liver, mouth, throat, larynx (the voice box), and esophagus; high blood pressure; and psychological disorders
- Unintentional injuries, such as motor-vehicle traffic crashes, falls, drowning, burns, and firearm injuries
- Violence, such as child maltreatment, homicide, and suicide
- Harm to a developing fetus, such as fetal alcohol spectrum disorders, if a woman drinks while pregnant
- Sudden infant death syndrome (SIDS)
- Alcohol abuse or dependence

I'm Young—Is Drinking Bad for My Health?

Yes.[7,8] Studies have shown that alcohol use by youth and young adults increases the risk of both fatal and nonfatal injuries.[9,10,11] Research has also shown that youth who use alcohol before age fifteen are five times more likely to become alcohol dependent than adults who begin drinking at age twenty-one.[12] Other consequences of youth alcohol use include increased risky sexual behaviors, poor school performance, and increased risk of suicide and homicide.[13,14,15]

Is It Okay to Drink When Pregnant?

No, there is no safe level of alcohol use during pregnancy. Women who are pregnant or plan on becoming pregnant should refrain from drinking alcohol.[16] Several conditions, including fetal alcohol syndrome disorders, have been linked to alcohol use during pregnancy. Women of childbearing age should also avoid binge drinking to reduce the risk of unintended pregnancy and potential exposure of a developing fetus to alcohol.

References

1. United States Department of Agriculture and United States Department of Health and Human Services. In: *Dietary Guidelines for Americans*. Chapter 9—Alcoholic Beverages. Washington, DC: US Government Printing Office; 2005, p. 43–46. Available at http://www.health.gov/DIETARYGUIDELINES/dga2005/document/html/chapter9.htm. Accessed March 28, 2008.

2. National Highway Traffic Safety Administration. Available at http://www.nhtsa.dot.gov/. Accessed March 28, 2008.

3. National Institute of Alcohol Abuse and Alcoholism. NIAAA council approves definition of binge drinking (PDF–1.6Mb) *NIAAA Newsletter* 2004;3:3.

4. *Diagnostic and Statistical Manual of Mental Disorders (DSM-IV)*, 4th edition, Text Revision. Washington, DC: American Psychiatric Association; 2000.

5. Centers for Disease Control and Prevention. Fetal alcohol spectrum disorders. Available at http://www.cdc.gov/ncbddd/fas/default.htm. Accessed March 31, 2008.

6. Substance Abuse and Mental Health Services Administration. Available at http://www.samhsa.gov/treatment/treatment_public_i.aspx. Accessed March 28, 2008.

7. National Research Council and Institute of Medicine. *Reducing Underage Drinking: A Collective Responsibility.** Committee

on Developing a Strategy to Reduce and Prevent Underage Drinking. Division of Behavioral and Social Sciences and Education. Washington, DC: The National Academies Press; 2004.

8. U.S. Department of Health and Human Services. *The Surgeon General's Call to Action to Prevent and Reduce Underage Drinking*. Rockville, MD: U.S. Department of Health and Human Services; 2007. Available at http://www.surgeongeneral.gov/topics/underagedrinking/. Accessed March 28, 2008.

9. Hingson RW, Heeren T, Jamanka A, Howland J. Age of onset and unintentional injury involvement after drinking. *JAMA* 2000; 284(12):1527–33.

10. Hingson RW, Heeren T, Winter M, Wechsler H. Magnitude of alcohol-related mortality and morbidity among U.S. college students ages 18–24: Changes from 1998 to 2001. *Annu Rev Public Health* 2005; 26:259–79.

11. Levy DT, Mallonee S, Miller TR, Smith GS, Spicer RS, Romano EO, Fisher DA. Alcohol involvement in burn, submersion, spinal cord, and brain injuries. *Medical Science Monitor* 2004;10(1): CR17–24.

12. Office of Applied Studies. The NSDUH Report: Alcohol dependence or abuse and age at first use. Rockville, MD: Substance Abuse and Mental Health Services Administration, October 2004. Available at http://www.oas.samhsa.gov/2k4/ageDependence/ageDependence.htm. Accessed March 31, 2008.

13. Substance Abuse and Mental Health Services Administration. A Comprehensive Plan for Preventing and Reducing Underage Drinking. Washington, DC: 2006. Available at http://www.stopalcoholabuse.gov/media/underagedrinking/pdf/underagerpttocongress.pdf (PDF). Accessed March 28, 2008.

14. Centers for Disease Control and Prevention (CDC). Alcohol-Related Disease Impact (ARDI). Atlanta, GA: CDC. Available at http://www.cdc.gov/alcohol/ardi.htm. Accessed March 28, 2008.

15. Miller JW, Naimi TS, Brewer RD, Jones SE. Binge drinking and associated health risk behaviors among high school students. *Pediatrics* 2007;119:76–85.

16. Department of Health and Human Services. U.S. Surgeon General Releases Advisory on Alcohol Use in Pregnancy; urges

women who are pregnant or who may become pregnant to abstain from alcohol. Released Monday, February 21, 2005. Available at http://www.hhs.gov/surgeongeneral/pressreleases/sg02222005.html. Accessed March 31, 2008.

Excessive Alcohol Use and Risks to Men's Health

Men are more likely than women to drink excessively. Excessive drinking is associated with significant increases in short-term risks to health and safety, and the risk increases as the amount of drinking increases. Men are also more likely than women to take other risks (e.g., drive fast or without a safety belt), when combined with excessive drinking, further increasing their risk of injury or death.[1,2,3,4]

Drinking Levels for Men

- Approximately 62 percent of adult men reported drinking alcohol in the last thirty days and were two times more likely to binge drink than women during the same time period.[5]
- Men average about 12.5 binge drinking episodes per person per year, while women average about 2.7 binge drinking episodes per year.[3]
- Most people who binge drink are not alcoholics or alcohol dependent.[6,7]
- It is estimated that about 17 percent of men and about 8 percent of women will meet criteria for alcohol dependence at some point in their lives.

Injuries and Deaths as a Result of Excessive Alcohol Use

- Men consistently have higher rates of alcohol-related deaths and hospitalizations than women.[1,9,10]
- Among drivers in fatal motor-vehicle traffic crashes, men are almost twice as likely as women to have been intoxicated (i.e., a blood alcohol concentration of 0.08 percent or greater).[11]
- Excessive alcohol consumption increases aggression and, as a result, can increase the risk of physically assaulting another person.[12]
- Men are more likely than women to commit suicide, and more likely to have been drinking prior to committing suicide.[13,14,15]

Reproductive Health and Sexual Function

Excessive alcohol use can interfere with testicular function and male hormone production, resulting in impotence, infertility, and reduction of male secondary sex characteristics such as facial and chest hair.[16, 17]

Excessive alcohol use is commonly involved in sexual assault. Impaired judgment caused by alcohol may worsen the tendency of some men to mistake a women's friendly behavior for sexual interest and misjudge their use of force. Also, alcohol use by men increases the chances of engaging in risky sexual activity, including unprotected sex, sex with multiple partners, or sex with a partner at risk for sexually transmitted diseases.[4]

Cancer

Alcohol consumption increases the risk of cancer of the mouth, throat, esophagus, liver, and colon in men.[18,19,20]

References

1. Centers for Disease Control and Prevention (CDC). Alcohol-Related Disease Impact (ARDI). Atlanta, GA: CDC. Available at http://www.cdc.gov/alcohol/ardi.htm. Accessed March 28, 2008.
2. Levy DT, Mallonee S, Miller TR, Smith GS, Spicer RS, Romano EO, Fisher DA. Alcohol involvement in burn, submersion, spinal cord, and brain injuries. *Med Sci Monit* 2004; 10(1):CR17–24.
3. Naimi TS, Brewer RD, Mokdad A, Clark D, Serdula MK, Marks JS. Binge drinking among US adults. *JAMA* 2003; 289(1):70–75.
4. Nolen-Hoeksema S. Gender differences in risk factors and consequences for alcohol use and problems. *Clinical Psychology Review* 2004;24:981.
5. Centers for Disease Control and Prevention. Behavioral Risk Factor Surveillance System prevalence data. Atlanta, GA: Centers for Disease Control and Prevention. Available at www.cdc.gov/brfss. Accessed March 28, 2008.
6. Dawson DA, Grant BF, LI T-K. Quantifying the risks associated with exceeding recommended drinking limits. *Alcohol Clin Exp Res* 2005;29:902–8.

7. Woerle S, Roeber J, Landen MG. Prevalence of alcohol dependence among excessive drinkers in New Mexico. *Alcohol Clin Exp Res* 2007;31:293–98.

8. Hasin DS, Stinson FS, Ogburn E, Grant BF. Prevalence, correlates, disability, and comorbidity of DSM-IV alcohol abuse and dependence in the United States. *Arch Gen Psychiatry* 2007; 64:830–42.

9. Minino AM, Heron MP, Murphy SL, Kochanek KD. Deaths: final data for 2004. *National Vital Statistics Report*, Volume 55, No. 19, August 21, 2007. Hyattsville, MD: Centers for Disease Control and Prevention, National Center for Health Statistics. Available at http://www.cdc.gov/nchs/data/nvsr/nvsr55/nvsr55_19.pdf (PDF). Accessed March 28, 2008.

10. Chen CM, Yi H. Trends in alcohol-related morbidity among short-stay community hospital discharges, United States, 1979–2005. Bethesda, MD: National Institutes of Health, National Institute on Alcohol Abuse and Alcoholism. NIAAA Surveillance Report #80; 2007. Available at http://pubs.niaaa.nih.gov/publications/surveillance80/HDS05.pdf (PDF). Accessed March 28, 2008.

11. National Highway Traffic Safety Administration. *Traffic Safety Facts 2006*. Washington, DC: U.S. Department of Transportation, National Highway Traffic Safety Administration, National Center for Statistics & Analysis. DOT HS 810 818; 2008. Available at http://www-nrd.nhtsa.dot.gov/CMSWeb/index.aspx. Accessed March 28, 2008.

12. Scott KD, Schafer J, Greenfield TK. The roles of alcohol in physical assault perpetration and victimization. *J Stud Alcohol* 1999;60:528–36.

13. Hayward l, Zubrick SR, Silburn S. Blood alcohol levels in suicide cases. *J Epidemiol Community Health* 1992; 46(3):256–60.

14. May PA, Van Winkle NW, Williams MB, McFeeley PJ, DeBruyn LM, Serna P. Alcohol and suicide death among American Indians of New Mexico: 1980–1998. *Suicide Life Threat Behav* 2002; 32(3):240–55.

15. Suokas J, Suominen K, Lonnqvist J. Chronic alcohol problems among suicide attempters—post-mortem findings of a 14-year follow-up. *Nord J Psychiatry* 2005;59(1):45–50.

16. Adler RA. Clinically important effects of alcohol on endocrine function. *Journal Clinical Endocr Metabol* 1992; 74(5):957–60.

17. Emanuele MA, Emanuele NV. Alcohol's effects on male reproduction. *Alcohol Research and Health* 1998; 22(3):195–201.

18. American Cancer Society. Alcohol and Cancer. Atlanta, GA: American Cancer Society; 2006. Available at http://www.cancer.org/downloads/PRO/alcohol.pdf*(PDF). Accessed March 28, 2008.

19. Donato F, Tagger A, Chiesa R, Ribero ML, Tomasoni V, Fasola M, et al. Hepatitis B and C virus infection, alcohol drinking and hepatocellular carcinoma: a case-control study in Italy. *Hepatology* 1997; 26(3):579–84.

20. Baan R, Straif K, Grosse Y, Secretan B, et al. on behalf of the WHO International Agency for Research on Cancer Monograph Working Group. Carcinogenicity of alcoholic beverages. *Lancet Oncol* 2007; 8:292–93.

Section 10.2

Health Risks of Smoking and How to Quit

"Health Effects of Cigarette Smoking" is excerpted from the Centers for the Disease Control and Prevention, January 23, 2008. "What Happens When You Quit Smoking?" is excerpted from "Smoking and How to Quit: What Happens When You Quit Smoking?" National Women's Health Information Center, March 19, 2008. "How to Quit" is reprinted from "Smoking and How to Quit: How to Quit," National Women's Health Information Center, March 19, 2008.

Health Effects of Cigarette Smoking

Smoking harms nearly every organ of the body, causing many diseases and reducing the health of smokers in general.[1] The adverse health effects from cigarette smoking account for an estimated 438,000 deaths, or nearly one of every five deaths, each year in the United

States.[2,3] More deaths are caused each year by tobacco use than by all deaths from human immunodeficiency virus (HIV), illegal drug use, alcohol use, motor vehicle injuries, suicides, and murders combined.[2,4]

Cancer

Cancer is the second leading cause of death and was among the first diseases causally linked to smoking.[1]

Smoking causes about 90 percent of lung cancer deaths in men and almost 80 percent of lung cancer deaths in women. The risk of dying from lung cancer is more than twenty-three times higher among men who smoke cigarettes, and about thirteen times higher among women who smoke cigarettes, compared with never smokers.[1]

Smoking causes cancers of the bladder, oral cavity, pharynx, larynx (voice box), esophagus, cervix, kidney, lung, pancreas, and stomach, and causes acute myeloid leukemia.[1]

Rates of cancers related to cigarette smoking vary widely among members of racial/ethnic groups, but are generally highest in African-American men.[5]

Cardiovascular Disease (Heart and Circulatory System)

Smoking causes coronary heart disease, the leading cause of death in the United States.[1] Cigarette smokers are two to four times more likely to develop coronary heart disease than nonsmokers.[6]

Cigarette smoking approximately doubles a person's risk for stroke.[7,8]

Cigarette smoking causes reduced circulation by narrowing the blood vessels (arteries). Smokers are more than ten times as likely as nonsmokers to develop peripheral vascular disease.[9]

Smoking causes abdominal aortic aneurysm.[1]

Respiratory Disease and Other Effects

Cigarette smoking is associated with a tenfold increase in the risk of dying from chronic obstructive lung disease.[7] About 90 percent of all deaths from chronic obstructive lung diseases are attributable to cigarette smoking.[1]

Cigarette smoking has many adverse reproductive and early childhood effects, including an increased risk for infertility, preterm delivery, stillbirth, low birth weight, and sudden infant death syndrome (SIDS).[1]

Postmenopausal women who smoke have lower bone density than women who never smoked. Women who smoke have an increased risk for hip fracture than never smokers.[10]

References

1. U.S. Department of Health and Human Services. *The Health Consequences of Smoking: A Report of the Surgeon General*. U.S. Department of Health and Human Services, Centers for Disease Control and Prevention, National Center for Chronic Disease Prevention and Health Promotion, Office on Smoking and Health, 2004 [cited 2006 Dec 5]. Available from: http://www.cdc.gov/tobacco/data_statistics/sgr/sgr_2004/index.htm.

2. Centers for Disease Control and Prevention. *Annual Smoking-Attributable Mortality, Years of Potential Life Lost, and Productivity Losses—United States, 1997–2001*. Morbidity and Mortality Weekly Report [serial online]. 2002;51(14):300–303 [cited 2006 Dec 5]. Available from: http://www.cdc.gov/mmwr/preview/mmwrhtml/mm5114a2.htm.

3. Centers for Disease Control and Prevention. *Health United States, 2003, With Chartbook on Trends in the Health of Americans*. (PDF–225KB) Hyattsville, MD: CDC, National Center for Health Statistics; 2003 [cited 2006 Dec 5]. Available from: http://www.cdc.gov/nchs/data/hus/tables/2003/03hus031.pdf.

4. McGinnis J, Foege WH. Actual Causes of Death in the United States. *Journal of the American Medical Association* 1993;270:2207–12.

5. Novotny TE, Giovino GA. Tobacco Use. In: Brownson RC, Remington PL, Davis JR (eds). *Chronic Disease Epidemiology and Control*. Washington, DC: American Public Health Association; 1998;117–148 [cited 2006 Dec 5].

6. U.S. Department of Health and Human Services. *Reducing the Health Consequences of Smoking—25 Years of Progress: A Report of the Surgeon General*. Atlanta, GA: U.S. Department of Health and Human Services, CDC; 1989. DHHS Pub. No. (CDC) 89–8411 [cited 2006 Dec 5]. Available from: http://profiles.nlm.nih.gov/NN/B/B/X/S/.

7. U.S. Department of Health and Human Services. *Tobacco Use Among U.S. Racial/Ethnic Minority Groups—African Americans, American Indians and Alaska Natives, Asian Americans and Pacific Islanders, and Hispanics: A Report of the Surgeon General*. Atlanta, GA: U.S. Department of Health and Human

Services, CDC; 1998 [cited 2006 Dec 5]. Available from: http://www.cdc.gov/tobacco/data_statistics/sgr/sgr_1998/index.htm.

8. Ockene IS, Miller NH. Cigarette Smoking, Cardiovascular Disease, and Stroke: A Statement for Healthcare Professionals From the American Heart Association. *Journal of American Health Association*. 1997; 96(9):3243–47 [cited 2006 Dec 5].

9. Fielding JE, Husten CG, Eriksen MP. Tobacco: Health Effects and Control. In: Maxcy KF, Rosenau MJ, Last JM, Wallace RB, Doebbling BN (eds.). *Public Health and Preventive Medicine*. New York: McGraw-Hill;1998;817–45 [cited 2006 Dec 5].

10. U.S. Department of Health and Human Services. *Women and Smoking: A Report of the Surgeon General*. Rockville, MD: U.S. Department of Health and Human Services, CDC; 2001 [cited 2006 Dec 5]. Available from: http://www.cdc.gov/tobacco/data_statistics/sgr/sgr_2001/index.htm.

What Happens When You Quit Smoking?

If you quit smoking right now, your body will begin to heal immediately:

- In twenty minutes your heart rate will drop.
- In twelve hours the carbon monoxide (a gas that can be toxic) in your blood will drop to normal.
- In two weeks to three months your heart attack risk will begin to drop and your lungs will be working better.
- In one to nine months your coughing and shortness of breath will decrease and your lungs will start to function better, lowering your risk of lung infection.
- In one year your risk for heart disease will be half that of a smoker.
- In five years your risk of having a stroke will be the same as that of someone who doesn't smoke.
- In ten years your risk of dying from lung cancer will be half that of a smoker. Your risk of cancer of the mouth, throat, esophagus, bladder, kidney, and pancreas will also decrease.
- In fifteen years your risk of heart disease will be the same as that of someone who doesn't smoke.

How to Quit

Make the Decision to Quit and Feel Great!

If you have made the decision to quit smoking, congratulations! Not only will you improve your own health, you will also protect the health of your loved ones by no longer exposing them to secondhand smoke.

We know how hard it can be to quit smoking. Did you know that many people try to quit two or three times before they give up smoking for good? Nicotine is a very addictive drug—as addictive as heroin and cocaine. The good news is that millions of people have given up smoking for good. It's hard work to quit, but you can do it! Freeing yourself of an expensive habit that is dangerous to your health and the health of others will make you feel great!

Many people who smoke worry that they will gain weight if they quit. In fact, nearly 80 percent of people who quit smoking do gain weight, but the average weight gain is just five pounds. Keep in mind, however, that 56 percent of people who continue to smoke will gain weight too. The bottom line: The health benefits of quitting far exceed any risks from the weight gain that may follow quitting.

Tips to Help You Quit

Research has shown that these five steps will help you to quit for good:

- **Pick a date to stop smoking:** Before that day, get rid of all cigarettes, ashtrays, and lighters everywhere you smoke. Do not allow anyone to smoke in your home. Write down why you want to quit and keep this list as a reminder.
- **Get support from your family, friends, and coworkers:** Studies have shown you will be more likely to quit if you have help. Let the people important to you know the date you will be quitting and ask them for their support. Ask them not to smoke around you or leave cigarettes out.
- **Find substitutes for smoking and vary your routine:** When you get the urge to smoke, do something to take your mind off smoking. Talk to a friend, go for a walk, or go to the movies. Reduce stress with exercise, meditation, hot baths, or reading. Try sugar-free gum or candy to help handle your cravings. Drink lots of water and juices. You might want to try changing your daily routine as well. Try drinking tea instead of coffee,

eating your breakfast in a different place, or taking a different route to work.

- **Talk to your doctor or nurse about medicines to help you quit:** Some people have withdrawal symptoms when they quit smoking. These symptoms can include depression, trouble sleeping, feeling irritable or restless, and trouble thinking clearly. There are medicines to help relieve these symptoms. Most medicines help you quit smoking by giving you small, steady doses of nicotine, the drug in cigarettes that causes addiction. Talk to your doctor or nurse to see if one of these medicines may be right for you:
    - *Nicotine patch:* Worn on the skin and supplies a steady amount of nicotine to the body through the skin
    - *Nicotine gum or lozenge:* Releases nicotine into the bloodstream through the lining in your mouth
    - *Nicotine nasal spray:* Inhaled through your nose and passes into your bloodstream
    - *Nicotine inhaler:* Inhaled through the mouth and absorbed in the mouth and throat
    - *Bupropion:* An antidepressant medicine that reduces nicotine withdrawal symptoms and the urge to smoke
    - *Varenicline (Chantix®):* A medicine that reduces nicotine withdrawal symptoms and the pleasurable effects of smoking
- **Be prepared for relapse:** Most people relapse, or start smoking again, within the first three months after quitting. Don't get discouraged if you relapse. Remember, many people try to quit several times before quitting for good. Think of what helped and didn't help the last time you tried to quit. Figuring these out before you try to quit again will increase your chances for success. Certain situations can increase your chances of smoking. These include drinking alcohol, being around other smokers, gaining weight, stress, or becoming depressed. Talk to your doctor or nurse for ways to cope with these situations.

Where to Get Help

Get more help if you need it. Join a quit-smoking program or support group to help you quit. These programs can help you handle withdrawal and stress and teach you skills to resist the urge to smoke. Contact your local hospital, health center, or health department for information about quit-smoking programs and support groups in your area.

Section 10.3

Controlling Blood Cholesterol

"About High Blood Cholesterol" and "High Blood Cholesterol Prevention" are reprinted from the Centers for Disease Control and Prevention, November 8, 2007.

About High Blood Cholesterol

Cholesterol is a waxy, fat-like substance found in your body. It is needed for the body to function normally and is found in all cells of the body. Your body makes enough cholesterol for its needs.

Cholesterol is carried in the blood in particles called lipoproteins. These particles are made up of cholesterol on the inside and protein on the outside. There are two kinds of lipoproteins:

- **Low-density lipoproteins (LDL):** These are the major type of lipoprotein that carries cholesterol in the bloodstream to the body. These are the type that can lead to a buildup of cholesterol in the arteries and lead to heart disease.
- **High-density lipoproteins (HDL):** These particles carry cholesterol back to the liver to remove it from the body. Higher levels of HDL are considered good.

An excess of either total or LDL cholesterol in the blood is a risk for heart disease and atherosclerosis. People can have an excess of cholesterol because of diet and because of the rate at which cholesterol is processed in the body. Most of the excess cholesterol comes from diet. Cholesterol can build up on the artery walls of your body. This buildup is called plaque. Over time, plaque can cause the arteries to become narrow, which is called atherosclerosis. As a result, less oxygen–rich blood can pass through. When the arteries that carry blood to the heart are affected, coronary artery disease can result. A heart attack occurs when a coronary artery becomes completely blocked. A coronary artery can become blocked either by plaque buildup or by a plaque that ruptures or bursts, which causes a clot. Angina can also develop because of plaque buildup. Angina happens when the heart does not receive enough oxygen-rich blood.

High blood cholesterol itself does not cause symptoms, so many people may not know that their cholesterol level is too high. Simple blood tests can be done to check your total, LDL, and HDL cholesterol levels and other types of fats in the blood (such as triglycerides). If it is found that your cholesterol is high, your doctor may prescribe various treatments depending on your risk for developing heart disease. These include lifestyle changes such as diet, weight control, and physical activity. Certain drugs can also be prescribed to manage your cholesterol. Lifestyle changes are usually still recommended with medications. All people can do things to help keep cholesterol within the normal range.

High Blood Cholesterol Prevention

High blood cholesterol is a major risk factor for heart disease. There are a number of things that can be done to maintain normal cholesterol levels and reduce the risk of developing heart disease. All people at any age can take steps to keep normal cholesterol levels. People with high total cholesterol, high LDL cholesterol, or low HDL cholesterol should talk with their doctor about the best way to control or improve their cholesterol.

What Affects Cholesterol Levels?

A number of things can affect the cholesterol levels in your blood. These include the following:

- **Diet:** Certain foods have types of fat that raise your cholesterol level. These types of fats include saturated fat, trans fatty acids or trans fats, and dietary cholesterol. Saturated fats come largely from animal fat in the diet, but also some vegetable oils such as palm oil. Trans fats are made when vegetable oil is hydrogenated to harden it. Research suggests that trans fatty acids can raise cholesterol levels. Dietary cholesterol is found in foods that come from animal sources such as egg yolks, meat, and dairy products.
- **Weight:** Being overweight tends to increase LDL levels, lowers HDL levels, and increases total cholesterol level.

- **Physical inactivity:** Lack of regular physical activity can lead to weight gain, which could raise your LDL cholesterol level.
- **Heredity:** High blood cholesterol can run in families. An inherited genetic condition results in very high LDL cholesterol levels. This condition is called familial hypercholesterolemia.
- **Age and sex:** As people get older, their LDL cholesterol levels tend to rise. Men tend to have lower HDL levels than women. Younger women tend to have lower LDL levels than men, but higher levels at older ages (after age fifty-five).

What Can You Do?

Have your cholesterol checked. There are usually no signs or symptoms of high blood cholesterol, so it is important to have your blood cholesterol checked. A simple blood test can be done by your doctor to check your blood cholesterol level. A lipoprotein profile can be done to measure several different kinds of cholesterol as well as triglycerides (another kind of fat found in the blood).

Desirable or optimal levels for adults with or without existing heart disease are as follows:

- Total cholesterol: Less than 200 mg/dL
- Low-density lipoprotein (LDL) cholesterol ("bad" cholesterol): Less than 100 mg/dL
- High-density lipoprotein (HDL) cholesterol ("good" cholesterol): 40 mg/dL or higher
- Triglycerides: Less than 150 mg/dL

If a full lipoprotein panel is not done, you doctor may check your total and HDL cholesterol with a simpler blood test. The National Cholesterol Education Program recommends that healthy adults have their cholesterol levels checked once every five years.

Maintain a healthy diet: An overall healthy diet can help to maintain normal blood cholesterol levels. Saturated fat, trans fats, and dietary cholesterol tend to raise blood cholesterol levels. Other types of fats, such as monounsaturated and polyunsaturated fats can help to lower blood cholesterol levels. Getting enough soluble fiber in the diet can also help to lower cholesterol. For some people, a diet that has too many carbohydrates can lower HDL (the good cholesterol) and raise triglycerides. Alcohol can also raise triglycerides, and excessive alcohol use can lead to high blood pressure, another risk factor for heart disease and stroke.

Maintain a healthy weight: Being overweight or obese can raise your bad cholesterol levels. Losing weight can help you lower your blood cholesterol levels. Healthy weight status in adults is usually assessed by using weight and height to compute a number called the "body mass index" (BMI). BMI is used because it relates to the amount of body fat for most people. An adult who has a BMI of 30 or higher is considered to be obese. Overweight is a BMI between 25 and 29.9. Normal weight is a BMI of 18.5 to 24.9. Proper diet and regular physical activity can help to maintain a healthy weight. Other measures of excess body fat may include waist measurements or waist and hip measurements.

Be active: Physical activity can help to maintain a healthy weight and lower blood cholesterol levels. The Surgeon General recommends that adults should engage in moderate-level physical activities for at least thirty minutes on most days of the week.

No tobacco: Smoking injures blood vessels and speeds up the process of hardening of the arteries. Further, smoking is a major risk for heart disease and stroke. If you don't smoke, don't start. Quitting smoking lowers one's risk of heart attack and stroke. Your doctor can suggest programs to help you quit smoking.

Medications: If you are found to have high blood cholesterol, your doctor may prescribe medications, in addition to lifestyle changes, to help bring it under control. The primary focus of treatment is to get LDL cholesterol under control. Your treatment plan and goal will depend on your LDL level and your level of risk for heart disease and stroke. Your risk for heart disease and stroke will be based on whether you also have other risk factors and may include your blood pressure level or high blood pressure treatment, smoking status, age, HDL level, family history of early heart disease, and existing cardiovascular disease or diabetes. People with existing cardiovascular disease or diabetes are considered high risk.

Several types of medicines help to lower cholesterol:

- Statin drugs lower LDL cholesterol by slowing down the production of cholesterol and by increasing the liver's ability to remove the LDL cholesterol already in the blood.

- Bile acid sequestrants help to lower LDL cholesterol by binding with cholesterol-containing bile acids in the intestines, and are then eliminated in the stool.
- Niacin, or nicotinic acid, is a B vitamin that can improve all lipoproteins. Nicotinic acid lowers total cholesterol, LDL cholesterol, and triglyceride levels, while raising HDL cholesterol levels. Because the levels needed are well above recommended dietary intake levels, niacin treatment for cholesterol should be done only under medical supervision because of possible adverse side effects.
- Fibrates are used mainly to lower triglycerides and, to a lesser extent, to increase HDL levels.

All drugs may have adverse side effects, so their use needs to be checked by your doctor on a regular basis. Once your blood cholesterol level is controlled, your doctor will want to monitor it. The lifestyle changes that your doctor recommends are just as important as taking your medicines as prescribed.

Genetic factors: Genes can play a role in high blood cholesterol. Very high blood cholesterol levels can be related to a condition known as familial hypercholesterolemia. It is also possible that high blood cholesterol levels within a family are due to factors such as common diet.

Section 10.4

Preventing High Blood Pressure

Excerpted from "High Blood Pressure," "About High Blood Pressure," and "Preventing and Controlling High Blood Pressure," Centers for Disease Control and Prevention, August 22, 2007.

It is estimated that one of three American adults has high blood pressure or hypertension. Having high blood pressure increases one's chance for developing heart disease, a stroke, and other serious conditions.

High blood pressure is sometimes called the "silent killer" because it usually has no noticeable warning signs or symptoms until other serious problems arise; therefore, many people do not know that they have it. All persons, including children, can develop high blood pressure. However, high blood pressure is easily detectable and usually can be controlled. Maintaining a healthy blood pressure is an important public health strategy. Therefore, it is important for you to know your blood pressure level and to check it regularly.

About High Blood Pressure

What Is High Blood Pressure?

Blood pressure is the force of blood against the artery walls. It is often written or stated as two numbers. The first or top number represents the pressure when the heart contracts. This is called systolic pressure. The second or bottom number represents the pressure when the heart rests between beats. This is called diastolic pressure.

Blood pressure is traditionally measured with a device called a sphygmomanometer. It measures blood pressure in millimeters of mercury (mmHg). An inflatable cuff is wrapped around the arm and is inflated to squeeze the blood vessels in the arm. The health care provider uses a stethoscope to listen to the pulse as the pressure is released in order to determine the systolic and diastolic pressure. Some blood pressure testing devices are now electronic and provide digital readouts of the blood pressure measurement and pulse rate.

Blood pressure normally rises and falls throughout the day. When it consistently stays too high for too long, it is called hypertension. The Seventh Joint National Committee on Prevention, Detection, Evaluation, and Treatment of High Blood Pressure notes these levels for defining normal and high blood pressure in adults:

- High blood pressure or hypertension for adults is defined as a systolic blood pressure of 140 mmHg or higher or a diastolic blood pressure of 90 mmHg or higher.
- Normal blood pressure is a systolic blood pressure of less than 120 mmHg and a diastolic blood pressure of less than 80 mmHg.
- Prehypertension is defined as a systolic blood pressure of 120–139 mmHg or a diastolic blood pressure of 80–89 mmHg. Persons with prehypertension are at increased risk to progress to hypertension.

If the systolic and diastolic blood pressure levels are in different categories, blood pressure status is defined according to the higher category. For example, a person with a high systolic pressure but a normal diastolic pressure will be considered to have high blood pressure (sometimes referred to as systolic hypertension). A person with a high diastolic pressure but a normal systolic pressure will be considered to have high blood pressure also (sometimes referred to as diastolic hypertension).

High blood pressure for adults will usually be measured on at least two different doctor visits before a diagnosis of high blood pressure is made.

More importantly, high blood pressure can be prevented or controlled through lifestyle changes and with medications when needed.

Types of High Blood Pressure

Essential hypertension: In most cases, high blood pressure does not have a specific treatable cause. This form is called essential hypertension.

Secondary hypertension: In a few cases, the cause of hypertension is some other underlying condition. This is called secondary hypertension. This may be due to kidney disorders, congenital abnormalities, or other conditions. Blood pressure usually returns to normal when the problem is corrected.

Pregnancy-related hypertension: Existing high blood pressure can predispose some women to develop problems when they become pregnant. This is called preexisting chronic hypertension. Also, some women first develop hypertension when they are pregnant. There are several types of this pregnancy-induced hypertension, sometimes called gestational hypertension. Either type of high blood pressure can harm the mother's kidneys and other organs, and it can cause low birth weight and early delivery.

Treatment of High Blood Pressure

High blood pressure can be treated with both lifestyle modifications, usually as the first step, and, if needed, medications. Lifestyle factors to treat high blood pressure include weight control, exercise, healthy diet, limiting alcohol use, and other lifestyle modifications.

There are several types of medications that are used to treat high blood pressure. Frequently, more than one type will be used. It is important to take these as prescribed. High blood pressure medicines fall into one of these types:

- Diuretics work in the kidney and flush excess water and sodium from the body. They are sometimes called "water pills."
- Beta blockers reduce nerve impulses to the heart and blood vessels that make the heart beat slower and with less force.
- Angiotensin-converting enzyme (ACE) inhibitors cause the blood vessels to relax. ACE inhibitors prevent the formation of a hormone called angiotensin II, which normally causes the blood vessels to narrow.
- Angiotensin antagonists shield the blood vessels from angiotensin II. As a result, the vessels become wider.
- Calcium channel blockers prevent calcium from entering the muscle cells of the heart and blood vessels. This causes the blood vessels to relax.
- Alpha-blockers reduce nerve impulses to the blood vessels, which allows the blood to pass more easily.
- Alpha-beta-blockers work the same way as alpha-blockers but also slow the heartbeat, as beta-blockers do. As a result, less blood is pumped through the vessels.
- Nervous system inhibitors relax blood vessels by controlling nerve impulses. This causes the blood vessels to become wider.

- Vasodilators directly open the blood vessels by relaxing the muscle in the vessel walls.

Outcomes of High Blood Pressure

High blood pressure is often called the "silent killer" because it usually has no noticeable warning signs or symptoms until other serious problems arise. Therefore, many people with high blood pressure do not know that they have it. High blood pressure is a major risk factor for heart disease, the leading cause of death in the United States. It can lead to hardened or stiffened arteries, which causes a decrease of blood flow to the heart muscle and other parts of the body. Reduced blood to the heart muscle can lead to angina (chest pain or damage to the heart muscle due to a lack of blood carrying oxygen to the heart muscle) or to a heart attack (caused by a chronic spasm or blockage of blood and oxygen to the heart).

High blood pressure is a major risk factor for heart failure, a serious condition where the heart cannot pump enough blood for the body's needs. It is also the major risk factor for stroke, which is the third leading cause of death in the United States. A stroke may be caused by a rupture or blockage of an artery that supplies blood and oxygen to the brain.

In addition, high blood pressure can result in damage to the eyes, including blindness. The blood vessels in the eyes can rupture or burst from high blood pressure, leading to impairment of sight.

High blood pressure can also result in kidney disease and kidney failure. The kidneys filter wastes from fluids in the body. High blood pressure can thicken and narrow the blood vessels of the kidneys, resulting in less fluid being filtered and wastes building up in the body. Also, diseases of the kidney can be a cause of high blood pressure.

Preventing and Controlling High Blood Pressure

There are several things that you can do to keep your blood pressure healthy. These actions should become part of your regular lifestyle. You should discuss with your health care provider the best ways for you to address these issues.

Maintain a healthy weight: Being overweight or obese can raise your blood pressure, and losing weight can help you lower your blood pressure. Healthy weight status in adults is usually assessed by using weight and height to compute a number called the "body mass index" (BMI). BMI is used because it relates to the amount of body fat for most people. An adult who has a BMI of 30 or higher is considered to be obese. Overweight is a BMI between 25 and 29.9. Normal weight is a BMI of 18 to 24.9. Proper diet and regular physical activity can help to maintain a healthy weight. Other measures of excess body fat may include waist measurements or waist and hip measurements.

Be active: Being physically inactive is related to high blood pressure, and physical activity can help to lower blood pressure. The Surgeon General recommends that adults should engage in moderate-level physical activities for at least thirty minutes on most days of the week.

Maintain a healthy diet: Along with healthy weight and regular physical activity, an overall healthy diet can help to maintain healthy blood pressure levels. This includes eating lots of fresh fruits and vegetables and lowering or cutting out salt or sodium and increasing potassium. High salt and sodium intake and a low potassium intake (due to not eating enough fruits and vegetables) can increase blood pressure. You need to watch the sodium that is already included in processed foods and to avoid adding sodium or salt in cooking or at the table. Low saturated fat and cholesterol are also part of an overall healthy diet. Recent studies such as the Dietary Approaches to Stop Hypertension (DASH) trial show that blood pressure can be significantly lowered through diet.

Moderate alcohol use: Excessive alcohol consumption is related to increased blood pressure. People who drink alcohol should do so in moderation. Based on current dietary guidelines, moderate drinking for women is defined as an average of one drink or less per day. Moderate drinking for men is defined as an average of two drinks or less per day.

Prevent and control diabetes: People with diabetes have a higher risk of high blood pressure, but they can also work to reduce their risk. Recent studies suggest that all people can take steps to reduce their risk of diabetes. These include a healthy diet, weight loss, and regular physical activity.

No tobacco: Smoking injures blood vessels and speeds up the process of hardening of the arteries. Further, smoking is a major risk for heart disease and stroke. If you don't smoke, don't start. Quitting smoking lowers one's risk of heart attack and stroke. Your doctor can suggest programs to help you quit smoking.

Medications: If you develop high blood pressure, your doctor may prescribe medications, in addition to lifestyle changes, to help bring it under control. Once your blood pressure is controlled, continuing your medication and doctor visits is critical to keep your blood pressure in check. The lifestyle changes noted above are just as important as taking your medicines as prescribed.

Genetic factors: Genes can play a role in high blood pressure. It is also possible that an increased risk of high blood pressure within a family is due to factors such as a common sedentary lifestyle or poor eating habits. Therefore, lifestyle factors should be considered for preventing and controlling high blood pressure.

Section 10.5

Managing Stress

Completely banishing stress from your life may never be an attainable goal. Nor, some would argue, should it be. If you consistently try your hardest and seek new endeavors, you will naturally feel challenged and sometimes even stressed. This is all part of personal growth. But sometimes stress threatens to overwhelm you.

Fortunately, there are steps you can take to minimize its negative toll, and to prevent it from getting a grip on you in the first place. These strategies provide you with a sense of control over your life and/or the situation. They also boost your mood and your confidence in handling a stressful situation.

Usually there is no one right or wrong way to cope with a stressful situation. The idea is to have as much information—as many "tools in your toolbox"—as possible.

For stressors that are uncontrollable, the key is to adapt your response to the needs of the situation and/or manage your cognitive or emotional responses in order to minimize stress. For example:

- Remind yourself that you successfully have handled similar situations in the past.
- Reassure yourself that you will be fine regardless of what happens.
- Find some humor in the situation.
- Reward yourself afterward with something enjoyable.
- Find a trusted friend to talk with about the experience.
- Use relaxation exercises to control your physical response to the situation.
- Make a list of similar situations and how you successfully managed them in the past.
- Ask others what they have done in similar situations to prepare yourself.
- Expect surprises in your life and in these situations, and don't let being stressed add to your stress.

For stressors you have some control over, you can do things to actively respond to the situation. For example:

- Make a list of stressors, so that you can prioritize them and tackle them one at a time, in order to minimize feelings of being overwhelmed.
- Change aspects of a stressful situation that give you problems. Rearrange your schedule, have a problem-solving discussion with the bothersome person, organize your workspace, schedule some time for a break, take a brief walk, or ask someone for help.
- Expect surprises in your life and in these situations, and don't let being stressed add to your stress.

Develop systematic problem-solving skills:

- Identify the stressful situation.
- Define it as an objective, solvable problem.
- Brainstorm solutions—don't evaluate them yet!

- Anticipate the possible outcomes of each solution.
- Choose a solution and act on it.
- Evaluate the results, and start over if necessary.
- Don't expect to be perfect. Give it your best shot and learn from the experiences.

Improve your coping skills. Practice assertive communication and problem solving. Find someone who successfully handles stress and imitate him or her. Surround yourself with confident and competent people. Take care of yourself physically; learn yoga, relaxation exercises, and deep muscle relaxation skills.

Plan and prepare in advance for problematic situations. For example, anticipate problems and develop a game plan for how to respond, including reminding yourself that the situation has occurred before and that you have survived it before.

Make lifestyle changes that are conducive to healthy and less stressful living. Exercise regularly, drink plenty of water, maintain a well-balanced diet and eat regular meals, try to balance work and personal life, schedule time for personal recreation, stay involved with family and friends, and limit social contact with people who are chronically negative.

There also are some medications that can calm the physiological response to stressful events. They do not teach you new coping skills to help you get through them. In the long term, learning relaxation skills, coping strategies, and how to think through problems are what will help you with the next unexpected situation.

If you find yourself unable to function at the level you used to or at the level you wish to, stress may be interfering with your life. If you find yourself worrying, feeling physical (muscle) tension, having rapid heart rate or doing a lot of "what-if-ing," or postponing work because you feel overwhelmed, talk to your family doctor or see a psychologist or psychiatrist to discuss your stress level and coping skills.

Chapter 11

Other Behaviors that Can Affect Your Health

Chapter Contents

Section 11.1

Aggressive Driving

Reprinted from "Stop Aggressive Driving Planner," National Highway Traffic Safety Administration, October 2000. Despite the older date of this document, the information presented here remains relevant.

Are You an Aggressive Driver?

Do you do the following:

- **Express frustration:** Taking out your frustrations on your fellow motorists can lead to violence or a crash.
- **Fail to pay attention when driving:** Reading, eating, drinking, or talking on the phone can be a major cause of roadway crashes.
- **Tailgate:** This is a major cause of crashes that can result in serious deaths or injuries.
- **Make frequent lane changes:** If you whip in and out of lanes to advance ahead, you can be a danger to other motorists.
- **Run red lights:** Do not enter an intersection on a yellow light. Remember flashing red lights should be treated as a stop sign.
- **Speed:** Going faster than the posted speed limit, being a "road racer," and going too fast for conditions are some examples of speeding.

Life in the Fast Lane

Plan ahead. Allow yourself extra time:

- **Concentrate:** Don't allow yourself to become distracted by talking on your cellular phone, eating, drinking, or putting on makeup.
- **Relax:** Tune the radio to your favorite relaxing music. Music can calm your nerves and help you to enjoy your time in the car.

- **Drive the posted speed limit:** Fewer crashes occur when vehicles are traveling at or about the same speed.
- **Identify alternate routes:** Try mapping out an alternate route. Even if it looks longer on paper, you may find it is less congested.
- **Use public transportation:** Public transportation can give you some much-needed relief from life behind the wheel.
- **Just be late:** If all else fails, just be late.

When Confronted with Aggressive Drivers

- **Get out of the way:** First and foremost make every attempt to get out of their way.
- **Put your pride aside:** Do not challenge them by speeding up or attempting to hold your own in your travel lane.
- **Avoid eye contact:** Eye contact can sometimes enrage an aggressive driver.
- **Gestures:** Ignore gestures and refuse to return them.
- **Report serious aggressive driving:** You or a passenger may call the police. But, if you use a cell phone, pull over to a safe location.

Section 11.2

Drug Abuse

"Commonly Abused Drugs" is adapted from "Drugs of Abuse/Uses and Effects," U.S. Department of Justice, June 2004. "Frequently Asked Questions about Drug Abuse" is excerpted from "Frequently Asked Questions," National Institute on Drug Abuse, August 13, 2008.

Commonly Abused Drugs

Commonly abused drugs include narcotics, such as heroin, morphine, oxycodone, and codeine; depressants, such as gamma hydroxybutyric acid (liquid ecstasy), benzodiazepines, barbiturates, and Quaaludes; stimulants, like cocaine and methamphetamines; hallucinogens, such as ecstasy, acid, phencyclidine hydrochloride (PCP), Psilocybe mushrooms, and peyote cactus; and cannabis, including marijuana and hashish.

Frequently Asked Questions about Drug Abuse

What Is Drug Addiction?

Drug addiction is a complex brain disease. It is characterized by drug craving, seeking, and use that can persist even in the face of extremely negative consequences. Drug seeking may become compulsive in large part as a result of the effects of prolonged drug use on brain functioning and, thus, on behavior. For many people, relapses are possible even after long periods of abstinence.

How Quickly Can I Become Addicted to a Drug?

There is no easy answer to this. If and how quickly you might become addicted to a drug depends on many factors, including the biology of your body. All drugs are potentially harmful and may have life-threatening consequences associated with their abuse. There are also vast differences among individuals in sensitivity to various drugs. While one person may use a drug one or many times and suffer no ill effects, another person may be particularly vulnerable and overdose with first use. There is no way of knowing in advance how someone may react.

How Do I Know If Someone Is Addicted to Drugs?

If a person is compulsively seeking and using a drug despite negative consequences, such as loss of job, debt, physical problems brought on by drug abuse, or family problems, then he or she probably is addicted. Seek professional help to determine if this is the case and, if so, the appropriate treatment.

What Are the Physical Signs of Abuse or Addiction?

The physical signs of abuse or addiction can vary depending on the person and the drug being abused. For example, someone who abuses marijuana may have a chronic cough or worsening of asthmatic symptoms. Each drug has short-term and long-term physical effects. Stimulants like cocaine increase heart rate and blood pressure, whereas opioids like heroin may slow the heart rate and reduce respiration.

Are There Effective Treatments for Drug Addiction?

Drug addiction can be effectively treated with behavioral-based therapies and, for addiction to some drugs such as heroin or nicotine, medications. Treatment will vary for each person depending on the type of drug(s) being used, and multiple courses of treatment may be needed to achieve success.

What Is Detoxification, or "Detox"?

Detoxification is the process of allowing the body to rid itself of a drug while managing the symptoms of withdrawal. It is often the first step in a drug treatment program and should be followed by treatment with a behavioral-based therapy and/or a medication, if available. Detox alone with no follow-up is not treatment.

What Is Withdrawal? How Long Does It Last?

Withdrawal is the variety of symptoms that occur after use of some addictive drugs is reduced or stopped. Length of withdrawal and symptoms vary with the type of drug. For example, physical symptoms of heroin withdrawal may include: restlessness, muscle and bone pain, insomnia, diarrhea, vomiting, and cold flashes. These physical symptoms may last for several days, but the general depression, or dysphoria (opposite of euphoria), that often accompanies heroin withdrawal may last for weeks. In many cases withdrawal can be easily treated with medications to ease the symptoms, but treating withdrawal is not the same as treating addiction.

Section 11.3

Anabolic Steroid Use

"Hormone Abuse Overview," © 2009 The Hormone Foundation (www.hormone.org).

Hormones are substances produced by glands (or organs) that travel to various sites in the body to affect bodily functions. Different types of steroid hormones, a class of hormones chemically similar to each other, have different functions. For example, the adrenal glands produce an anti-inflammatory steroid similar to cortisone. Cortisone may be prescribed to treat asthma, rashes, and various kinds of swelling or inflammation.

Another kind of steroid is called an anabolic steroid. The term "anabolic" means building up of a bodily substance. Anabolic steroids are related to the major male hormone testosterone, which is produced in the testes in men and in the adrenal glands in both men and women. These chemicals are recognized for their effects on building up muscle.

Synthetic (laboratory-made) anabolic steroids have some accepted uses as prescribed medications, but they are best used in specific situations calling for that type of hormone therapy and for a limited period of time. For example, anabolic steroids can help in rebuilding tissues that have become weakened because of serious injury or illness. They also can be used to treat certain types of anemia and breast cancer.

Anabolic steroids also are helpful in treating men who have a low level of testosterone and those with a rare genetic problem that causes episodes of swelling, called angioedema.

While anabolic steroids serve a clearly defined role in healing, these powerful drugs are creating serious health risks, especially for our nation's youth. The abuse of steroids, in fact, is evolving into a major health problem in the United States.

Steroids attract many young people and adults, who take these drugs to enhance athletic performance and improve their body image. Even though they may take steroids with good intentions, they may not understand that the drugs are potentially harmful and can cause a hormone imbalance leading to considerable health problems, including permanent undesirable sexual changes for both men and women. Anabolic steroids should never be taken except by prescription when under a doctor's care.

Steroid use among professional and Olympic athletes is believed to be widespread. Some athletes use steroids to build muscle mass and to speed recovery time from training and injuries. Others use them to improve their physical appearance. Athletes may continue using anabolic steroids because of a feeling of confidence and even euphoria (extreme feeling of well-being) that may result.

However, a number of unhealthy and damaging effects may result from the use of anabolic steroids that can lead to both emotional and physical problems. Studies have shown that abuse of steroids can increase aggressive behavior, cause mood swings, and impair judgment. More recently, studies have reported an association between steroid use and later abuse of other harmful drugs. Other reported effects include male-pattern baldness, acne, and blood-filled liver cysts that can rupture, causing death. Using steroids can increase the risk of heart disease, stimulate the growth of certain cancers, and worsen other medical problems.

Steroids taken orally (by mouth) have been linked to liver disease. Steroids taken by injection (by needle) can increase the risk of infectious diseases such as hepatitis or acquired immunodeficiency syndrome (AIDS). In one study, 25 percent of steroid users shared needles.

Equally troubling, anabolic steroids can retard growth. Young, developing bodies are particularly sensitive to steroids and some of the side effects may be permanent. In addition to stunting growth in adolescents whose bones should still be growing, steroids can trigger the growth of breasts in males. This can happen because the chemical structure of certain anabolic steroids is converted to the female hormone estrogen by a chemical reaction in the body.

On the other hand, females may develop a deeper voice, an enlarged clitoris, and facial hair growth. Women and girls also may experience the loss of scalp hair. These are potentially permanent side effects.

Although long-term studies are scarce, experts believe that some harmful effects may not appear until many years after the abuse of these drugs.

High-profile athletes who use steroids often become role models to children and teens because of the athletes' physical appearance and success in sports. The use of performance-enhancing substances among adult sports figures then influences the behavior of some teens, who begin to use steroids themselves. Although sports can build skills in cooperation and competition, and sports performance can enhance self-esteem, use of anabolic steroids harms young athletes' bodies as well as their minds.

In 2007, the Centers for Disease Control and Prevention (CDC) found that 3.9 percent of high school students in the United State reported using anabolic steroids without a prescription. Among high school males, 5.1 percent admitted using illegal anabolic steroids; among females, the rate was 2.7 percent.

Although males are more likely to have used illegal steroids without a prescription than females, girls are also at risk. For young women, body image is a powerful persuader, often based on inappropriate entertainment and media models. These drugs can help to decrease body fat, which is their appeal. But their side effects are serious and unattractive: facial hair, acne, male-pattern baldness, masculine appearance, and deeper voice, among others.

Easy access to performance-enhancing drugs, combined with the pressures of popular culture, presents a complex and serious problem. Because not enough research is done in this area, we still do not know how great the problem is throughout society and what the effects of steroid abuse ultimately will be.

Section 11.4

Dangers of Tanning and Ultraviolet Rays

This chapter begins with "Protect Yourself from the Sun," excerpted from the Centers for Disease Control and Prevention, May 17, 2007. Text under the heading "The Truth about Indoor Tanning" is reprinted from www.osteopathic.org, with the consent of the American Osteopathic Association. © 2008 American Osteopathic Association.

Protect Yourself from the Sun

Summer is a great time to have fun outdoors. It's also a time to take precautions to avoid sunburns, which can increase your risk of skin cancer.

Skin cancer is the most common form of cancer in the United States. Exposure to the sun's ultraviolet (UV) rays appears to be the most important environmental factor involved with developing skin cancer. During the summer months, UV radiation tends to be greater.

To help prevent skin cancer while still having fun outdoors, regularly use sun protective practices such as the following:

- Seek shade, especially during midday hours (10:00 a.m. to 4:00 p.m.), when UV rays are strongest and do the most damage.
- Cover up with clothing to protect exposed skin.
- Get a hat with a wide brim to shade the face, head, ears, and neck.
- Grab shades that wrap around and block as close to 100 percent of both ultraviolet A (UVA) and ultraviolet B (UVB) rays as possible.
- Rub on sunscreen with sun protective factor (SPF) 15 or higher, and both UVA and UVB protection.

It's always wise to choose more than one way to cover up when you're in the sun. Use sunscreen, and put on a T-shirt. Seek shade, and grab your sunglasses. Wear a hat, but rub on sunscreen too. Combining these sun protective actions helps protect your skin from the sun's damaging UV rays.

UV rays reach you on cloudy and hazy days, as well as bright and sunny days. UV rays will also reflect off any surface like water, cement, sand, and snow. Additionally, UV rays from artificial sources of light, like tanning beds, cause skin cancer and should be avoided.

Most forms of skin cancer can be cured. However, the best way to avoid skin cancer is to protect your skin from the sun.

Remember, when in the sun, seek shade, cover up, get a hat, wear sunglasses, and use sunscreen!

The Truth about Indoor Tanning

As the temperatures rise and shorts replace pants, pale winter skin may sway some to consider the speedy effects of indoor tanning to achieve a bronze summer glow. However, indoor tanning is even more dangerous than outdoor sun exposure.

"The myth of health associated with a suntan is simply that—a myth," explains Craig Wax, D.O., an osteopathic family physician practicing in Mullica Hill, New Jersey. "Some people expose themselves to the sun for the vitamin D. The amount of vitamin D made available is minimal compared with the risk of skin cancer with prolonged exposure."

He further explains that tanning is the body's way of protecting itself against ultraviolet (UV) ray exposure. The brown pigment melanin produced by skin is spread throughout the exposed areas. This pigment only minimally protects the skin against further damage from UV radiation.

Despite this information, the use of indoor tanning devices which emit ultraviolet light, both in tanning salons and at home, has never been more popular. The industry serves twenty-eight million people; generates $5 billion a year; and is represented by 30,000 tanning facilities across the country, according to the Skin Cancer Foundation.

"Many patients consider indoor tanning to be a safer alternative to sun tanning," he explains. "But it is just the opposite; tanning beds emit up to twice as much skin damaging radiation."

Dr. Wax explains that overexposure to UV rays can cause eye injury, premature wrinkling and aging of the skin, light-induced skin rashes, and increased chances of developing skin cancer.

"Young women are prone to use tanning salons," explains Dr. Wax, "because while the aging effects and skin cancer might take years to surface, the perceived social value of a tan is immediate." He warns that the dangers of tanning are serious and increase the potential for skin cancer, including:

- **Malignant melanoma:** The deadliest form of skin cancer, often surfacing as a flat or slightly raised discolored patch that has irregular borders. This is the result of intense exposure in childhood, resulting in multiple sunburns.
- **Basal cell carcinoma (BCC):** The most common form of skin cancer, BCC can be identified by an open sore, a red patch of skin, a shiny bump, a pink growth, or scar-like area. This type of skin cancer follows a similar pattern to melanoma and is best identified by a physician.

Dr. Wax further explains that the health risks associated with UV radiation are even more likely with smoking, the use of birth control pills, anti-depressants, acne medication, ingredients found in anti-dandruff shampoos, lime oil, and some cosmetics.

"If you or someone you know is using an indoor tanning device, it is important to educate them on the hazards of tanning," explains Dr. Wax.

Further, he explains that if skin shows signs of possible cancer, it is important to consult a physician immediately.

Section 11.5

Unsafe Sex

Excerpted from "Safe Sex," © 2009 A.D.A.M., Inc.
Reprinted with permission.

Safe sex means taking precautions during sex that can keep you from getting a sexually transmitted disease (STD), or from giving an STD to your partner. These diseases include genital herpes, genital warts, human immunodeficiency virus (HIV), chlamydia, gonorrhea, syphilis, hepatitis B and C, and others.

An STD is a contagious disease that can be transferred to another person through sexual intercourse or other sexual contact. Many of the organisms that cause sexually transmitted diseases live on the penis, vagina, anus, mouth, and the skin of surrounding areas.

Most of the diseases are transferred by direct contact with a sore on the genitals or mouth. However, some organisms can be transferred in body fluids without causing a visible sore. They can be transferred to another person during oral, vaginal, or anal intercourse.

Some STDs can also be transferred by nonsexual contact with infected tissues or fluids, such as infected blood. For example, sharing needles when using IV (in the vein) drugs is a major cause of HIV and hepatitis B transmission. An STD can also be transmitted through contaminated blood transfusions and blood products, through the placenta from the mother to the fetus, and sometimes through breastfeeding.

The following factors increase your risk of getting a sexually transmitted disease (STD):

- Not knowing whether a partner has an STD or not
- Having a partner with a past history of any STD
- Having sex without a male or female condom
- Using drugs or alcohol in a situation where sex might occur
- If your partner is an IV drug user
- Having anal intercourse

Drinking alcohol or using drugs increases the likelihood that you will participate in high-risk sex. In addition, some diseases can be transferred through the sharing of used needles or other drug paraphernalia.

Abstinence is an absolute answer to preventing STDs. However, abstinence is not always a practical or desirable option.

Next to abstinence, the least risky approach is to have a mutually monogamous sexual relationship with someone you know is free of any STD. Ideally, before having sex with a new partner, each of you should get screened for STDs, especially HIV and hepatitis B, and share the test results with each another.

Use condoms to avoid contact with semen, vaginal fluids, or blood. Both male and female condoms dramatically reduce the chance you will get or spread an STD. However, condoms must be used properly:

- Keep in mind that STDs can still be spread, even if you use a condom, because a condom does not cover surrounding skin areas. But a condom definitely reduces your risk.
- Lubricants may help reduce the chance a condom will break. Use only water-based lubricants, because oil-based or petroleum-type lubricants can cause latex to weaken and tear. Using condoms with nonoxynol-9 (a spermicide) can help prevent pregnancy, but may increase the chance of HIV transmission because the spermicide can irritate the vaginal walls.
- The condom should be in place from the beginning to end of sexual activity and should be used every time you have sex.
- Use latex condoms for vaginal, anal, and oral intercourse.

Here are additional safe-sex steps:

- **Be responsible:** If you have an STD, like HIV or herpes, advise any prospective sexual partner. Allow him or her to decide what to do. If you mutually agree on engaging in sexual activity, use latex condoms and other measures to protect the partner.
- **If pregnant, take precautions:** If you have an STD, learn about the risk to the infant before becoming pregnant. Ask your provider how to prevent the fetus from becoming infected. HIV-positive women should not breastfeed their infant.
- **Know your partner:** Before having sex, first establish a committed relationship that allows trust and open communication.

You should be able to discuss past sexual histories, any previous STDs or IV drug use. You should not feel coerced or forced into having sex.

- **Stay sober:** Alcohol and drugs impair your judgment, communication abilities, and ability to properly use condoms or lubricants.

In summary, safe sex requires prior planning and good communication between partners. Given that, couples can enjoy the pleasures of a sexual relationship while reducing the potential risks involved.

References

Cohn SE. Sexually transmitted diseases, HIV, and AIDS in women. *Med Clin North Am.* 2003; 87(5): 971–95.

Greydanus DE. Contraception for college students. *Pediatr Clin North Am.* 2005; 52(1): 135–61, ix.

Polizzotto MJ. Prevention of sexually transmitted diseases. *Clin Fam Pract.* 2005; 7(1): 1–12.

Workowski KA, Berman SM. Centers for Disease Control and Prevention (CDC). Clinical prevention guidance. Sexually transmitted diseases treatment guidelines. *MMWR Morb Mortal Wkly Rep.* 2006;4; 55(RR-11):2–6.

Part Two

Leading Causes of Death in Men

Chapter 12

Causes of Death: A Statistical Overview

Chapter Contents

Section 12.1

Leading Causes of Death for Men of All Ages

Reprinted from "Leading Causes of Death in Males, United States, 2004," Centers for Disease Control and Prevention, September 10, 2007.

Below are the leading causes of death in males for 2004.

Table 12.1. All Males, All Ages

Rank	Cause of Death	Percentage
1	Heart disease	27.2
2	Cancer	24.3
3	Unintentional injuries	6.1
4	Stroke	5.0
5	Chronic lower respiratory diseases	5.0
6	Diabetes	3.0
7	Influenza and pneumonia	2.3
8	Suicide	2.2
9	Kidney disease	1.7
10	Alzheimer disease	1.6

Note regarding Tables 12.2 through 12.6: Percentage is the percentage of total deaths in the race category due to the disease indicated. The white, black, American Indian/Alaska native, and Asian/Pacific Islander race groups include persons of Hispanic and non-Hispanic origin. Persons of Hispanic origin may be of any race.

Table 12.2. White Males, All Ages

Rank	Cause of Death	Percentage
1	Heart disease	27.7
2	Cancer	24.6
3	Unintentional injuries	6.1
4	Chronic lower respiratory diseases	5.3
5	Stroke	4.9
6	Diabetes	2.8
7	Influenza and pneumonia	2.3
8	Suicide	2.3
9	Alzheimer disease	1.7
10	Kidney disease	1.6

Table 12.3. Black Males, All Ages

Rank	Cause of Death	Percentage
1	Heart disease	24.8
2	Cancer	22.2
3	Unintentional injuries	5.9
4	Stroke	5.2
5	Homicide	4.7
6	Diabetes	3.8
7	Human immunodeficiency virus (HIV) disease	3.3
8	Chronic lower respiratory diseases	2.8
9	Kidney disease	2.4
10	Influenza and pneumonia	1.9

Table 12.4. American Indian or Alaska Native Males, All Ages (*continued on next page*)

Rank	Cause of Death	Percentage
1	Heart disease	20.1
2	Cancer	17.4
3	Unintentional injuries	14.2
4	Diabetes	5.1
5	Chronic liver disease	4.5

Table 12.4. American Indian or Alaska Native Males, All Ages (*continued*)

Rank	Cause of Death	Percentage
6	Suicide	4.3
7	Stroke	3.4
8	Chronic lower respiratory diseases	3.3
9	Homicide	2.5
10	Influenza and pneumonia	2.0

Table 12.5. Asian or Pacific Islander Males, All Ages

Rank	Cause of Death	Percentage
1	Cancer	26.7
2	Heart disease	25.4
3	Stroke	7.6
4	Unintentional injuries	5.5
5	Chronic lower respiratory diseases	3.5
6	Diabetes	3.3
7	Influenza and pneumonia	2.8
8	Suicide	2.5
9	Kidney disease	1.7
10	Homicide	1.2

Table 12.6. Hispanic Males, All Ages

Rank	Cause of Death	Percentage
1	Heart disease	21.9
2	Cancer	19.0
3	Unintentional injuries	11.4
4	Stroke	4.7
5	Diabetes	4.2
6	Homicide	4.1
7	Chronic liver disease	3.5
8	Suicide	2.7
9	Chronic lower respiratory diseases	2.4
10	Perinatal conditions	2.2

Section 12.2

A Statistical Look at Cancer in Men

Reprinted from "Cancer among Men," Centers for Disease Control and Prevention, October 4, 2007.

Three most common cancers among men (the numbers in parentheses are the rates per 100,000 persons):

- Prostate cancer (145.3): First among men of all races and Hispanic origin
- Lung cancer (85.3): Second among white (84.4), black (104.5), Asian/Pacific Islander (49.7), and American Indian/Alaska Native (51.1) men; third among Hispanic men (48.5)
- Colorectal cancer (58.2): Second among Hispanic men (50.3); third among white (57.0), black (67.6), Asian/Pacific Islander (42.0), and American Indian/Alaska Native (32.6) men

Leading causes of cancer death among men:

- Lung cancer (70.3): First among men of all racial and Hispanic origin
- Prostate cancer (25.4): Second among white (23.4), black (56.1), American Indian/Alaska Native (16.5), and Hispanic (19.3) men
- Colorectal cancer (21.6): Third among men of all races and Hispanic origin
- Liver cancer: Second among Asian/Pacific Islander men (15.1).

Note: The combined rate for all races is presented when the ranking of cancer sites did not differ across race and ethnicity; race- or ethnicity-specific rates are presented when ranking differed by race or ethnicity.

Section 12.3

Homicide Statistics

Reprinted from "Homicide Trends in the U.S.: Trends by Gender," U.S. Department of Justice, July 11, 2007.

Most victims and perpetrators in homicides are male:

- Male offender/Male victim: 65.3 percent
- Male offender/Female victim: 22.7 percent
- Female offender/Male victim: 9.6 percent
- Female offender/Female victim: 2.4 percent

Both male and female offenders are more likely to target male victims than female victims.

Victimization rates for both males and females have declined in recent years:

- Males were almost four times more likely than females to be murdered in 2005.
- In 2005 rates for females reached their lowest point recorded; rates for males increased slightly from the low point recorded in 2000.

Offending rates for both males and females followed the same pattern as victimization rates:

- Males were almost ten times more likely than females to commit murder in 2005.
- The offending rates for females declined since the early 1980s but stabilized after 1999. Offending rates for males peaked in the early 1990s, fell to record lows, and stabilized in recent years.

The gender distribution of homicide victims and offenders differs by type of homicide:

- For the years 1976 to 2005 combined, among all homicide victims, females are particularly at risk for intimate killings and sex-related homicides.

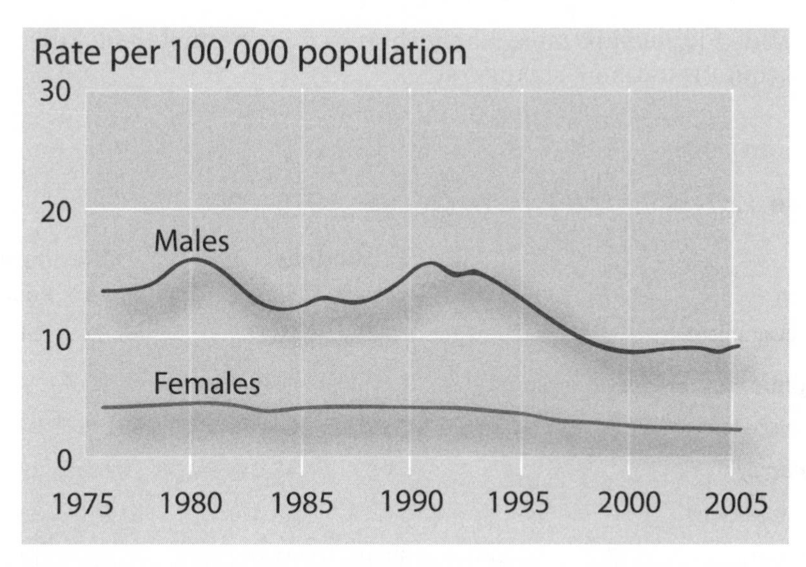

Figure 12.1. *Homicide victimization by gender, 1976–2005*

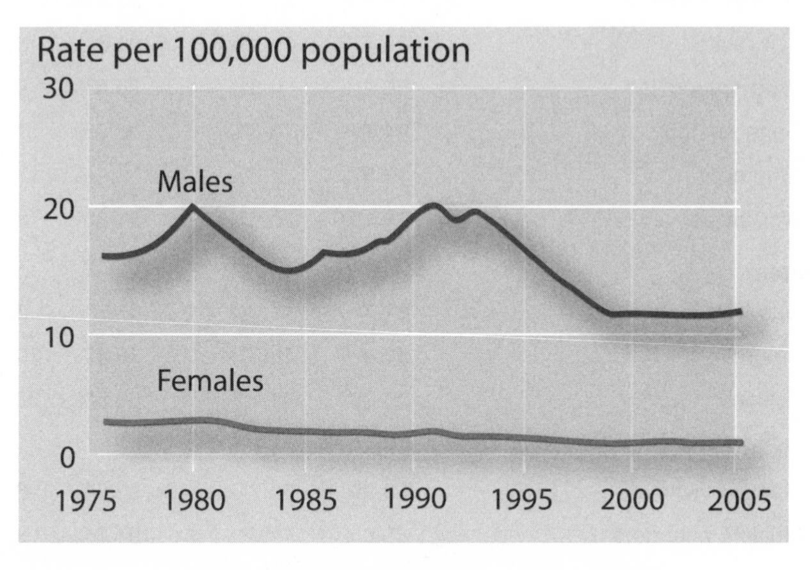

Figure 12.2. *Homicide offending by gender, 1976–2005*

The relationship between the victim and the offender differs for female and male victims:

- Female victims are more likely than male victims to be killed by an intimate or family member.
- Male victims are more likely than female victims to be killed by acquaintances or strangers.

Table 12.7. Homicide Type by Gender, 1976–2005

	Victims		Offenders	
	Male	**Female**	**Male**	**Female**
All homicides	76.5%	23.5%	88.8%	11.2%
Victim/offender relationship				
Intimate	35.2%	64.8%	65.5%	34.5%
Family	51.5%	48.5%	70.8%	29.2%
Infanticide	54.6%	45.4%	61.8%	38.2%
Eldercide	58.1%	41.9%	85.2%	14.8%
Circumstances				
Felony murder	78.4%	21.6%	93.2%	6.8%
Sex related	18.8%	81.2%	93.6%	6.4%
Drug related	90.2%	9.8%	95.5%	4.5%
Gang related	94.7%	5.3%	98.3%	1.7%
Argument	77.8%	22.2%	85.6%	14.4%
Workplace	79.1%	20.9%	91.3%	8.7%
Weapon				
Gun homicide	82.7%	17.3%	91.3%	8.7%
Arson	56.4%	43.6%	79.1%	20.9%
Poison	55.3%	44.7%	63.5%	36.5%
Multiple victims or offenders				
Multiple victims	63.3%	36.7%	93.5%	6.5%
Multiple offenders	85.6%	14.4%	91.6%	8.4%

Table 12.8. Victim Offender Relationship by Victim Gender, 1976–2005

	Percentage of homicide victims by gender	
Victim/Offender relationship	**Male**	**Female**
Total	100.0 %	100.0 %
Intimate	5.0%	30.0%
Spouse	3.0	18.3
Ex-spouse	0.2	1.4
Boyfriend/Girlfriend	1.8	10.4
Other family	6.8%	11.8%
Parent	1.3	2.8
Child	2.1	5.4
Sibling	1.2	0.9
Other family	2.2	2.8
Acquaintance/Known	35.3%	21.8%
Neighbor	1.1	1.3
Employee/er	0.1	0.1
Friend/Acquaintance	29.4	17.0
Other Known	4.6	3.4
Stranger	15.5%	8.7%
Undetermined	37.4%	27.6%

Source: FBI, Supplementary Homicide Reports, 1976–2005.

Note: The victims of the September 11, 2001, terrorist attacks are not included in this analysis.

Chapter 13

Heart Disease

Chapter Contents

Section 13.1

Men and Heart Disease

Excerpted from "Men and Heart Disease Fact Sheet," Centers for Disease Control and Prevention, June 6, 2008.

Facts on Heart Disease in Men

In 2005, 322,841 men died from heart disease, the leading cause of death for men in the United States.[1]

The age-adjusted death rate for heart disease in men was 260 per 100,000 population in 2005.[1]

About 9.4 percent of all white men, 7.1 percent of black men, and 5.6 percent of Mexican American men live with coronary heart disease.[2]

The average age of a first heart attack for men is sixty-six years.[7]

Almost half of men who have a heart attack under age sixty-five die within eight years.[4]

Results from the Framingham Heart Study suggest that men have a 49 percent lifetime risk of developing coronary heart disease after the age of forty.[4]

Between 70 and 89 percent of sudden cardiac events occur in men.[4]

Major risk factors for heart disease include high blood pressure, high blood cholesterol, tobacco use, diabetes, physical inactivity, and poor nutrition.[5]

In a large study of blood pressure treatment and control, an average reduction of 12 to 13 mm Hg in systolic blood pressure over four years of follow-up was associated with a 21 percent reduction in coronary heart disease, 37 percent reduction in stroke, and 13 percent reduction in all-cause mortality rates.[6]

Studies suggest that a 10 percent decrease in total cholesterol levels may reduce the development of coronary heart disease by as much as 30 percent.[3]

In this section, the term "heart disease" refers to the broadest category of "disease of the heart" as defined by the International Classification of Diseases and used by the Center for Disease Control's (CDC's) National Center for Health Statistics. This category includes acute rheumatic fever, chronic rheumatic heart disease, hypertensive heart disease, coronary heart disease, pulmonary heart disease, congestive heart failure, and any other heart condition or disease.

References

1. National Center for Health Statistics. Health, United States, 2007 with *Chartbook on Trends in the Health of Americans*. Hyatsville, MD: 2007.
2. American Heart Association. *Heart Disease and Stroke Statistics—2008 Update*. Dallas, Texas: American Heart Association, 2008.
3. Cohen, JD. A population-based approach to cholesterol control. *American Journal of Medicine* 1997:102:23–25.
4. Hurst W. *The Heart, Arteries, and Veins*. 10th ed. New York: McGraw Hill; 2002.
5. Preventing chronic diseases: Investing wisely in health preventing heart disease and stroke. July 2005. Centers for Disease Control and Prevention. February 6, 2006. http://www.cdc.gov/nccdphp/publications/factsheets/Prevention/cvh.htm
6. He J, Whelton PK. Elevated systolic blood pressure and risk of cardiovascular and renal disease: overview of evidence from observational epidemiologic studies and randomized controlled trials. *Am Heart J*. 1999; 138(3 Pt 2):211–19.
7. American Heart Association. *Heart Disease and Stroke Statistics—2005 Update*. Dallas, Texas: American Heart Association, 2005.

Section 13.2

Coronary Artery Disease

Excerpted from "Coronary Artery Disease," National Heart Lung and Blood Institute, National Institutes of Health, June 2008.

What Is Coronary Artery Disease?

Coronary artery disease (CAD) is a condition in which plaque builds up inside the coronary arteries. These arteries supply your heart muscle with oxygen-rich blood.

Plaque is made up of fat, cholesterol, calcium, and other substances found in the blood. When plaque builds up in the arteries, the condition is called atherosclerosis.

Plaque narrows the arteries and reduces blood flow to your heart muscle. It also makes it more likely that blood clots will form in your arteries. Blood clots can partially or completely block blood flow.

Overview

When your coronary arteries are narrowed or blocked, oxygen-rich blood can't reach your heart muscle. This can cause angina or a heart attack.

Angina is chest pain or discomfort that occurs when not enough oxygen-rich blood is flowing to an area of your heart muscle. Angina may feel like pressure or squeezing in your chest. The pain also may occur in your shoulders, arms, neck, jaw, or back.

A heart attack occurs when blood flow to an area of your heart muscle is completely blocked. This prevents oxygen-rich blood from reaching that area of heart muscle and causes it to die. Without quick treatment, a heart attack can lead to serious problems and even death.

Over time, CAD can weaken the heart muscle and lead to heart failure and arrhythmias. Heart failure is a condition in which your heart can't pump enough blood throughout your body. Arrhythmias are problems with the speed or rhythm of your heartbeat.

Outlook

CAD is the most common type of heart disease. It's the leading cause of death in the United States for both men and women. Lifestyle changes, medicines, and/or medical procedures can effectively prevent or treat CAD in most people.

What Causes Coronary Artery Disease?

Research suggests that coronary artery disease (CAD) starts when certain factors damage the inner layers of the coronary arteries. These factors include the following:

- Smoking
- High amounts of certain fats and cholesterol in the blood
- High blood pressure
- High amounts of sugar in the blood due to insulin resistance or diabetes

When damage occurs, your body starts a healing process. Excess fatty tissues release compounds that promote this process. This healing causes plaque to build up where the arteries are damaged.

The buildup of plaque in the coronary arteries may start in childhood. Over time, plaque can narrow or completely block some of your coronary arteries. This reduces the flow of oxygen-rich blood to your heart muscle.

Plaque also can crack, which causes blood cells called platelets to clump together and form blood clots at the site of the cracks. This narrows the arteries more and worsens angina or causes a heart attack.

Who Is at Risk for Coronary Artery Disease?

Certain traits, conditions, or habits may raise your chance of developing CAD. These conditions are known as risk factors.

You can control most risk factors and help prevent or delay CAD. Other risk factors can't be controlled.

Major Risk Factors

Many factors raise the risk of developing CAD. The more risk factors you have, the greater chance you have of developing CAD:

- **Unhealthy blood cholesterol levels:** This includes high low-density lipoprotein (LDL) cholesterol (sometimes called bad cholesterol) and low high-density lipoprotein (HDL) cholesterol (sometimes called good cholesterol).
- **High blood pressure:** Blood pressure is considered high if it stays at or above 140/90 mmHg over a period of time.
- **Smoking:** This can damage and tighten blood vessels, raise cholesterol levels, and raise blood pressure. Smoking also doesn't allow enough oxygen to reach the body's tissues.
- **Insulin resistance:** This condition occurs when the body can't use its own insulin properly. Insulin is a hormone that helps move blood sugar into cells where it's used.
- **Diabetes:** This is a disease in which the body's blood sugar level is high because the body doesn't make enough insulin or doesn't use its insulin properly.
- **Overweight or obesity:** Overweight is having extra body weight from muscle, bone, fat, and/or water. Obesity is having a high amount of extra body fat.
- **Metabolic syndrome:** Metabolic syndrome is the name for a group of risk factors linked to overweight and obesity that raise your chance for heart disease and other health problems, such as diabetes and stroke.
- **Lack of physical activity:** Lack of activity can worsen other risk factors for CAD.
- **Age:** As you get older, your risk for CAD increases. Genetic or lifestyle factors cause plaque to build in your arteries as you age. By the time you're middle-aged or older, enough plaque has built up to cause signs or symptoms. In men, the risk for CAD increases after age forty-five. In women, the risk for CAD risk increases after age fifty-five.
- **Family history of early heart disease:** Your risk increases if your father or a brother was diagnosed with CAD before fifty-five years of age, or if your mother or a sister was diagnosed with CAD before sixty-five years of age.

Although age and a family history of early heart disease are risk factors, it doesn't mean that you will develop CAD if you have one or both.

Making lifestyle changes and/or taking medicines to treat other risk factors can often lessen genetic influences and prevent CAD from developing, even in older adults.

Emerging Risk Factors

Scientists continue to study other possible risk factors for CAD.

High levels of a protein called C-reactive protein (CRP) in the blood may raise the risk for CAD and heart attack. High levels of CRP are proof of inflammation in the body. Inflammation is the body's response to injury or infection. Damage to the arteries' inner walls seems to trigger inflammation and help plaque grow.

Research is under way to find out whether reducing inflammation and lowering CRP levels also can reduce the risk of developing CAD and having a heart attack.

High levels of fats called triglycerides in the blood also may raise the risk of CAD, particularly in women.

Other Factors that Affect Coronary Artery Disease

Other factors also may contribute to CAD. These include the following:

- **Sleep apnea:** Sleep apnea is a disorder in which your breathing stops or gets very shallow while you're sleeping. Untreated sleep apnea can raise your chances of having high blood pressure, diabetes, and even a heart attack or stroke.
- **Stress:** Research shows that the most commonly reported "trigger" for a heart attack is an emotionally upsetting event—particularly one involving anger.
- **Alcohol:** Heavy drinking can damage the heart muscle and worsen other risk factors for heart disease. Men should have no more than two drinks containing alcohol a day. Women should have no more than one drink containing alcohol a day.

What Are the Signs and Symptoms of Coronary Artery Disease?

A common symptom of coronary artery disease (CAD) is angina. Angina is chest pain or discomfort that occurs when your heart muscle doesn't get enough oxygen-rich blood.

Angina may feel like pressure or a squeezing pain in your chest. You also may feel it in your shoulders, arms, neck, jaw, or back. This pain tends to get worse with activity and go away when you rest. Emotional stress also can trigger the pain.

Another common symptom of CAD is shortness of breath. This symptom happens if CAD causes heart failure. When you have heart failure, your heart can't pump enough blood throughout your body. Fluid builds up in your lungs, making it hard to breathe.

The severity of these symptoms varies. The symptoms may get more severe as the buildup of plaque continues to narrow the coronary arteries.

Some people who have CAD have no signs or symptoms. This is called silent CAD. It may not be diagnosed until a person show signs and symptoms of a heart attack, heart failure, or an arrhythmia (an irregular heartbeat).

Heart Attack

A heart attack happens when an area of plaque in a coronary artery breaks apart, causing a blood clot to form.

The blood clot cuts off most or all blood to the part of the heart muscle that's fed by that artery. Cells in the heart muscle die because they don't receive enough oxygen-rich blood. This can cause lasting damage to your heart.

The most common symptom of heart attack is chest pain or discomfort. Most heart attacks involve discomfort in the center of the chest that lasts for more than a few minutes or goes away and comes back. The discomfort can feel like pressure, squeezing, fullness, or pain. It can be mild or severe. Heart attack pain can sometimes feel like indigestion or heartburn.

Heart attacks also can cause upper body discomfort in one or both arms, the back, neck, jaw, or stomach. Shortness of breath or fatigue (tiredness) often may occur with or before chest discomfort. Other symptoms of heart attack are nausea (feeling sick to your stomach), vomiting, lightheadedness or fainting, and breaking out in a cold sweat.

Heart Failure

Heart failure is a condition in which your heart can't pump enough blood to your body. Heart failure doesn't mean that your heart has stopped or is about to stop working. It means that your heart can't fill with enough blood or pump with enough force, or both.

This causes you to have shortness of breath and fatigue that tends to increase with activity. Heart failure also can cause swelling in your feet, ankles, legs, and abdomen.

Arrhythmia

An arrhythmia is a problem with the speed or rhythm of the heartbeat. When you have an arrhythmia, you may notice that your heart is skipping beats or beating too fast. Some people describe arrhythmias as a fluttering feeling in their chests. These feelings are called palpitations.

Some arrhythmias can cause your heart to suddenly stop beating. This condition is called sudden cardiac arrest (SCA). SCA can make you faint and it can cause death if it's not treated right away.

How Is Coronary Artery Disease Diagnosed?

Your doctor will diagnose coronary artery disease (CAD) based on the following things:

- Your medical and family histories
- Your risk factors
- The results of a physical exam and diagnostic tests and procedures

Diagnostic Tests and Procedures

No single test can diagnose CAD. If your doctor thinks you have CAD, he or she will probably do one or more of the following tests.

Electrocardiogram (EKG): An EKG is a simple test that detects and records the electrical activity of your heart. An EKG shows how fast your heart is beating and whether it has a regular rhythm. It also shows the strength and timing of electrical signals as they pass through each part of your heart. Certain electrical patterns that the EKG detects can suggest whether CAD is likely. An EKG also can show signs of a previous or current heart attack.

Stress testing: During stress testing, you exercise to make your heart work hard and beat fast while heart tests are performed. If you can't exercise, you're given medicine to speed up your heart rate.

When your heart is beating fast and working hard, it needs more blood and oxygen. Arteries narrowed by plaque can't supply enough oxygen-rich blood to meet your heart's needs. A stress test can show possible signs of CAD, such as the following:

- Abnormal changes in your heart rate or blood pressure

- Symptoms such as shortness of breath or chest pain
- Abnormal changes in your heart rhythm or your heart's electrical activity

During the stress test, if you can't exercise for as long as what's considered normal for someone your age, it may be a sign that not enough blood is flowing to your heart. But other factors besides CAD can prevent you from exercising long enough (for example, lung diseases, anemia, or poor general fitness).

Some stress tests use a radioactive dye, sound waves, positron emission tomography (PET), or cardiac magnetic resonance imaging (MRI) to take pictures of your heart when it's working hard and when it's at rest.

These imaging stress tests can show how well blood is flowing in the different parts of your heart. They also can show how well your heart pumps blood when it beats.

Echocardiography: This test uses sound waves to create a moving picture of your heart. Echocardiography provides information about the size and shape of your heart and how well your heart chambers and valves are working.

The test also can identify areas of poor blood flow to the heart, areas of heart muscle that aren't contracting normally, and previous injury to the heart muscle caused by poor blood flow.

Chest x-ray: A chest x ray takes a picture of the organs and structures inside the chest, including your heart, lungs, and blood vessels. A chest x ray can reveal signs of heart failure, as well as lung disorders and other causes of symptoms that aren't due to CAD.

Blood tests: Blood tests check the levels of certain fats, cholesterol, sugar, and proteins in your blood. Abnormal levels may show that you have risk factors for CAD.

Electron-beam computed tomography (EBCT): This test finds and measures calcium deposits (called calcifications) in and around the coronary arteries. The more calcium detected, the more likely you are to have CAD. EBCT isn't used routinely to diagnose CAD, because its accuracy isn't yet known.

Coronary angiography and cardiac catheterization: Your doctor may ask you to have coronary angiography if other tests or factors show that you're likely to have CAD. This test uses dye and special x-rays to show the insides of your coronary arteries.

To get the dye into your coronary arteries, your doctor will use a procedure called cardiac catheterization. A long, thin, flexible tube called a catheter is put into a blood vessel in your arm, groin (upper thigh), or neck. The tube is then threaded into your coronary arteries, and the dye is released into your bloodstream. Special x-rays are taken while the dye is flowing through your coronary arteries.

Cardiac catheterization is usually done in a hospital. You're awake during the procedure. It usually causes little to no pain, although you may feel some soreness in the blood vessel where your doctor put the catheter.

How Is Coronary Artery Disease Treated?

Treatment for coronary artery disease (CAD) may include lifestyle changes, medicines, and medical procedures. The goals of treatments are as follows:

- To relieve symptoms
- To reduce risk factors in an effort to slow, stop, or reverse the buildup of plaque
- To lower the risk of blood clots forming, which can cause a heart attack
- To widen or bypass clogged arteries
- To prevent complications of CAD

Lifestyle Changes

Making lifestyle changes can often help prevent or treat CAD. For some people, these changes may be the only treatment needed:

- Follow a heart healthy eating plan to prevent or reduce high blood pressure and high blood cholesterol and to maintain a healthy weight.
- Increase your physical activity. Check with your doctor first to find out how much and what kinds of activity are safe for you.
- Lose weight, if you're overweight or obese.
- Quit smoking, if you smoke. Avoid exposure to secondhand smoke.
- Learn to cope with and reduce stress.

Medicines

You may need medicines to treat CAD if lifestyle changes aren't enough. Medicines used to treat CAD include anticoagulants, aspirin and other antiplatelet medicines, angiotensin-converting enzyme (ACE) inhibitors, beta blockers, calcium channel blockers, nitroglycerin, glycoprotein IIb-IIIa, statins, and fish oil and other supplements high in omega-3 fatty acids.

Medical Procedures

You may need a medical procedure to treat CAD. Both angioplasty and coronary artery bypass grafting (CABG) are used as treatments.

Angioplasty opens blocked or narrowed coronary arteries. During angioplasty, a thin tube with a balloon or other device on the end is threaded through a blood vessel to the narrowed or blocked coronary artery. Once in place, the balloon is inflated to push the plaque outward against the wall of the artery. This widens the artery and restores the flow of blood.

Angioplasty can improve blood flow to your heart, relieve chest pain, and possibly prevent a heart attack. Sometimes a small mesh tube called a stent is placed in the artery to keep it open after the procedure.

In CABG, arteries or veins from other areas in your body are used to bypass (that is, go around) your narrowed coronary arteries. CABG can improve blood flow to your heart, relieve chest pain, and possibly prevent a heart attack.

You and your doctor can discuss which treatment is right for you.

Cardiac Rehabilitation

Your doctor may prescribe cardiac rehabilitation (rehab) for angina or after CABG, angioplasty, or a heart attack. Cardiac rehab, when combined with medicine and surgical treatments, can help you recover faster, feel better, and develop a healthier lifestyle. Almost everyone with CAD can benefit from cardiac rehab.

Living With Coronary Artery Disease

Doing physical activity regularly, taking prescribed medicines, following a heart healthy eating plan, and watching your weight can help control CAD.

See your doctor regularly to keep track of your blood pressure and blood cholesterol and blood sugar levels. Talk to your doctor about how often you should schedule office visits or blood tests. Between those visits, call your doctor if you develop any new symptoms or if your symptoms worsen.

Let the people you see regularly know you're at risk for a heart attack. They can seek emergency care if you suddenly faint, collapse, or develop other severe symptoms.

You may feel depressed or anxious if you've been diagnosed with CAD and/or had a heart attack. You may worry about heart problems or making lifestyle changes that are necessary for your health. Your doctor may recommend medicine, professional counseling, or relaxation therapy if you have depression or anxiety.

Section 13.3

Heart Attack

Excerpted from "What Is a Heart Attack," National Heart Lung and Blood Institute, National Institutes of Health, March 2008.

What Is a Heart Attack?

A heart attack occurs when blood flow to a section of heart muscle becomes blocked. If the flow of blood isn't restored quickly, the section of heart muscle becomes damaged from lack of oxygen and begins to die.

Heart attack is a leading killer of both men and women in the United States. But fortunately, today there are excellent treatments for heart attack that can save lives and prevent disabilities. Treatment is most effective when started within one hour of the beginning of symptoms. If you think you or someone you're with is having a heart attack, call 9–1–1 right away.

Overview

Heart attacks occur most often as a result of a condition called coronary artery disease (CAD). In CAD, a fatty material called plaque builds up over many years on the inside walls of the coronary arteries (the arteries that supply blood and oxygen to your heart). Eventually, an area of plaque can rupture, causing a blood clot to form on the surface of the plaque. If the clot becomes large enough, it can mostly or completely block the flow of oxygen-rich blood to the part of the heart muscle fed by the artery.

During a heart attack, if the blockage in the coronary artery isn't treated quickly, the heart muscle will begin to die and be replaced by scar tissue. This heart damage may not be obvious, or it may cause severe or long-lasting problems.

Severe problems linked to heart attack can include heart failure and life-threatening arrhythmias (irregular heartbeats). Heart failure is a condition in which the heart can't pump enough blood throughout the body. Ventricular fibrillation is a serious arrhythmia that can cause death if not treated quickly.

Get Help Quickly

Acting fast at the first sign of heart attack symptoms can save your life and limit damage to your heart. Treatment is most effective when started within one hour of the beginning of symptoms.

The most common heart attack signs and symptoms are as follows:

- Chest discomfort or pain—uncomfortable pressure, squeezing, fullness, or pain in the center of the chest that can be mild or strong. This discomfort or pain lasts more than a few minutes or goes away and comes back.
- Upper body discomfort in one or both arms, the back, neck, jaw, or stomach.
- Shortness of breath may occur with or before chest discomfort.
- Other signs include nausea (feeling sick to your stomach), vomiting, lightheadedness or fainting, or breaking out in a cold sweat.

If you think you or someone you know may be having a heart attack:

- Call 9–1–1 within a few minutes—five at the most—of the start of symptoms.
- If your symptoms stop completely in less than five minutes, still call your doctor.
- Only take an ambulance to the hospital. Going in a private car can delay treatment.

- Take a nitroglycerin pill if your doctor has prescribed this type of medicine.

Outlook

Each year, about 1.1 million people in the United States have heart attacks, and almost half of them die. CAD, which often results in a heart attack, is the leading killer of both men and women in the United States.

Many more people could recover from heart attacks if they got help faster. Of the people who die from heart attacks, about half die within an hour of the first symptoms and before they reach the hospital.

Section 13.4

Heart Failure

Reprinted from "Heart Failure: Frequently Asked Questions," NIH Senior Health, December 28, 2007.

What is heart failure?

In heart failure, the heart cannot pump enough blood through the body. Heart failure develops over time as the pumping action of the heart gets weaker. Heart failure does not mean that the heart has stopped working or is about to stop working.

When the heart is weakened by heart failure, blood and fluid can back up into the lungs and fluid builds up in the feet, ankles, and legs. People with heart failure often experience tiredness and shortness of breath.

What causes heart failure?

Heart failure is caused by other diseases and conditions that damage the heart muscle. It is most commonly caused by coronary artery disease, including heart attack. Diabetes and high blood pressure also contribute to heart failure risk. People who have had a heart attack are at high risk of developing heart failure.

What are the symptoms of heart failure?

The most common symptoms of heart failure include shortness of breath or difficulty breathing, feeling tired, and swelling. Swelling is caused by fluid buildup in the body and can lead to weight gain and frequent urination, as well as coughing.

How common is heart failure?

Approximately five million people in the United States have heart failure. It contributes to three hundred thousand deaths each year. It is the number one cause of hospitalizations for people over the age of sixty-five.

Who is at greatest risk?

Heart failure is most common in people over sixty-five. African Americans are more likely to have heart failure and to suffer more severely from it. African Americans are more likely to develop symptoms at an earlier age, have their heart failure get worse faster, have more hospital visits, and die from heart failure. High blood cholesterol, high blood pressure, and diabetes are risk factors for coronary artery disease and heart failure.

Do men or women have a higher risk of heart failure?

Men have a higher rate of heart failure than women, but because women usually live longer, the condition affects more women in their seventies and eighties.

How can heart failure be prevented?

Keeping your cholesterol and blood pressure levels healthy and keeping diabetes in check can help prevent coronary artery disease and heart failure. You can prevent heart disease by losing weight if you are overweight, quitting smoking, and limiting the amount of alcohol you drink. Doctors also recommend that you eat a diet low in salt because salt can cause extra fluid to build up in your body.

What are the tests for heart failure?

There is not one specific test to diagnose heart failure. Because the symptoms are common for other conditions, your doctor will determine if you have heart failure by doing a detailed medical history, an examination, and several tests. During a physical exam, a doctor will listen for abnormal heart sounds and lung sounds that indicate fluid buildup, as well as look for signs of swelling.

If there are signs of heart failure, the doctor may order several tests, including the following:

- An electrocardiogram (EKG) to measure the rate and regularity of the heartbeat
- A chest x-ray to evaluate the heart and lungs
- A B-type natriuretic peptide (BNP) blood test to measure the level of a hormone called BNP that increases when heart failure is present

How is heart failure treated?

Treatment for heart failure includes lifestyle changes, medications, and specialized care for those in advanced stages of the disease. Lifestyle changes may mean reducing salt and fluid intake, and adopting a plan to lose weight.

Medications for the management of heart failure include diuretics to reduce fluid buildup, angiotensin-converting enzyme (ACE) inhibitors to lower blood pressure, beta blockers to slow the heart rate, and digoxin to help the heart beat stronger and pump more blood. For severe heart failure, patients may require additional oxygen, a mechanical heart pump, or transplantation.

What research is being conducted on heart failure?

Scientists are trying to determine the best way to prevent and treat heart failure. For example, a recent study by the National Heart, Lung, and Blood Institute found that implantable defibrillators can prolong the lives of some heart failure patients.

Researchers are also looking at genetics in relation to heart failure treatments. One study is investigating whether patients who have certain genetic markers may respond better to beta blockers than those who do not.

Section 13.5

Cardiac Arrest

"Sudden Cardiac Arrest Facts," © 2008 Sudden Cardiac Arrest Association (www.suddencardiacarrest.org). Reprinted with permission.

What Is Sudden Cardiac Arrest?

Sudden cardiac arrest (SCA) is a leading cause of death in the United States, killing more than 325,000 people each year. That's more than the total death rate for breast cancer, lung cancer, and human immunodeficiency virus (HIV)/acquired immunodeficiency syndrome (AIDS) combined. During SCA, heart function ceases abruptly and without warning. When this occurs, the heart is no longer able to pump blood to the rest of the body, and in over 90 percent of victims, death occurs. This is usually caused when the electrical impulses in the affected heart become rapid (ventricular tachycardia, or "VT") or chaotic (ventricular fibrillation, or "VF"), or both. These irregular heart rhythms are arrhythmias. The general public and media often mistakenly refer to SCA as a "massive heart attack."

SCA is an electrical problem, whereby the arrhythmia prevents the heart from pumping blood to the brain and vital organs. There is an immediate cessation of the heart. In most cases, there are no warning signs or symptoms. A heart attack is a "plumbing" problem caused by one or more blockages in the heart's blood vessels, preventing proper flow, and the heart muscle dies. Symptoms include chest pain, radiating pain in left arm, between shoulder blades, and/or jaw, difficulty breathing, dizziness, nausea and vomiting, and sweating. In some cases, a heart attack may lead to a sudden cardiac arrest event.

Resuscitation from SCA

When someone collapses from SCA, immediate cardiopulmonary resuscitation (CPR) and use of an automated external defibrillator (AED) are essential for any chance of recovery. The AED analyzes the heart rhythm of the victim, and if necessary, a computerized command will instruct the user to press a button to deliver an appropriate shock to restore the normal operation of the heart. These devices are fail-safe and will not cause injury to the user, nor will they deliver a shock if none is needed. For patients in "VF," studies show that if early defibrillation is provided within the first minute, the odds are 90 percent that the victim's life can be saved. After that, the rate of survival drops 10 percent with every minute. As many as 30 to 50 percent would likely survive if CPR and AEDs were used within five minutes of collapse.

Many heart failure patients who have either suffered an SCA or are at risk have surgery to implant a small device called an implantable cardioverter defibrillator, or ICD. ICDs are designed to recognize certain types of arrhythmias and correct them with a shock. Ninety-five percent of lethal ventricular arrhythmias were shown to be effectively terminated by ICDs.

Who Is at Risk for SCA?

SCA can strike persons of any age, gender, race, and even those who seem in good health, as evidenced by world-class professional athletes at the peak of fitness. Many patients who may be at risk are not being identified, screened, and given options for medical treatment. If someone has any of the following risk factors or symptoms, he or she should discuss with a doctor whether further heart testing and/or evaluation by an electrophysiologist (EP) or cardiologist is necessary:

- History of early heart disease, heart attack, or cardiac death in the family
- Unexplained fainting or near fainting or palpitations
- Chest pain, shortness of breath, or fainting with exertion (such as during sports)
- Heart failure or heart attack
- Weak heart muscle or a cardiac ejection fraction (EF) of less than 40 percent (EF refers to the percentage of blood that is pumped out of the heart's main pumping chamber during each heartbeat)
- Cardiac risk factors such as high blood pressure, diabetes, obesity, smoking, or high cholesterol

Prevention

About 80 percent of SCA victims have signs of coronary heart disease. Leading a heart healthy lifestyle is important in preventing coronary artery disease and other heart conditions:

- Learn CPR and the use of an AED.
- Activate 911 immediately in an emergency.
- Help your community by advocating placement of AEDs in public places.
- Know your personal and family health history that may identify risk factors.

Chapter 14

Prostate Cancer

What is cancer?

The body is made up of many types of cells. Normally, cells grow, divide, and produce more cells as needed to keep the body healthy. Sometimes, however, the process goes wrong—cells become abnormal and form more cells in an uncontrolled way. These extra cells form a mass of tissue, called a growth or tumor. Tumors can be benign, which means not cancerous, or malignant, which means cancerous.

What is prostate cancer?

The prostate is a male sex gland, about the size of a large walnut. It is located below the bladder and in front of the rectum. The prostate's main function is to make fluid for semen, a white substance that carries sperm.

Prostate cancer occurs when a malignant tumor forms in the tissue of the prostate. In its early stage, prostate cancer needs the male hormone testosterone to grow and survive.

How common is prostate cancer among men in the United States?

Prostate cancer is one of the most common types of cancer among American men. It is a slow-growing disease that mostly affects older

---

Reprinted from "Prostate Cancer: Frequently Asked Questions," NIH Senior Health, March 28, 2007.

men. In fact, more than 65 percent of all prostate cancers are found in men over the age of sixty-five. The disease rarely occurs in men younger than forty years of age.

What is metastatic prostate cancer?

Sometimes, cancer cells break away from the malignant tumor in the prostate and enter the bloodstream or the lymphatic system and travel to other organs in the body.

When cancer spreads from its original location in the prostate to another part of the body such as the bone, it is called metastatic prostate cancer, not bone cancer. Doctors sometimes call this "distant" disease.

Can a man survive prostate cancer?

Yes. Today, more men are surviving prostate cancer than ever before. In fact, the number of deaths from prostate cancer has been declining since the early 1990s. If found early, the disease can very likely be cured.

What causes prostate cancer?

Scientists don't know exactly what causes prostate cancer. They cannot explain why one man gets prostate cancer and another does not. However, they have been able to identify some risk factors that are associated with the disease. A risk factor is anything that increases your chances of getting a disease.

What is the most important risk factor for prostate cancer?

Age is the most important risk factor for prostate cancer. The disease is extremely rare in men under age forty, but the risk increases greatly with age. More than 65 percent of cases are diagnosed in men over age sixty-five. The average age at the time of diagnosis is seventy.

Are there other major risk factors for prostate cancer besides age?

Yes. Race is another major risk factor. In the United States, this disease is much more common in African American men than in any other group of men. It is least common in Asian and American Indian men. A man's risk for developing prostate cancer is higher if his father or brother has had the disease.

Diet also may play a role. There is some evidence that a diet high in animal fat may increase the risk of prostate cancer and a diet high in fruits and vegetables may decrease the risk. Studies to find out whether men can reduce their risk of prostate cancer by taking certain dietary supplements are ongoing.

Are conditions like an enlarged prostate or obesity risk factors for prostate cancer?

Scientists have wondered whether an enlarged prostate, a condition also known as benign prostatic hyperplasia or BPH, might increase the risk for prostate cancer.

They have also studied obesity, lack of exercise, smoking, radiation exposure, and a sexually transmitted virus to see if they might increase risk. But at this time, there is little evidence that any of these factors contribute to an increased risk.

What are the symptoms of prostate cancer?

- A need to urinate frequently, especially at night
- Difficulty starting urination or holding back urine
- Inability to urinate
- Weak or interrupted flow of urine

If prostate cancer develops and is not treated, it can cause these symptoms:

- Painful or burning urination
- Difficulty in having an erection
- Painful ejaculation
- Blood in urine or semen
- Pain or stiffness in the lower back, hips, or upper thighs

Are there other conditions that have symptoms like prostate cancer?

Yes. Any of the symptoms caused by prostate cancer may also be due to enlargement of the prostate, which is not cancer. If you have any of the symptoms mentioned above, see your doctor or a urologist right away to find out if you need treatment. A urologist is a doctor who specializes in treating diseases of the genitourinary system.

What tests are available for men who have prostate problems?

Doctors use the following tests to detect prostate abnormalities, but these tests cannot show whether abnormalities are cancer or another, less serious condition. The results from these tests will help the doctor decide whether to check the patient further for signs of cancer:

- **Digital rectal exam:** The doctor inserts a lubricated, gloved finger into the rectum and feels the prostate through the rectal wall to check for hard or lumpy areas. A recent study revealed that men with low prostate specific antigen levels, or PSA, may still have prostate cancer.
- **Blood test for prostate specific antigen or PSA:** A lab measures the levels of PSA in a blood sample. The level of PSA may rise in men who have prostate cancer, an enlarged prostate, or infection in the prostate.

If initial tests show that prostate cancer might be present, what happens next?

The doctor may order other exams, including ultrasound and x-rays, to learn more about the cause of the symptoms. But to confirm the presence of cancer, doctors must perform a biopsy. During a biopsy, the doctor uses needles to remove small tissue samples from the prostate and then looks at the samples under a microscope.

If a biopsy shows that cancer is present, the doctor will report on the grade of the tumor. Doctors describe a tumor as low-, medium-, or high-grade cancer, based on the way it appears under the microscope.

If prostate cancer is found, how do doctors describe how far the cancer has spread?

If cancer is found in the prostate, the doctor needs to stage the disease. Staging is a careful attempt to find out whether the cancer has spread and, if so, what parts of the body are affected. The doctor also needs to find out the grade of the cancer. The grade tells how closely the tumor resembles normal tissue.

There are four stages used to describe prostate cancer. Doctors may refer to the stages using Roman numerals I–IV or capital letters A–D. The higher the stage, the more advanced the cancer. Following are the main features of each stage:

- **Stage I or stage A:** The cancer is too small to be felt during a rectal exam and causes no symptoms. The doctor may find it by accident when performing surgery for another reason, usually an enlarged prostate. There is no evidence that the cancer has spread outside the prostate. A sub-stage, T1c, is a tumor identified by needle biopsy because of elevated PSA.
- **Stage II or stage B:** The tumor is still confined to the prostate but involves more tissue within the prostate. The cancer is large enough to be felt during a rectal exam, or it may be found through a biopsy that is done because of a high PSA level. There is no evidence that the cancer has spread outside the prostate.
- **Stage III or stage C:** The cancer has spread outside the prostate to nearby tissues. The person may be experiencing symptoms, such as problems with urination.
- **Stage IV or stage D:** The cancer has spread to lymph nodes or to other parts of the body. There may be problems with urination, fatigue, and weight loss.

If I do need to seek treatment for prostate cancer, what are some of my options?

There are a number of ways to treat prostate cancer, and the doctor will develop a treatment to fit each man's needs. The choice of treatment mostly depends on the stage of the disease and the grade of the tumor. But doctors also consider a man's age, general health, and his feelings about the treatments and their possible side effects.

Treatment for prostate cancer may involve watchful waiting, surgery, radiation therapy, or hormonal therapy. Some men receive a combination of therapies. A cure is probable for men whose prostate cancer is diagnosed early.

What are some of the side effects of these treatments?

Surgery, radiation therapy, and hormonal therapy all have the potential to disrupt sexual desire or performance for a short while or permanently. Discuss your concerns with your health care provider.

Several options are available to help you manage sexual problems related to prostate cancer treatment.

What is "watchful waiting" and why would I choose it as a treatment?

With watchful waiting, a man's condition is closely monitored, but treatment does not begin until symptoms appear or change. The doctor may suggest watchful waiting for some men who have prostate cancer that is found at an early stage and appears to be growing slowly.

Also, watchful waiting may be advised for older men or men with other serious medical problems. For these men, the risks and possible side effects of surgery, radiation therapy, or hormonal therapy may outweigh the possible benefits. Doctors monitor these patients with regular check-ups. If symptoms appear or get worse, the doctor may recommend active treatment.

What types of surgery are available for men with prostate cancer?

Surgery is a common treatment for early stage prostate cancer. It is used to remove the cancer. The surgeon may remove the entire prostate—a type of surgery called radical prostatectomy—or, in a few cases, remove only part of it.

Sometimes the surgeon will also remove nearby lymph nodes. Side effects may include lack of sexual function, which is called impotence, or problems holding urine, which is called incontinence.

How is radiation used to treat prostate cancer?

Radiation therapy uses high-energy x-rays to kill cancer cells and shrink tumors. Doctors may recommend it instead of surgery or after surgery to destroy any cancer cells that may remain in the area. In advanced stages, the doctor may recommend it to relieve pain or other symptoms. Radiation can cause problems with impotence and bowel function.

The radiation may come from a machine, which is external radiation, or from tiny radioactive seeds placed inside or near the tumor, which is internal radiation. Men who receive only the radioactive seeds usually have small tumors. Some men receive both kinds of radiation therapy.

For external radiation therapy, patients go to the hospital or clinic—usually five days a week for several weeks. Internal radiation may require patients to stay in the hospital for a short time.

How is hormonal therapy used to treat prostate cancer?

Hormonal therapy deprives cancer cells of the male hormones they need to grow and survive. This treatment is often used for prostate cancer that has spread to other parts of the body. Sometimes doctors use hormonal therapy to try to keep the cancer from coming back after surgery or radiation treatment. Side effects can include impotence, hot flashes, loss of sexual desire, and thinning of bones.

What kinds of follow-up treatment could I have?

Regardless of the type of treatment you receive, you will be closely monitored to see how well the treatment is working. Monitoring may include the following:

- A PSA blood test, usually every three months to one year
- A bone scan and/or computed tomography (CT) scan to see if the cancer has spread
- A complete blood count to monitor for signs and symptoms of anemia
- Looking for signs or symptoms that the disease might be progressing, such as fatigue, increased pain, or decreased bowel and bladder function

What kinds of treatments for prostate cancer are being developed?

Through research, doctors are trying to find new, more effective ways to treat prostate cancer. Cryosurgery—destroying cancer by freezing it—is under study as an alternative to surgery and radiation therapy. To avoid damaging healthy tissue, the doctor places an instrument known as a cryoprobe in direct contact with the tumor to freeze it.

Doctors are studying new ways of using radiation therapy and hormonal therapy, too. Studies have shown that hormonal therapy given after radiation therapy can help certain men whose cancer has spread to nearby tissues.

Scientists are also testing the effectiveness of chemotherapy and biological therapy for men whose cancer does not respond or stops responding to hormonal therapy.

They are also exploring new ways to schedule and combine various treatments. For example, they are studying hormonal therapy to find out if using it to shrink the tumor before a man has surgery or radiation might be a useful approach. They are also testing combinations of hormone therapy and vaccines to prevent recurrence of prostate cancer.

Are there genes that put me at greater risk of getting prostate cancer?

Researchers are studying changes in genes that may increase the risk for developing prostate cancer. Some studies are looking at the genes of men who were diagnosed with prostate cancer at a relatively young age, less than fifty-five years old, and the genes of families who have several members with the disease. Other studies are trying to identify which genes, or arrangements of genes, are most likely to lead to prostate cancer.

Much more work is needed, however, before scientists can say exactly how genetic changes relate to prostate cancer. At the moment, no genetic risk has been firmly established.

Are there other options for someone with prostate cancer?

Some prostate cancer patients take part in studies of new treatments. These studies—called clinical trials—are designed to find out whether a new treatment is safe and effective. Often, clinical trials compare a new treatment with a standard one so that doctors can learn which is more effective. People with prostate cancer who are interested in taking part in a clinical trial should talk with their doctor.

What role do diet and dietary supplements play in prostate cancer?

Diet may play a role. There is some evidence that a diet high in animal fat may increase the risk of prostate cancer and a diet high in fruits and vegetables may decrease the risk.

Researchers are also looking at diets that are low in fat and high in soy, fruits, vegetables, and other food products to see if they might prevent a recurrence of prostate cancer. In addition, recent studies suggest that a diet that regularly includes tomato-based foods may help protect men from prostate cancer.

Studies to find out whether men can reduce their risk of prostate cancer by taking certain dietary supplements are ongoing.

These studies include the use of dietary supplements such as vitamin E and selenium. At the moment, no dietary factor has been proven to change your risk of developing prostate cancer or to alter the course of the disease after diagnosis.

Who can provide emotional support for someone dealing with prostate cancer?

Living with a serious disease such as cancer is not easy. Some people find they need help coping with the emotional as well as the practical aspects of their disease. Patients often get together in support groups where they can share what they have learned about coping with their disease and the effects of treatment. Patients may want to talk with a member of their health care team about finding a support group.

People living with cancer may worry about caring for their families, keeping their jobs, or continuing daily activities. Concerns about treatments and managing side effects, hospital stays, and medical bills are also common. Doctors, nurses, dietitians, and other members of the health care team can answer questions about treatment, working, or other activities.

Meeting with a social worker, counselor, or member of the clergy can be helpful to those who want to talk about their feelings or discuss their concerns. Often, a social worker can suggest resources for help with rehabilitation, emotional support, financial aid, transportation, or home care.

It is natural for a man and his partner to be concerned about the effects of prostate cancer and its treatment on their sexual relationship. They may want to talk with the doctor about possible side effects and whether these are likely to be temporary or permanent. Whatever the outlook, it is usually helpful for patients and their partners to talk about their concerns and help one another find ways to be intimate during and after treatment.

Chapter 15

Lung Cancer

What is cancer?

The body is made up of many types of cells. Normally, cells grow, divide, and produce more cells as needed to keep the body healthy and functioning properly.

Sometimes, however, the process goes wrong—cells become abnormal and form more cells in an uncontrolled way. These extra cells form a mass of tissue, called a growth or tumor. Tumors can be benign, meaning not cancerous, or malignant, meaning cancerous.

What is lung cancer?

Lung cancer occurs when malignant tumors form in the tissue of the lung. The lungs are a pair of sponge-like organs. The right lung has three sections, called lobes, and is larger than the left lung, which has two lobes.

Are there different types of lung cancer?

There are two major types of lung cancer—non–small cell lung cancer and small cell lung cancer. Each type of lung cancer grows and spreads in different ways, and each is treated differently.

Excerpted from "Lung Cancer: Frequently Asked Questions," NIH Senior Health, March 23, 2007.

Non–small cell lung cancer is more common than small cell lung cancer. It generally grows and spreads slowly. Small cell lung cancer, sometimes called oat cell cancer, grows more quickly and is more likely to spread to other organs in the body.

How does smoking affect lung cancer rates?

In 1965, about 42 percent of all adults smoked, but by 2005 only 21 percent did. During that time, there has been a sharp drop in lung cancer deaths among men, mainly because fewer men are smoking.

Smoking rates, which were dropping, have stopped declining in recent years. Smoking by young people actually increased by 73 percent in the 1990s.

Also, more women are getting lung cancer than ever before and more are dying from it, mainly because more young women are smoking. Many smoking education programs now focus on reversing the increase in the number of women and young people who smoke.

What is the main cause of lung cancer?

Cigarette smoking is the number one cause of lung cancer. Scientists have reported widely on the link between cancer and smoking since the 1960s. Since then, study after study has provided more proof that cigarette smoking is the primary cause of lung cancer.

Before cigarette smoking became popular in the early part of the twentieth century, doctors rarely, if ever, saw patients with lung cancer. But today, lung cancer is the leading cause of death by cancer. Nearly 90 percent of people with lung cancer developed it because they smoked cigarettes.

Using tobacco products has been shown to cause cancer. In fact, smoking tobacco, using smokeless tobacco, and being exposed regularly to secondhand tobacco smoke are responsible for a large number of cancer deaths in the U.S. each year.

What are the risks of getting lung cancer if you are a smoker?

If you smoke cigarettes, you are at much higher risk for lung cancer than a person who has never smoked. The risk of dying from lung cancer is twenty-three times higher for men who smoke and thirteen times higher for women who smoke than for people who have never smoked.

Stopping smoking greatly reduces your risk for developing lung cancer. But after you stop, the risk goes down slowly. Ten years after the last cigarette, the risk of dying from lung cancer drops by 50 percent.

Can smoking cigars and pipes lead to lung cancer?

Smoking cigars and pipes also puts you at risk for lung cancer. Cigar and pipe smokers have a higher risk of lung cancer than nonsmokers. Even cigar and pipe smokers who do not inhale are at increased risk for lung, mouth, and other types of cancer.

Can secondhand smoke cause a nonsmoker to get lung cancer?

Some studies suggest that nonsmokers who are exposed to environmental tobacco smoke, also called secondhand smoke, are at increased risk of lung cancer. Secondhand smoke is the smoke that nonsmokers are exposed to when they share air space with someone who is smoking. Each year, about three thousand nonsmoking adults die of lung cancer as a result of breathing secondhand smoke.

Can exposure to radon lead to lung cancer?

Exposure to radon can put a person at risk for lung cancer, too. People who work in mines may be exposed to this invisible, odorless, and radioactive gas that occurs naturally in soil and rocks. It is also found in houses in some parts of the country. A kit available at most hardware stores allows homeowners to measure radon levels in their homes.

Is there a risk of lung cancer from exposure to asbestos?

Another substance that can contribute to lung cancer is asbestos. Asbestos is used in shipbuilding, asbestos mining and manufacturing, insulation work, and brake repair. If inhaled, asbestos particles can lodge in the lungs, damaging cells and increasing the risk for lung cancer.

What are the possible signs of lung cancer?

The possible signs of lung cancer are as follows:

- A cough that doesn't go away and gets worse over time

- Constant chest pain
- Coughing up blood
- Shortness of breath, wheezing, or hoarseness
- Repeated problems with pneumonia or bronchitis
- Swelling of the neck and face
- Loss of appetite or weight loss
- Fatigue

What are the chances of developing a second lung cancer?

A person who has had lung cancer once is more likely to develop a second lung cancer compared to a person who has never had lung cancer. Quitting smoking after lung cancer is diagnosed may prevent the development of a second lung cancer.

How does a doctor usually detect lung cancer?

Seeing a spot on a chest x-ray is usually how a doctor first suspects that lung cancer may be present. Doctors may also use imaging methods such as a computed tomography (CT) scan or a positron emission tomography (PET) scan to look for signs of cancer.

A CT scan, is a series of detailed pictures of areas inside the body. A PET scan is a computerized image of the metabolic activity of body tissues.

Are there new ways to detect lung cancer before it starts to spread?

One screening method that shows promise detecting lung cancer before it has spread is spiral computerized tomography, or spiral CT. Spiral CT can scan the lungs from the neck to the diaphragm in less than twenty seconds, or a single breath-hold. Preliminary studies show that it may help doctors find small tumors, but questions remain about the technology's risk and benefits as a screening tool.

In the summer of 2002, the National Cancer Institute launched a $200 million trial called the National Lung Screening Trial to determine if spiral CT is better than conventional x-ray at finding dangerous lung cancers and distinguishing between cancers and noncancerous changes in the lungs.

The NLST isn't the only study looking at the benefits of spiral CT and chest x-ray. Recent reports in two medical journals have reported conflicting information about whether spiral CT is better than chest x-ray at improving survival rates or reducing mortality. The only way to get a sure answer is to conduct a randomized clinical trial to examine the two methods. The results of the NLST, which is the only randomized clinical trial in the United States looking at this issue, will be available by 2009.

How does a doctor confirm that someone has lung cancer?

To confirm that a person has lung cancer, the doctor must examine fluid or tissue from the lung. This is done through a biopsy—the removal of a small sample of fluid or tissue for examination under a microscope by a pathologist. A biopsy can show whether a person has cancer. A number of procedures may be used to obtain this tissue:

- **Bronchoscopy:** The doctor puts a bronchoscope—a thin, lighted tube—into the mouth or nose and down through the windpipe to look into the breathing passages. Through this tube, the doctor can collect cells or small samples of tissue.
- **Needle aspiration:** The doctor numbs the chest area and inserts a thin needle into the tumor to remove a sample of tissue.
- **Thoracentesis:** Using a needle, the doctor removes a sample of the fluid that surrounds the lungs to check for cancer cells.
- **Thoracotomy:** Surgery to open the chest is sometimes needed to diagnose lung cancer. This procedure is a major operation performed in a hospital.

How does a doctor determine how far a lung cancer has progressed?

Once lung cancer has been found, it is usually staged. Staging means determining how far the cancer has progressed. Through staging, the doctor can tell if the cancer has spread and, if so, to what parts of the body. Lung cancer often spreads to the brain or bones. Knowing the stage of the disease helps the doctor plan treatment.

Small cell lung cancer is divided into two stages. Limited stage is generally cancer confined to the chest and extensive stage is cancer that has spread outside the chest.

Non–small cell lung cancer is divided into four stages, I–IV. Most patients with stage I and II non–small cell tumors and some patients with stage III tumors can undergo surgery with the goal of cure. Stage IV denotes cancer that has spread to other sites in the body, most often bone, brain, or liver. Most stage IV cancers cannot be cured, although treatment may be available to help prolong life.

What tests do doctors use to stage lung cancer?

Doctors can perform several tests to stage lung cancer. Staging means finding out how far the cancer has progressed. The following tests are used to stage lung cancer:

- Computed axial tomography or CAT scan is a computer linked to an x-ray machine that creates a series of detailed pictures of areas inside the body.
- Magnetic resonance imaging, or MRI, is a powerful magnet linked to a computer that makes detailed pictures of areas inside the body.
- Radionuclide scanning uses a mildly radioactive substance to show whether cancer has spread to other organs, such as the liver.
- A bone scan uses a small amount of a radioactive substance to show whether cancer has spread to the bones.
- A mediastinoscopy or mediastinotomy can help show whether the cancer has spread to the lymph nodes in the chest by removing a tissue sample. The patient receives a general anesthetic for this procedure.

What are the standard treatments for lung cancer?

Surgery is an operation to remove the cancer. Depending on the location of the tumor, the surgeon may remove a small part of the lung, a lobe of the lung, or the entire lung.

Chemotherapy uses anti-cancer drugs to kill cancer cells throughout the body. Doctors use chemotherapy to control cancer growth and relieve symptoms. Anti-cancer drugs are given by injection; through a catheter, a long thin tube temporarily placed in a large vein; or in pill form.

Radiation therapy uses high-energy beams to kill cancer cells and shrink tumors. An external machine delivers radiation to a limited area, affecting cancer cells only in that area. Doctors may use radiation therapy before surgery to shrink a tumor or after surgery to destroy any cancer cells remaining in the treated area.

Photodynamic therapy, a newer technique, is laser therapy that is used in combination with a chemical to kill cancer cells. Doctors may use it to reduce symptoms of lung cancer, such as bleeding, or to treat very small tumors.

What are some common ways to treat non–small cell lung cancer?

Doctors treat patients with non–small cell lung cancer in several ways, and surgery is a common treatment. Cryosurgery, a treatment that freezes and destroys cancer tissue, may be used to control symptoms in the later stages of non–small cell lung cancer. Doctors may also use radiation therapy and chemotherapy to slow the progress of the disease and to manage symptoms.

What is the best way to treat small cell lung cancer?

Small cell lung cancer spreads quickly. In many cases, cancer cells have already spread to other parts of the body when the disease is diagnosed. In order to reach cancer cells throughout the body, doctors almost always use chemotherapy.

What new procedures have been developed to treat lung cancer?

Researchers continue to look at new ways to combine, schedule, and sequence the use of chemotherapy, surgery, and radiation to treat lung cancer. For instance, in one large study, patients with non–small cell lung cancer that had spread to nearby tissues or lymph nodes took radiation and chemotherapy at the same time instead of sequentially. Their five-year survival rates rose from about 6 percent to 16 percent.

Another study compared treatments given to two groups of people with small cell lung cancer. One group had chemotherapy plus two daily radiation treatments. The other had chemotherapy with only one daily radiation treatment. Researchers found that the group receiving two daily radiation treatments with their chemotherapy had better survival rates.

Are there any new chemotherapy drugs available to treat lung cancer?

Newer chemotherapy drugs, known by the brand names Navelbine®, Taxol®, Taxotere®, Gemzar®, Hycamtin®, and Camptosar® have produced improved response rates in tests of each drug alone. Various combinations of the new drugs with traditional agents, such as cisplatin and carboplatin, are now either in clinical trials or have reported early results of the trials.

Other researchers are working to develop drugs called "molecularly targeted agents," which kill cancer cells by targeting key molecules involved in cancer cell growth. One of these drugs, called Avastin®, helped patients live a few months longer when it was combined with traditional chemotherapy.

Are there other options for someone with lung cancer?

Some lung cancer patients take part in studies of new treatments. These studies, called clinical trials, are designed to find out whether a new treatment is safe and effective. Often, clinical trials compare a new treatment with a standard one so that doctors can learn which is more effective. People with lung cancer who are interested in taking part in a clinical trial should talk with their doctor.

Chapter 16

Colorectal Cancer

What is colorectal cancer?

Cancer of the colon or rectum is called colorectal cancer. The colon and the rectum are part of the large intestine, which is part of the digestive system. Colorectal cancer occurs when malignant tumors form in the lining of the large intestine, also called the large bowel.

How common is colorectal cancer?

Colorectal cancer accounts for almost 10 percent of all cancer deaths in the United States. The risk of developing colorectal cancer rises after age fifty. It is common in both men and women.

What are some of the risk factors for colorectal cancer?

Studies show that the following risk factors can increase a person's chances of developing colorectal cancer: age, polyps, diet, personal history, family history, and ulcerative colitis.

If I have a polyp, does that mean I'm going to get colorectal cancer?

Polyps are benign, or noncancerous, growths on the inner wall of the colon and rectum. They are fairly common in people over age fifty.

Excerpted from "Colorectal Cancer: Frequently Asked Questions," NIH Senior Health, April 30, 2007.

Some types of polyps increase a person's risk of developing colorectal cancer. Not all polyps become cancerous, but nearly all colon cancers start as polyps.

Does the condition known as ulcerative colitis increase my risk of getting colorectal cancer?

Yes. Ulcerative colitis is a condition in which there is a chronic break in the lining of the colon. It has been associated with an increased risk of colon cancer.

Does diet play a role in colorectal cancer?

Diet may be associated with a risk of developing colorectal cancer. Colorectal cancer occurs more frequently in populations that consume a diet high in fat, protein, calories, alcohol, and both red and white meat, and low in calcium and folate, than in populations that consume a low-fat, high-fiber diet.

If a family member had colorectal cancer, what are the chances I will have the disease?

Parents, siblings, or children of a person who has had colorectal cancer are somewhat more likely to develop this type of cancer themselves. This is especially true if the relative had the cancer at a young age. If many family members have had colorectal cancer, the chances increase even more.

What are possible signs of colorectal cancer?

Possible signs of colorectal cancer include the following:

- A change in the frequency of bowel movements
- Diarrhea, constipation, or feeling that the bowel does not empty completely
- Either bright red or very dark blood in the stool
- Stools that are narrower than usual
- General abdominal discomfort such as frequent gas pains, bloating, fullness, and/or cramps
- Weight loss with no known reason

- Constant tiredness
- Vomiting

What are some of the tools used to detect colorectal cancer?

Here are some of the tools used to detect colorectal cancer:

- A fecal occult blood test, or FOBT, is a test used to check for hidden blood in the stool. Sometimes cancers or polyps can bleed, and FOBT can detect small amounts of bleeding.
- A sigmoidoscopy is an examination of the rectum and lower colon—or sigmoid colon—using a lighted instrument called a sigmoidoscope.
- A colonoscopy is an examination of the rectum and entire colon using a lighted instrument called a colonoscope.
- A double contrast barium enema, or DCBE, is a series of x-rays of the colon and rectum. The patient is given an enema with a solution that contains barium, a substance that outlines the colon and rectum on the x-rays.

Does the U.S. government have any specific recommendations about getting tested for colorectal cancer?

Yes. In July 2002, the U.S. Preventive Services Task Force made its strongest ever recommendation for colorectal cancer screening: it urged all adults age fifty and over to get screened, or tested, for the disease. The task force noted that various screening tests are available, making it possible for patients and their clinicians to decide which test is best for each person.

If colorectal cancer is found, how do doctors describe how far the cancer has spread?

Doctors use the following stages to describe how the cancer spreads:

- **Stage 0:** The cancer is very early. It is found only in the innermost lining of the colon or rectum.
- **Stage I:** The cancer involves more of the inner wall of the colon or rectum.

- **Stage II:** The cancer has spread outside the colon or rectum to nearby tissue, but not to the lymph nodes. Lymph nodes are small, bean-shaped structures that are part of the body's immune system.
- **Stage III:** The cancer has spread to nearby lymph nodes, but not to other parts of the body.
- **Stage IV:** The cancer has spread to other parts of the body. Colorectal cancer tends to spread to the liver and/or lungs.
- **Recurrent:** Recurrent cancer means the cancer has come back after treatment. The disease may recur in the colon or rectum or in another part of the body.

What are the standard methods for treating colorectal cancer?

The three standard treatments for colon cancer are surgery, chemotherapy, and radiation. Surgery, however, is the most common treatment for all stages of colon cancer. Surgery is an operation to remove the cancer. A doctor may remove the cancer using several types of surgery. For rectal cancer, radiation treatment also is an option.

What types of surgery are available for someone with colorectal cancer?

Several types of surgery are available for someone with colorectal cancer. If the cancer is found at a very early stage, the doctor may remove it without cutting through the abdominal wall. Instead, the doctor may put a tube up the rectum into the colon and cut the cancer out. This is called a local excision.

If the cancer is found in a polyp, which is a small bulging piece of tissue, the operation is called a polypectomy.

If the cancer is larger, the surgeon will remove the cancer and a small amount of healthy tissue around it. This is called a colectomy. The surgeon may then sew the healthy parts of the colon together. Usually, the surgeon will also remove lymph nodes near the colon and examine them under a microscope to see whether they contain cancer.

If the doctor is not able to sew the two ends of the colon back together, an opening called a stoma is made on the abdomen for waste to pass out of the body before it reaches the rectum. This procedure is called a colostomy.

Sometimes the colostomy is needed only until the lower colon has healed, and then it can be reversed. But if the doctor needs to remove the entire lower colon, the colostomy may be permanent.

Are there any treatments that follow surgery?

Even if the doctor removes all the cancer that can be seen at the time of the operation, some patients may receive chemotherapy after surgery to kill any cancer cells that are left. Chemotherapy treatment after surgery—to increase the chances of a cure—is called adjuvant therapy.

Researchers have found that patients who received adjuvant therapy usually survived longer and went for longer periods of time without a recurrence of colon cancer than patients treated with surgery alone.

Patients age seventy and older benefited from adjuvant treatment as much as their younger counterparts. In fact, adjuvant therapy is equally as effective—and no more toxic—for patients seventy and older as it is for younger patients, provided the older patients have no other serious diseases.

What are some of the side effects of treatment for colorectal cancer?

For surgery, the main side effects are short-term pain and tenderness around the area of the operation. For chemotherapy, the side effects depend on which drugs you take and what the dosages are. Most often the side effects include nausea, vomiting, and hair loss. For radiation therapy, fatigue, loss of appetite, nausea, and diarrhea may occur.

Are there therapies that use a person's own immune system to fight colorectal cancer?

Yes. One treatment, biological therapy, stimulates the immune system's ability to fight cancer. In this therapy, substances made by the body or in a laboratory are used to boost, direct, or restore the body's natural defenses against disease.

Another term for biological therapy is immunotherapy. At the moment, biological therapies are not standard therapy. They are experimental treatments.

What are some of the newest drugs doctors use to combat colorectal cancer?

Various drugs are under study as possible treatments for colorectal cancer. In May 2002 researchers found that a drug regimen consisting of oxaliplatin, 5-fluorouracil, and leucovorin can improve outcomes for patients with colorectal cancer.

A 2005 study found that patients who took the drug Avastin® with their standard chemotherapy treatment had a longer survival than those who did not take Avastin. The generic name for Avastin is bevacizumab.

Scientists are also working on new vaccines and monoclonal antibodies that may improve how patients' immune systems respond to colorectal cancers. Monoclonal antibodies are a single type of antibody that researchers make in large amounts in a laboratory.

Are there tools that are better at finding colorectal cancer early?

Scientists are looking at the role that sigmoidoscopy and colonoscopy may play in reducing deaths from colorectal cancer through early detection.

Two studies reported in the July 20, 2000, issue of the *New England Journal of Medicine* showed that colonoscopy can find many precancerous polyps that sigmoidoscopy misses. However, more studies are needed to find out if colonoscopy can actually reduce the number of deaths from colorectal cancer.

Are there any drugs available that can help prevent colorectal cancer?

Scientists are doing research on chemoprevention—the use of drugs to prevent cancer from developing in the first place. For example, researchers have found that anti-inflammatory drugs helped keep intestinal tumors from forming, but serious side effects have been noted so researchers are proceeding cautiously.

Studies have shown that non-steroidal anti-inflammatory drugs can keep large bowel polyps from forming. Bowel polyps can start out benign, or noncancerous, but can become cancerous.

Are there genes that put me at greater risk of getting colorectal cancer?

Researchers are working hard to understand and identify the genes involved in colorectal cancer. Hereditary nonpolyposis colorectal cancer, or HNPCC, is one condition that causes people to develop colorectal cancer at a young age. The discovery of four genes involved with this disease has provided crucial clues about the role of DNA repair in colorectal and other cancers.

Are there other options for someone with colorectal cancer?

Some colorectal cancer patients take part in studies of new treatments. These studies, called clinical trials, are designed to find out whether a new treatment is safe and effective.

Chapter 17

Liver Cancer

The Liver

The liver is the largest organ in the body. It is found behind the ribs on the right side of the abdomen. The liver has two parts, a right lobe and a smaller left lobe.

The liver has many important functions that keep a person healthy. It removes harmful material from the blood. It makes enzymes and bile that help digest food. It also converts food into substances needed for life and growth.

The liver gets its supply of blood from two vessels. Most of its blood comes from the hepatic portal vein. The rest comes from the hepatic artery.

Understanding Liver Cancer

Most primary liver cancers begin in hepatocytes (liver cells). This type of cancer is called hepatocellular carcinoma or malignant hepatoma.

When liver cancer spreads (metastasizes) outside the liver, the cancer cells tend to spread to nearby lymph nodes and to the bones and lungs. When this happens, the new tumor has the same kind of abnormal cells as the primary tumor in the liver. For example, if liver cancer spreads to the bones, the cancer cells in the bones are actually

---

Excerpted from "What You Need to Know about Liver Cancer," National Cancer Institute, September 16, 2002. Revised by David A. Cooke, M.D., March 2009.

liver cancer cells. The disease is metastatic liver cancer, not bone cancer. It is treated as liver cancer, not bone cancer. Doctors sometimes call the new tumor "distant" disease.

Similarly, cancer that spreads to the liver from another part of the body is different from primary liver cancer. The cancer cells in the liver are like the cells in the original tumor. When cancer cells spread to the liver from another organ (such as the colon, lung, or breast), doctors may call the tumor in the liver a secondary tumor. In the United States, secondary tumors in the liver are far more common than primary tumors.

Liver Cancer: Who's at Risk?

Studies have shown the following risk factors:

- **Chronic liver infection (hepatitis):** Certain viruses can infect the liver. The infection may be chronic. (It may not go away.) The most important risk factor for liver cancer is a chronic infection with the hepatitis B virus or the hepatitis C virus. These viruses can be passed from person to person through blood (such as by sharing needles) or sexual contact. An infant may catch these viruses from an infected mother. Liver cancer can develop after many years of infection with the virus. These infections may not cause symptoms, but blood tests can show whether either virus is present. If so, the doctor may suggest treatment. Also, the doctor may discuss ways of avoiding infecting other people. In people who are not already infected with hepatitis B virus, hepatitis B vaccine can prevent chronic hepatitis B infection and can protect against liver cancer. Researchers are now working to develop a vaccine to prevent hepatitis C infection.
- **Cirrhosis:** Cirrhosis is a disease that develops when liver cells are damaged and replaced with scar tissue. Cirrhosis may be caused by alcohol abuse, certain drugs and other chemicals, and certain viruses or parasites. About 5 percent of people with cirrhosis develop liver cancer.
- **Aflatoxin:** Liver cancer can be caused by aflatoxin, a harmful substance made by certain types of mold. Aflatoxin can form on peanuts, corn, and other nuts and grains. In Asia and Africa, aflatoxin contamination is a problem. However, the U.S. Food and Drug Administration (FDA) does not allow the sale of foods that have high levels of aflatoxin.

- **Being male:** Men are twice as likely as women to get liver cancer.
- **Family history:** People who have family members with liver cancer may be more likely to get the disease.
- **Age:** In the United States, liver cancer occurs more often in people over age sixty than in younger people.

The more risk factors a person has, the greater the chance that liver cancer will develop. However, many people with known risk factors for liver cancer do not develop the disease.

People who think they may be at risk for liver cancer should discuss this concern with their doctor. The doctor may plan a schedule for checkups.

Symptoms

Liver cancer is sometimes called a "silent disease" because in an early stage it often does not cause symptoms. But, as the cancer grows, symptoms may include the following:

- Pain in the upper abdomen on the right side; the pain may extend to the back and shoulder
- Swollen abdomen (bloating)
- Weight loss
- Loss of appetite and feelings of fullness
- Weakness or feeling very tired
- Nausea and vomiting
- Yellow skin and eyes, and dark urine from jaundice
- Fever

These symptoms are not sure signs of liver cancer. Other liver diseases and other health problems can also cause these symptoms. Anyone with these symptoms should see a doctor as soon as possible. Only a doctor can diagnose and treat the problem.

Diagnosis

If a patient has symptoms that suggest liver cancer, the doctor performs one or more of the following procedures:

- **Physical exam:** The doctor feels the abdomen to check the liver, spleen, and nearby organs for any lumps or changes in their shape or size. The doctor also checks for ascites, an abnormal buildup of fluid in the abdomen. The doctor may examine the skin and eyes for signs of jaundice.
- **Blood tests:** Many blood tests may be used to check for liver problems. One blood test detects alpha-fetoprotein (AFP). High AFP levels could be a sign of liver cancer. Other blood tests can show how well the liver is working.
- **Computed tomography (CT) scan:** An x-ray machine linked to a computer takes a series of detailed pictures of the liver and other organs and blood vessels in the abdomen. The patient may receive an injection of a special dye so the liver shows up clearly in the pictures. From the CT scan, the doctor may see tumors in the liver or elsewhere in the abdomen.
- **Ultrasound test:** The ultrasound device uses sound waves that cannot be heard by humans. The sound waves produce a pattern of echoes as they bounce off internal organs. The echoes create a picture (sonogram) of the liver and other organs in the abdomen. Tumors may produce echoes that are different from the echoes made by healthy tissues.
- **Magnetic resonance imaging (MRI):** A powerful magnet linked to a computer is used to make detailed pictures of areas inside the body. These pictures are viewed on a monitor and can also be printed.
- **Angiogram:** For an angiogram, the patient may be in the hospital and may have anesthesia. The doctor injects dye into an artery so that the blood vessels in the liver show up on an x-ray. The angiogram can reveal a tumor in the liver.
- **Biopsy:** In some cases, the doctor may remove a sample of tissue. A pathologist uses a microscope to look for cancer cells in the tissue. The doctor may obtain tissue in several ways. One way is by inserting a thin needle into the liver to remove a small amount of tissue. This is called fine-needle aspiration. The doctor may use CT or ultrasound to guide the needle. Sometimes the doctor obtains a sample of tissue with a thick needle (core biopsy) or by inserting a thin, lighted tube (laparoscope) into a small incision in the abdomen. Another way is to remove tissue during an operation.

Staging

If liver cancer is diagnosed, the doctor needs to know the stage, or extent, of the disease to plan the best treatment. Staging is an attempt to find out the size of the tumor, whether the disease has spread, and if so, to what parts of the body. Careful staging shows whether the tumor can be removed with surgery. This is very important because most liver cancers cannot be removed with surgery.

The doctor may determine the stage of liver cancer at the time of diagnosis, or the patient may need more tests. These tests may include imaging tests, such as a CT scan, MRI, angiogram, or ultrasound. Imaging tests can help the doctor find out whether the liver cancer has spread. The doctor also may use a laparoscope to look directly at the liver and nearby organs.

Treatment

At this time, liver cancer can be cured only when it is found at an early stage (before it has spread) and only if the patient is healthy enough to have an operation. However, treatments other than surgery may be able to control the disease and help patients live longer and feel better. When a cure or control of the disease is not possible, some patients and their doctors choose palliative therapy. Palliative therapy aims to improve the quality of a person's life by controlling pain and other problems caused by the disease.

Treatment Choices

The doctor can describe treatment choices and discuss the results expected with each treatment option. The doctor and patient can work together to develop a treatment plan that fits the patient's needs.

Cancer of the liver is very hard to control with current treatments. For that reason, many doctors encourage patients with liver cancer to consider taking part in a clinical trial. Clinical trials are research studies testing new treatments. They are an important option for people with all stages of liver cancer.

The choice of treatment depends on the condition of the liver; the number, size, and location of tumors; and whether the cancer has spread outside the liver. Other factors to consider include the patient's age, general health, concerns about the treatments and their possible side effects, and personal values.

Usually, the most important factor is the stage of the disease. The stage is based on the size of the tumor, the condition of the liver, and whether the cancer has spread. The following are brief descriptions of the stages of liver cancer and the treatments most often used for each stage. For some patients, other treatments may be appropriate.

Localized Resectable Cancer

Localized resectable liver cancer is cancer that can be removed during surgery. There is no evidence that the cancer has spread to the nearby lymph nodes or to other parts of the body. Lab tests show that the liver is working well.

Surgery to remove part of the liver is called partial hepatectomy. The extent of the surgery depends on the size, number, and location of the tumors. It also depends on how well the liver is working. The doctor may remove a wedge of tissue that contains the liver tumor, an entire lobe, or an even larger portion of the liver.

In a partial hepatectomy, the surgeon leaves a margin of normal liver tissue. This remaining healthy tissue takes over the functions of the liver.

For a few patients, liver transplantation may be an option. For this procedure, the transplant surgeon removes the patient's entire liver (total hepatectomy) and replaces it with a healthy liver from a donor. A liver transplant is an option only if the disease has not spread outside the liver and only if a suitable donated liver can be found. While the patient waits for a donated liver to become available, the health care team monitors the patient's health and provides other treatments, as necessary.

Localized Unresectable Cancer

Localized unresectable liver cancer cannot be removed by surgery even though it has not spread to the nearby lymph nodes or to distant parts of the body. Surgery to remove the tumor is not possible because of cirrhosis (or other conditions that cause poor liver function), the location of the tumor within the liver, or other health problems.

Patients with localized unresectable cancer may receive other treatments to control the disease and extend life:

- **Radiofrequency ablation:** The doctor uses a special probe to kill the cancer cells with heat. The probe contains tiny electrodes that destroy the cancer cells. Sometimes the doctor can insert the probe directly through the skin. Only local anesthesia is needed. In other cases, the doctor may insert the probe through a small incision in the abdomen or may make a wider incision to open the abdomen. These procedures are done in the hospital with general anesthesia. Other therapies that use heat to destroy liver tumors include laser or microwave therapy.

- **Percutaneous ethanol injection:** The doctor injects alcohol (ethanol) directly into the liver tumor to kill cancer cells. The doctor uses ultrasound to guide a small needle. The procedure may be performed once or twice a week. Usually local anesthesia is used, but if the patient has many tumors in the liver, general anesthesia may be needed.

- **Cryosurgery:** The doctor makes an incision into the abdomen and inserts a metal probe to freeze and kill cancer cells. The doctor may use ultrasound to help guide the probe.

- **Hepatic arterial infusion:** The doctor inserts a tube (catheter) into the hepatic artery, the major artery that supplies blood to the liver. The doctor then injects an anticancer drug into the catheter. The drug flows into the blood vessels that go to the tumor. Because only a small amount of the drug reaches other parts of the body, the drug mainly affects the cells in the liver. Hepatic arterial infusion also can be done with a small pump. The doctor implants the pump into the body during surgery. The pump continuously sends the drug to the liver.

- **Chemoembolization:** The doctor inserts a tiny catheter into an artery in the leg. Using x-rays as a guide, the doctor moves the catheter into the hepatic artery. The doctor injects an anticancer drug into the artery and then uses tiny particles to block the flow of blood through the artery. Without blood flow, the drug stays in the liver longer. Depending on the type of particles used, the blockage may be temporary or permanent. Although the hepatic artery is blocked, healthy liver tissue continues to receive blood from the hepatic portal vein, which carries blood from the stomach and intestine. Chemoembolization requires a hospital stay.

- **Total hepatectomy with liver transplantation:** If localized liver cancer is unresectable because of poor liver function, some patients may be able to have a liver transplant. While the patient waits for a donated liver to become available, the health care team monitors the patient's health and provides other treatments, as necessary.

Advanced Cancer

Advanced cancer is cancer that is found in both lobes of the liver or that has spread to other parts of the body. Although advanced liver cancer cannot be cured, some patients receive anticancer therapy to try to slow the progress of the disease. Others discuss the possible benefits and side effects and decide they do not want to have anti-cancer therapy. In either case, patients receive palliative care to reduce their pain and control other symptoms.

Treatment for advanced liver cancer may involve chemotherapy, radiation therapy, or both:

- Chemotherapy uses drugs to kill cancer cells. The patient may receive one drug or a combination of drugs. The doctor may use chemoembolization or hepatic arterial infusion. Or the doctor may give systemic therapy, meaning that the drugs are injected into a vein and flow through the bloodstream to nearly every part of the body. The doctor may call this intravenous or IV chemotherapy. Usually chemotherapy is an outpatient treatment given at the hospital, clinic, or at the doctor's office. However, depending on which drugs are given and the patient's general health, the patient may need to stay in the hospital.
- Radiation therapy (also called radiotherapy) uses high-energy rays to kill cancer cells. Radiation therapy is local therapy, meaning that it affects cancer cells only in the treated area. A large machine outside the body directs radiation to the tumor area.

Recurrent Cancer

Recurrent cancer means the disease has come back after the initial treatment. Even when a tumor in the liver seems to have been completely removed or destroyed, the disease sometimes returns because undetected cancer cells remained somewhere in the body after treatment. Most recurrences occur within the first two years of treatment. The patient may have surgery or a combination of treatments for recurrent liver cancer.

Side Effects of Treatment

Because cancer treatment may damage healthy cells and tissues, unwanted side effects often occur. Side effects depend on many factors, including the type and extent of the treatment. Side effects may not be the same for each person, and they may even change from one treatment session to the next. The health care team will explain the possible side effects of treatment and how they will help the patient manage them.

Surgery

It takes time to heal after surgery, and the time needed to recover is different for each person. Patients are often uncomfortable during the first few days. However, medicine can usually control their pain. Patients should feel free to discuss pain relief with the doctor or nurse. It is common to feel tired or weak for a while. Also, patients may have diarrhea and a feeling of fullness in the abdomen. The health care team watches the patient for signs of bleeding, infection, liver failure, or other problems requiring immediate treatment.

After a liver transplant, the patient may need to stay in the hospital for several weeks. During that time, the health care team checks for signs of how well the patient's body is accepting the new liver. The patient takes drugs to prevent the body from rejecting the new liver. These drugs may cause puffiness in the face, high blood pressure, or an increase in body hair.

Cryosurgery

Because a smaller incision is needed for cryosurgery than for traditional surgery, recovery after cryosurgery is generally faster and less painful. Also, infection and bleeding are not as likely.

Percutaneous Ethanol Injection

Patients may have fever and pain after percutaneous ethanol injection. The doctor can suggest medicines to relieve these problems.

Chemoembolization and Hepatic Arterial Infusion

Chemoembolization and hepatic arterial infusion cause fewer side effects than systemic chemotherapy because the drugs do not flow through the entire body. Chemoembolization sometimes causes nausea, vomiting, fever, and abdominal pain. The doctor can give medications to help lessen these problems. Some patients may feel very tired for several weeks after the treatment.

Side effects from hepatic arterial infusion include infection and problems with the pump device. Sometimes the device may have to be removed.

Systemic Chemotherapy

The side effects of chemotherapy depend mainly on the drugs and the doses the patient receives. As with other types of treatment, side effects are different for each patient.

Systemic chemotherapy affects rapidly dividing cells throughout the body, including blood cells. Blood cells fight infection, help the blood to clot, and carry oxygen to all parts of the body. When anticancer drugs damage blood cells, patients are more likely to get infections, may bruise or bleed easily, and may have less energy. Cells in hair roots and cells that line the digestive tract also divide rapidly. As a result, patients may lose their hair and may have other side effects such as poor appetite, nausea and vomiting, or mouth sores. Usually, these side effects go away gradually during the recovery periods between treatments or after treatment is complete. The health care team can suggest ways to relieve side effects.

Recently, new classes of chemotherapy agents have shown promise in treatment of liver cancer. These drugs are given systemically, but are more targeted in their effects. Many of these agents disrupt systems in cancer cells that allow for growth and spread, and their side effects may be less severe than those of traditional agents. Their roles in treatment of this cancer are still being defined, but they appear promising.

Radiation Therapy

The side effects of radiation therapy depend mainly on the treatment dose and the part of the body that is treated. Patients are likely to become very tired during radiation therapy, especially in the later weeks of treatment. Resting is important, but doctors usually advise patients to try to stay as active as they can.

Radiation therapy to the chest and abdomen may cause nausea, vomiting, diarrhea, or urinary discomfort. Radiation therapy also may cause a decrease in the number of healthy white blood cells, cells that help protect the body against infection. Although the side effects of radiation therapy can be distressing, the doctor can usually treat or control them.

The Promise of Cancer Research

Laboratory scientists are studying the liver to learn more about what may cause liver cancer and how liver cancer cells work. They are looking for new therapies to kill cancer cells.

Doctors in hospitals and clinics are conducting many types of clinical trials. These are research studies in which people take part voluntarily. In these trials, researchers are studying ways to treat liver cancer that have shown promise in laboratory studies. Research has led to advances in treatment methods, but controlling liver cancer remains a challenge. Scientists continue to search for more effective ways to treat this disease.

Patients who join clinical trials have the first chance to benefit from new treatments. They also make an important contribution to medical science. Although clinical trials may pose some risks, researchers take very careful steps to protect people.

Currently, clinical trials involve chemotherapy, chemoembolization, and radiofrequency ablation for the treatment of liver cancer. Another approach under study is biological therapy, which uses the body's natural ability (immune system) to fight cancer. Biological therapy is being studied in combination with chemotherapy.

Chapter 18

Other Cancers of Special Concern to Men

Chapter Contents

Section 18.1

Penile Cancer

Excerpted from PDQ® Cancer Information Summary. National Cancer Institute; Bethesda, MD. Penile Cancer Treatment (PDQ®): Patient Version. Updated June 2008. Available at: http://cancergov. Accessed September 1, 2008.

Penile cancer is a disease in which malignant (cancer) cells form in the tissues of the penis.

The penis is a rod-shaped male reproductive organ that passes sperm and urine from the body. It contains two types of erectile tissue (spongy tissue with blood vessels that fill with blood to make an erection):

- **Corpora cavernosa:** The two columns of erectile tissue that form most of the penis.
- **Corpus spongiosum:** The single column of erectile tissue that forms a small portion of the penis. The corpus spongiosum surrounds the urethra (the tube through which urine and sperm pass from the body).

The erectile tissue is wrapped in connective tissue and covered with skin. The glans (head of the penis) is covered with loose skin called the foreskin.

Human papillomavirus infection may increase the risk of developing penile cancer. Anything that increases your chance of getting a disease is called a risk factor. Circumcision may help prevent infection with the human papillomavirus (HPV). A circumcision is an operation in which the doctor removes part or all of the foreskin from the penis. Many boys are circumcised shortly after birth. Men who were not circumcised at birth may have a higher risk of developing penile cancer.

Other risk factors for penile cancer include the following:

- Being age sixty or older
- Having phimosis (a condition in which the foreskin of the penis cannot be pulled back over the glans)

- Having poor personal hygiene
- Having many sexual partners
- Using tobacco products

Possible signs of penile cancer include sores, discharge, and bleeding. These and other symptoms may be caused by penile cancer. Other conditions may cause the same symptoms. A doctor should be consulted if any of the following problems occur:

- Redness, irritation, or a sore on the penis
- A lump on the penis

Tests that examine the penis are used to detect (find) and diagnose penile cancer. The following tests and procedures may be used:

- **Physical exam and history:** An exam of the body to check general signs of health, including checking the penis for signs of disease, such as lumps or anything else that seems unusual. A history of the patient's health habits and past illnesses and treatments will also be taken.
- **Biopsy:** The removal of cells or tissues so they can be viewed under a microscope by a pathologist to check for signs of cancer.

The prognosis (chance of recovery) and treatment options depend on the following:

- The stage of the cancer
- The location and size of the tumor
- Whether the cancer has just been diagnosed or has recurred (come back)

Stages of Penile Cancer

After penile cancer has been diagnosed, tests are done to find out if cancer cells have spread within the penis or to other parts of the body.

The process used to find out if cancer has spread within the penis or to other parts of the body is called staging. The information gathered from the staging process determines the stage of the disease. It is important to know the stage in order to plan treatment.

The following stages are used for penile cancer:

- **Stage 0 (carcinoma in situ):** In stage 0, abnormal cells are found on the surface of the skin of the penis. These abnormal cells may become cancer and spread into nearby normal tissue. Stage 0 is also called carcinoma in situ.
- **Stage I:** In stage I, cancer has formed and spread to connective tissue just under the skin of the penis.
- **Stage II:** In stage II, cancer has spread to connective tissue just under the skin of the penis and to one lymph node in the groin or to erectile tissue (spongy tissue that fills with blood to make an erection) and possibly to one lymph node in the groin.
- **Stage III:** In stage III, cancer has spread to connective tissue or erectile tissue of the penis and to more than one lymph node on one or both sides of the groin; or to the urethra or prostate and possibly to one or more lymph nodes on one or both sides of the groin.
- **Stage IV:** In stage IV, cancer has spread to tissues near the penis and may have spread to lymph nodes in the groin or pelvis; spread to anywhere in or near the penis and to one or more lymph nodes deep in the pelvis or groin; or spread to distant parts of the body.

Recurrent Penile Cancer

Recurrent penile cancer is cancer that has recurred (come back) after it has been treated. The cancer may come back in the penis or in other parts of the body.

Treatment Option Overview

Different types of treatments are available for patients with penile cancer. Some treatments are standard (the currently used treatment), and some are being tested in clinical trials. A treatment clinical trial is a research study meant to help improve current treatments or obtain information on new treatments for patients with cancer. When clinical trials show that a new treatment is better than the standard treatment, the new treatment may become the standard treatment. Patients may want to think about taking part in a clinical trial. Some clinical trials are open only to patients who have not started treatment.

Three types of standard treatment are used.

Surgery

Surgery is the most common treatment for all stages of penile cancer. A doctor may remove the cancer using one of the following operations:

- **Mohs microsurgery:** A procedure in which the tumor is cut from the skin in thin layers. During the surgery, the edges of the tumor and each layer of tumor removed are viewed through a microscope to check for cancer cells. Layers continue to be removed until no more cancer cells are seen. This type of surgery removes as little normal tissue as possible and is often used to remove cancer on the skin. It is also called Mohs surgery.
- **Laser surgery:** A surgical procedure that uses a laser beam (a narrow beam of intense light) as a knife to make bloodless cuts in tissue or to remove a surface lesion such as a tumor.
- **Cryosurgery:** A treatment that uses an instrument to freeze and destroy abnormal tissue. This type of treatment is also called cryotherapy.
- **Circumcision:** Surgery to remove part or all of the foreskin of the penis.
- **Wide local excision:** Surgery to remove only the cancer and some normal tissue around it.
- **Amputation of the penis:** Surgery to remove part or all of the penis. If part of the penis is removed, it is a partial penectomy. If all of the penis is removed, it is a total penectomy.

Lymph nodes in the groin may be taken out during surgery.

Even if the doctor removes all the cancer that can be seen at the time of the surgery, some patients may be given chemotherapy or radiation therapy after surgery to kill any cancer cells that are left. Treatment given after the surgery, to increase the chances of a cure, is called adjuvant therapy.

Radiation Therapy

Radiation therapy is a cancer treatment that uses high-energy x-rays or other types of radiation to kill cancer cells or keep them from growing. There are two types of radiation therapy. External radiation therapy uses a machine outside the body to send radiation toward the cancer. Internal radiation therapy uses a radioactive substance sealed in needles, seeds, wires, or catheters that are placed directly into or near the cancer. The way the radiation therapy is given depends on the type and stage of the cancer being treated.

Chemotherapy

Chemotherapy is a cancer treatment that uses drugs to stop the growth of cancer cells, either by killing the cells or by stopping them from dividing. When chemotherapy is taken by mouth or injected into a vein or muscle, the drugs enter the bloodstream and can reach cancer cells throughout the body (systemic chemotherapy). When chemotherapy is placed directly onto the skin (topical chemotherapy) or into the spinal column, an organ, or a body cavity such as the abdomen, the drugs mainly affect cancer cells in those areas (regional chemotherapy). The way the chemotherapy is given depends on the type and stage of the cancer being treated.

Topical chemotherapy may be used to treat stage 0 penile cancer.

Experimental Treatments

New types of treatment are being tested in clinical trials.

Biologic therapy: Biologic therapy is a treatment that uses the patient's immune system to fight cancer. Substances made by the body or made in a laboratory are used to boost, direct, or restore the body's natural defenses against cancer. This type of cancer treatment is also called biotherapy or immunotherapy. Topical biologic therapy may be used to treat stage 0 penile cancer.

Radiosensitizers: Radiosensitizers are drugs that make tumor cells more sensitive to radiation therapy. Combining radiation therapy with radiosensitizers helps kill more tumor cells.

Sentinel lymph node biopsy followed by surgery: Sentinel lymph node biopsy is the removal of the sentinel lymph node during surgery. The sentinel lymph node is the first lymph node to receive lymphatic drainage from a tumor. It is the first lymph node the cancer is likely to spread to from the tumor. A radioactive substance and/or blue dye is injected near the tumor. The substance or dye flows through the lymph ducts to the lymph nodes. The first lymph node to receive the substance or dye is removed. A pathologist views the tissue under a microscope to look for cancer cells. If cancer cells are not found, it may not be necessary to remove more lymph nodes. After the sentinel lymph node biopsy, the surgeon removes the cancer.

Patients may want to think about taking part in a clinical trial.

For some patients, taking part in a clinical trial may be the best treatment choice. Clinical trials are part of the cancer research process. Clinical trials are done to find out if new cancer treatments are safe and effective or better than the standard treatment.

Many of today's standard treatments for cancer are based on earlier clinical trials. Patients who take part in a clinical trial may receive the standard treatment or be among the first to receive a new treatment.

Patients who take part in clinical trials also help improve the way cancer will be treated in the future. Even when clinical trials do not lead to effective new treatments, they often answer important questions and help move research forward.

Patients can enter clinical trials before, during, or after starting their cancer treatment. Some clinical trials only include patients who have not yet received treatment. Other trials test treatments for patients whose cancer has not gotten better. There are also clinical trials that test new ways to stop cancer from recurring (coming back) or reduce the side effects of cancer treatment.

Follow-up

Follow-up tests may be needed. Some of the tests that were done to diagnose the cancer or to find out the stage of the cancer may be repeated. Some tests will be repeated in order to see how well the treatment is working. Decisions about whether to continue, change, or stop treatment may be based on the results of these tests. This is sometimes called re-staging.

Some of the tests will continue to be done from time to time after treatment has ended. The results of these tests can show if your condition has changed or if the cancer has recurred (come back). These tests are sometimes called follow-up tests or check-ups.

Section 18.2

Testicular Cancer

Excerpted from "Testicular Cancer: Questions and Answers," National Cancer Institute, May 24, 2005.

What is testicular cancer?

Testicular cancer is a disease in which cells become malignant (cancerous) in one or both testicles.

The testicles (also called testes or gonads) are a pair of male sex glands. They produce and store sperm and are the main source of testosterone (male hormones) in men. These hormones control the development of the reproductive organs and other male physical characteristics. The testicles are located under the penis in a sac-like pouch called the scrotum.

Based on the characteristics of the cells in the tumor, testicular cancers are classified as seminomas or nonseminomas. Other types of cancer that arise in the testicles are rare and are not described here. Seminomas may be one of three types: classic, anaplastic, or spermatocytic. Types of nonseminomas include choriocarcinoma, embryonal carcinoma, teratoma, and yolk sac tumors. Testicular tumors may contain both seminoma and nonseminoma cells.

Testicular cancer accounts for only 1 percent of all cancers in men in the United States. About 8,000 men are diagnosed with testicular cancer and about 390 men die of this disease each year.[1] Testicular cancer occurs most often in men between the ages of twenty and thirty-nine, and is the most common form of cancer in men between the ages of fifteen and thirty-four. It is most common in white men, especially those of Scandinavian descent. The testicular cancer rate has more than doubled among white men in the past forty years, but has only recently begun to increase among black men. The reason for the racial differences in incidence is not known.

What are the risk factors for testicular cancer?

The exact causes of testicular cancer are not known. However, studies have shown that several factors increase a man's chance of developing this disease:

- **Undescended testicle (cryptorchidism):** Normally, the testicles descend from inside the abdomen into the scrotum before birth. The risk of testicular cancer is increased in males with a testicle that does not move down into the scrotum. This risk does not change even after surgery to move the testicle into the scrotum. The increased risk applies to both testicles.
- **Congenital abnormalities:** Men born with abnormalities of the testicles, penis, or kidneys, as well as those with inguinal hernia (hernia in the groin area, where the thigh meets the abdomen), may be at increased risk.
- **History of testicular cancer:** Men who have had testicular cancer are at increased risk of developing cancer in the other testicle.
- **Family history of testicular cancer:** The risk for testicular cancer is greater in men whose brother or father has had the disease.

How is testicular cancer detected? What are symptoms of testicular cancer?

Most testicular cancers are found by men themselves. Also, doctors generally examine the testicles during routine physical exams. Between regular checkups, if a man notices anything unusual about his testicles, he should talk with his doctor. Men should see a doctor if they notice any of the following symptoms:

- A painless lump or swelling in a testicle
- Pain or discomfort in a testicle or in the scrotum
- Any enlargement of a testicle or change in the way it feels
- A feeling of heaviness in the scrotum
- A dull ache in the lower abdomen, back, or groin
- A sudden collection of fluid in the scrotum

These symptoms can be caused by cancer or by other conditions. It is important to see a doctor to determine the cause of any of these symptoms.

How is testicular cancer diagnosed?

To help find the cause of symptoms, the doctor evaluates a man's general health. The doctor also performs a physical exam and may order laboratory and diagnostic tests. These tests include the following:

- Blood tests that measure the levels of tumor markers. Tumor markers are substances often found in higher-than-normal amounts when cancer is present. Tumor markers such as alpha-fetoprotein (AFP), beta-human chorionic gonadotropin (ßHCG), and lactate dehydrogenase (LDH) may suggest the presence of a testicular tumor, even if it is too small to be detected by physical exams or imaging tests.
- Ultrasound, a test in which high-frequency sound waves are bounced off internal organs and tissues. Their echoes produce a picture called a sonogram. Ultrasound of the scrotum can show the presence and size of a mass in the testicle. It is also helpful in ruling out other conditions, such as swelling due to infection or a collection of fluid unrelated to cancer.
- Biopsy (microscopic examination of testicular tissue by a pathologist) to determine whether cancer is present. In nearly all cases of suspected cancer, the entire affected testicle is removed through an incision in the groin. This procedure is called radical inguinal orchiectomy. In rare cases (for example, when a man has only one testicle), the surgeon performs an inguinal biopsy, removing a sample of tissue from the testicle through an incision in the groin and proceeding with orchiectomy only if the pathologist finds cancer cells. (The surgeon does not cut through the scrotum to remove tissue. If the problem is cancer, this procedure could cause the disease to spread.)

If testicular cancer is found, more tests are needed to find out if the cancer has spread from the testicle to other parts of the body. Determining the stage (extent) of the disease helps the doctor to plan appropriate treatment.

How is testicular cancer treated? What are the side effects of treatment?

Although the incidence of testicular cancer has risen in recent years, more than 95 percent of cases can be cured. Treatment is more likely to be successful when testicular cancer is found early. In addition, treatment can often be less aggressive and may cause fewer side effects.

Most men with testicular cancer can be cured with surgery, radiation therapy, and/or chemotherapy. The side effects depend on the type of treatment and may be different for each person.

Seminomas and nonseminomas grow and spread differently and are treated differently. Nonseminomas tend to grow and spread more quickly; seminomas are more sensitive to radiation. If the tumor contains both seminoma and nonseminoma cells, it is treated as a nonseminoma. Treatment also depends on the stage of the cancer, the patient's age and general health, and other factors. Treatment is often provided by a team of specialists, which may include a surgeon, a medical oncologist, and a radiation oncologist.

The three types of standard treatment are described below.

Surgery: Surgery to remove the testicle through an incision in the groin is called a radical inguinal orchiectomy. Men may be concerned that losing a testicle will affect their ability to have sexual intercourse or make them sterile (unable to produce children). However, a man with one healthy testicle can still have a normal erection and produce sperm. Therefore, an operation to remove one testicle does not make a man impotent (unable to have an erection) and seldom interferes with fertility (the ability to produce children). For cosmetic purposes, men can have a prosthesis (an artificial testicle) placed in the scrotum at the time of their orchiectomy or at any time afterward.

Some of the lymph nodes located deep in the abdomen may also be removed (lymph node dissection). This type of surgery does not usually change a man's ability to have an erection or an orgasm, but it can cause problems with fertility if it interferes with ejaculation. Patients may wish to talk with their doctor about the possibility of removing the lymph nodes using a special nerve-sparing surgical technique that may preserve the ability to ejaculate normally.

Radiation therapy: Radiation therapy (also called radiotherapy) uses high-energy rays to kill cancer cells and shrink tumors. It is a local therapy, meaning that it affects cancer cells only in the treated areas. External radiation (from a machine outside the body), aimed at the lymph nodes in the abdomen, is used to treat seminomas. It is usually given after surgery. Because nonseminomas are less sensitive to radiation, men with this type of cancer usually do not undergo radiation therapy.

Radiation therapy affects normal as well as cancerous cells. The side effects of radiation therapy depend mainly on the treatment dose. Common side effects include fatigue, skin changes at the site where the treatment is given, loss of appetite, nausea, and diarrhea. Radiation therapy interferes with sperm production, but many patients regain their fertility over a period of one to two years.

Chemotherapy: Chemotherapy is the use of anticancer drugs to kill cancer cells. When chemotherapy is given to testicular cancer patients, it is usually given as adjuvant therapy (after surgery) to destroy cancerous cells that may remain in the body. Chemotherapy may also be the initial treatment if the cancer is advanced; that is, if it has spread outside the testicle at the time of the diagnosis. Most anticancer drugs are given by injection into a vein.

Chemotherapy is a systemic therapy, meaning drugs travel through the bloodstream and affect normal as well as cancerous cells throughout the body. The side effects depend largely on the specific drugs and the doses. Common side effects include nausea, hair loss, fatigue, diarrhea, vomiting, fever, chills, coughing/shortness of breath, mouth sores, or skin rash. Other side effects include dizziness, numbness, loss of reflexes, or difficulty hearing. Some anticancer drugs also interfere with sperm production. Although the reduction in sperm count is permanent for some patients, many others recover their fertility.

Some men with advanced or recurrent testicular cancer may undergo treatment with very high doses of chemotherapy. These high doses of chemotherapy kill cancer cells, but they also destroy the bone marrow, which makes and stores blood cells. Such treatment can be given only if patients undergo a bone marrow transplant. In a transplant, bone marrow stem cells are removed from the patient before chemotherapy is administered. These cells are frozen temporarily and then thawed and returned to the patient through a needle (like a blood transfusion) after the high-dose chemotherapy has been administered.

Men with testicular cancer should discuss their concerns about sexual function and fertility with their doctor. It is important to know that men with testicular cancer often have fertility problems even before their cancer is treated. If a man has preexisting fertility problems, or if he is to have treatment that might lead to infertility, he may want to ask the doctor about sperm banking (freezing sperm before treatment for use in the future). This procedure allows some men to have children even if the treatment causes loss of fertility.

Is follow-up treatment necessary? What does it involve?

Regular follow-up exams are extremely important for men who have been treated for testicular cancer. Like all cancers, testicular cancer can recur (come back). Men who have had testicular cancer should see their doctor regularly and should report any unusual symptoms right away. Follow-up varies for different types and stages of testicular cancer. Generally, patients are checked frequently by their doctor and have regular blood tests to measure tumor marker levels. They also have regular x-rays and computed tomography, also called CT scans or CAT scans (detailed pictures of areas inside the body created by a computer linked to an x-ray machine). Men who have had testicular cancer have an increased likelihood of developing cancer in the remaining testicle. Patients treated with chemotherapy may have an increased risk of certain types of leukemia, as well as other types of cancer. Regular follow-up care ensures that changes in health are discussed and that problems are treated as soon as possible.

Are clinical trials (research studies) available for men with testicular cancer?

Yes. Participation in clinical trials is an important treatment option for many men with testicular cancer. To develop new treatments, and better ways to use current treatments, the National Cancer Institute (NCI) is sponsoring clinical trials (research studies with people) in many hospitals and cancer centers around the country. Clinical trials are a critical step in the development of new methods of treatment. Before any new treatment can be recommended for general use, doctors conduct clinical trials to find out whether the treatment is safe for patients and effective against the disease.

People interested in taking part in a clinical trial should talk with their doctor.

Reference

1. American Cancer Society, Inc. *Cancer Facts and Figures 2005.* Atlanta: American Cancer Society, Inc., 2005. Also available at http://www.cancer.org/downloads/STT/CAFF2005f4PWSecured .pdf on the Internet.

Section 18.3

Breast Cancer in Men

PDQ® Cancer Information Summary. National Cancer Institute; Bethesda, MD. Male Breast Cancer Treatment (PDQ®): Patient Version. Updated July 2008. Available at: http://cancergov. Accessed September 1, 2008.

General Information about Male Breast Cancer

Male breast cancer is a disease in which malignant (cancer) cells form in the tissues of the breast.

Breast cancer may occur in men. Men at any age may develop breast cancer, but it is usually detected (found) in men between sixty and seventy years of age. Male breast cancer makes up less than 1 percent of all cases of breast cancer.

The following types of breast cancer are found in men:

- **Infiltrating ductal carcinoma:** Cancer that has spread beyond the cells lining ducts in the breast. Most men with breast cancer have this type of cancer.
- **Ductal carcinoma in situ:** Abnormal cells that are found in the lining of a duct; also called intraductal carcinoma.
- **Inflammatory breast cancer:** A type of cancer in which the breast looks red and swollen and feels warm.
- **Paget disease of the nipple:** A tumor that has grown from ducts beneath the nipple onto the surface of the nipple.

Lobular carcinoma in situ (abnormal cells found in one of the lobes or sections of the breast), which sometimes occurs in women, has not been seen in men.

Risk Factors

Anything that increases your risk of getting a disease is called a risk factor. Having a risk factor does not mean that you will get cancer; not having risk factors doesn't mean that you will not get cancer.

People who think they may be at risk should discuss this with their doctor. Risk factors for breast cancer in men may include the following:

- Being exposed to radiation
- Having a disease related to high levels of estrogen in the body, such as cirrhosis (liver disease) or Klinefelter syndrome (a genetic disorder)
- Having several female relatives who have had breast cancer, especially relatives who have an alteration of the BRCA2 gene

Male breast cancer is sometimes caused by inherited gene mutations (changes).

The genes in cells carry the hereditary information that is received from a person's parents. Hereditary breast cancer makes up approximately 5 to 10 percent of all breast cancer. Some altered genes related to breast cancer are more common in certain ethnic groups. Men who have an altered gene related to breast cancer have an increased risk of developing this disease.

Tests have been developed that can detect altered genes. These genetic tests are sometimes done for members of families with a high risk of cancer.

Symptoms and Diagnosis

Men with breast cancer usually have lumps that can be felt.

Lumps and other symptoms may be caused by male breast cancer. Other conditions may cause the same symptoms. A doctor should be seen if changes in the breasts are noticed.

Tests that examine the breasts are used to detect (find) and diagnose breast cancer in men. The following tests and procedures may be used:

- **Biopsy:** The removal of cells or tissues so they can be viewed under a microscope by a pathologist to check for signs of cancer. The following are different types of biopsies:
    - **Fine-needle aspiration (FNA) biopsy:** The removal of tissue or fluid using a thin needle.
    - **Core biopsy:** The removal of tissue using a wide needle.
    - **Excisional biopsy:** The removal of an entire lump of tissue.

- **Estrogen and progesterone receptor test:** A test to measure the amount of estrogen and progesterone (hormones) receptors in cancer tissue. If cancer is found in the breast, tissue from the tumor is checked in the laboratory to find out whether estrogen and progesterone could affect the way cancer grows. The test results show whether hormone therapy may stop the cancer from growing.
- **HER2 test:** A test to measure the amount of HER2 in cancer tissue. HER2 is a growth factor protein that sends growth signals to cells. When cancer forms, the cells may make too much of the protein, causing more cancer cells to grow. If cancer is found in the breast, tissue from the tumor is checked in the laboratory to find out if there is too much HER2 in the cells. The test results show whether monoclonal antibody therapy may stop the cancer from growing.

Prognosis

Survival for men with breast cancer is similar to that for women with breast cancer when their stage at diagnosis is the same. Breast cancer in men, however, is often diagnosed at a later stage. Cancer found at a later stage may be less likely to be cured.

The prognosis (chance of recovery) and treatment options depend on the following:

- The stage of the cancer (whether it is in the breast only or has spread to other places in the body)
- The type of breast cancer
- Estrogen-receptor and progesterone-receptor levels in the tumor tissue
- Whether the cancer is also found in the other breast
- The patient's age and general health

Stages of Male Breast Cancer

After breast cancer has been diagnosed, tests are done to find out if cancer cells have spread within the breast or to other parts of the body. This process is called staging. The information gathered from the staging process determines the stage of the disease. It is important to know the stage in order to plan treatment. Breast cancer in men is staged the same as it is in women. The spread of cancer from the breast to lymph nodes and other parts of the body appears to be similar in men and women.

Recurrent Male Breast Cancer

Recurrent breast cancer is cancer that has recurred (come back) after it has been treated. The cancer may come back in the breast, in the chest wall, or in other parts of the body.

Treatment Option Overview

Different types of treatment are available for men with breast cancer. Some treatments are standard (the currently used treatment), and some are being tested in clinical trials. A treatment clinical trial is a research study meant to help improve current treatments or obtain information on new treatments for patients with cancer. When clinical trials show that a new treatment is better than the standard treatment, the new treatment may become the standard treatment.

For some patients, taking part in a clinical trial may be the best treatment choice. Many of today's standard treatments for cancer are based on earlier clinical trials. Patients who take part in a clinical trial may receive the standard treatment or be among the first to receive a new treatment.

Patients who take part in clinical trials also help improve the way cancer will be treated in the future. Even when clinical trials do not lead to effective new treatments, they often answer important questions and help move research forward.

Some clinical trials only include patients who have not yet received treatment. Other trials test treatments for patients whose cancer has not gotten better. There are also clinical trials that test new ways to stop cancer from recurring (coming back) or reduce the side effects of cancer treatment.

Choosing the most appropriate cancer treatment is a decision that ideally involves the patient, family, and health care team.

Four types of standard treatment are used to treat men with breast cancer.

Surgery: Surgery for men with breast cancer is usually a modified radical mastectomy (removal of the breast, many of the lymph nodes under the arm, the lining over the chest muscles, and sometimes part of the chest wall muscles).

Breast-conserving surgery, an operation to remove the cancer but not the breast itself, is also used for some men with breast cancer. A lumpectomy is done to remove the tumor (lump) and a small amount of normal tissue around it. Radiation therapy is given after surgery to kill any cancer cells that are left.

Chemotherapy: Chemotherapy is a cancer treatment that uses drugs to stop the growth of cancer cells, either by killing the cells or by stopping them from dividing. When chemotherapy is taken by mouth or injected into a vein or muscle, the drugs enter the bloodstream and can reach cancer cells throughout the body (systemic chemotherapy). When chemotherapy is placed directly into the spinal column, an organ, or a body cavity such as the abdomen, the drugs mainly affect cancer cells in those areas (regional chemotherapy). The way the chemotherapy is given depends on the type and stage of the cancer being treated.

Hormone therapy: Hormone therapy is a cancer treatment that removes hormones or blocks their action and stops cancer cells from growing. Hormones are substances made by glands in the body and circulated in the bloodstream. Some hormones can cause certain cancers to grow. If tests show that the cancer cells have places where hormones can attach (receptors), drugs, surgery, or radiation therapy are used to reduce the production of hormones or block them from working.

Radiation therapy: Radiation therapy is a cancer treatment that uses high-energy x-rays or other types of radiation to kill cancer cells or keep them from growing. There are two types of radiation therapy. External radiation therapy uses a machine outside the body to send radiation toward the cancer. Internal radiation therapy uses a radioactive substance sealed in needles, seeds, wires, or catheters that are placed directly into or near the cancer. The way the radiation therapy is given depends on the type and stage of the cancer being treated.

New types of treatment are being tested in clinical trials.

Monoclonal antibodies as adjuvant therapy: Monoclonal antibody therapy is a cancer treatment that uses antibodies made in the laboratory from a single type of immune system cell. These antibodies can identify substances on cancer cells or normal substances that may help cancer cells grow. The antibodies attach to the substances and kill the cancer cells, block their growth, or keep them from spreading. Monoclonal antibodies are given by infusion. They may be used alone or to carry drugs, toxins, or radioactive material directly to cancer cells. Monoclonal antibodies are also used in combination with chemotherapy as adjuvant therapy (treatment given after surgery to increase the chances of a cure).

Trastuzumab (Herceptin®) is a monoclonal antibody that blocks the effects of the growth factor protein HER2.

Treatment Options for Male Breast Cancer

Breast cancer in men is treated the same as breast cancer in women.

Initial Surgery

Treatment for men diagnosed with breast cancer is usually modified radical mastectomy. Breast-conserving surgery with lumpectomy may be used for some men.

Adjuvant Therapy

Therapy given after an operation when cancer cells can no longer be seen is called adjuvant therapy. Even if the doctor removes all the cancer that can be seen at the time of the operation, the patient may be given radiation therapy, chemotherapy, hormone therapy, and/or monoclonal antibody therapy after surgery to try to kill any cancer cells that may be left:

- **Node-negative:** For men whose cancer is node-negative (cancer has not spread to the lymph nodes), adjuvant therapy should be considered on the same basis as for a woman with breast cancer because there is no evidence that response to therapy is different for men and women.
- **Node-positive:** For men whose cancer is node-positive (cancer has spread to the lymph nodes), adjuvant therapy may include chemotherapy plus tamoxifen (to block the effect of estrogen), other hormone therapy, or a clinical trial of trastuzumab (Herceptin).

These treatments appear to increase survival in men, as they do in women. The patient's response to hormone therapy depends on whether there are hormone receptors (proteins) in the tumor. Most breast cancers in men have these receptors. Hormone therapy is usually recommended for male breast cancer patients, but it can have many side effects, including hot flashes and impotence (the inability to have an erection adequate for sexual intercourse).

Distant Metastases

Treatment for men with distant metastases (cancer that has spread to other parts of the body) may be hormone therapy, chemotherapy, or both. Hormone therapy may include the following:

- Orchiectomy (the removal of the testicles to decrease hormone production).
- Luteinizing hormone-releasing hormone agonist with or without total androgen blockade (to decrease the production of sex hormones).
- Tamoxifen for cancer that is estrogen-receptor positive.
- Progesterone (a female hormone).
- Aromatase inhibitors (to lessen the amount of estrogen produced).

Hormone therapies may be used in sequence (one after the other). Standard chemotherapy regimens may be used if hormone therapy does not work. Men usually respond to therapy in the same way as women who have breast cancer.

Treatment Options for Locally Recurrent Male Breast Cancer

For men with locally recurrent disease (cancer that has come back in a limited area after treatment), treatment is usually either surgery combined with chemotherapy or radiation therapy combined with chemotherapy.

Chapter 19

Accidents and Injuries

Chapter Contents

Section 19.1

Safe Steps to Reduce Falls

Millions of Americans are only a step away from becoming victims of the leading cause of unintentional home injuries—falls.

According to The State of Home Safety in America™ (2004) conducted by the Home Safety Council, falls are by far the leading cause of unintentional home injury death. Falls account for an average of 5.1 million injuries and nearly 6,000 deaths each year. The vast majority of fall deaths occur among people age sixty-five and older and fall death rates are higher for males.

In an effort to reduce injuries among people of all ages, the Home Safety Council encourages families to identify and correct potential falling hazards in and around the home.

Home Safety "Walk-Through"

Walk through your home to identify and remedy potential falling hazards. What to look for:

- Prevent falls:
  - Have handrails on both sides of stairs and steps. Make sure handrails go from the top to the bottom of stairs.
  - Have lots of lights at the top and bottom of the stairs.
  - It is easy to trip on small rugs. Tape them to the floor or do not use them at all.
  - Keep the stairs clear.
  - Have nightlights in the bedroom, hall, and bathroom.
  - Have a mat or non-slip strips in the tub and shower.
  - Have a bath mat with a nonskid bottom on the bathroom floor.

- Have grab bars in the tub and shower.
- Wipe up spills when they happen.

- Protect young children:
  - Always watch young children.
  - Use safety gates at the top and bottom of stairs.
  - Window guards can keep a child from falling out the window. Have window guards on upstairs windows.
  - Cover the ground under playground equipment with a thick layer (nine to twelve inches) of mulch, wood chips, or other safety material.
- Outdoors:
  - Put bright lights over all porches and walkways.
  - Have handrails on both sides of the stairs.
  - Put ladders away after using them. Store ladders on their sides, in a shed or garage.
  - Keep sidewalks and paths clear, so you don't trip.
  - Fix broken or chipped steps and walkways as soon as possible.

Section 19.2

Preventing Fire-Related Injuries

"Fire Deaths and Injuries: An Overview" is reprinted from "Fire Deaths and Injuries Fact Sheet," Centers for Disease Control and Prevention, August 8, 2008. "Fire Prevention Tips" is reprinted from "Think Safe Be Safe: Fire Prevention Tips," © 2008 Home Safety Council (www .homesafetycouncil.org). Reprinted with permission.

Fire Deaths and Injuries: An Overview

Deaths from fires and burns are the fifth most common cause of unintentional injury deaths in the United States (CDC 2005) and the third leading cause of fatal home injury (Runyan 2004). The United States mortality rate from fires ranks sixth among the twenty-five developed countries for which statistics are available (International Association for the Study of Insurance Economics 2003).

Although the number of fatalities and injuries caused by residential fires has declined gradually over the past several decades, many residential fire-related deaths remain preventable and continue to pose a significant public health problem.

Occurrence and Consequences

On average in the United States in 2006, someone died in a fire about every 162 minutes, and someone was injured every 32 minutes (Karter 2007).

Four out of five U.S. fire deaths in 2005 occurred in homes (Karter 2007).

In 2006, fire departments responded to 412,500 home fires in the United States, which claimed the lives of 2,580 people (not including firefighters) and injured another 12,925, not including firefighters (Karter 2007).

Most victims of fires die from smoke or toxic gases and not from burns (Hall 2001).

Smoking is the leading cause of fire-related deaths (Ahrens 2003).

Cooking is the primary cause of residential fires (Ahrens 2003).

Costs

In 2005, residential fires caused nearly $7 billion in property damage (Karter 2007).

Fire and burn injuries represent 1 percent of the incidence of injuries and 2 percent of the total costs of injuries, or $7.5 billion each year (Finkelstein et al. 2006):

- Males account for $4.8 billion (64 percent) of the total costs of fire/burn injuries.
- Females account for $2.7 billion (36 percent) of the total costs of fire/burn injuries.
- Fatal fire and burn injuries cost $3 billion, representing 2 percent of the total costs of all fatal injuries.
- Hospitalized fire and burn injuries total $1 billion, or 1 percent of the total cost of all hospitalized injuries.
- Nonhospitalized fire and burn injuries cost $3 billion, or 2 percent of the total cost of all nonhospitalized injuries.

Groups at Risk

Groups at increased risk of fire-related injuries and deaths include the following:

- Children age four and under (CDC 1998)
- Older Adults ages sixty-five and older (CDC 1998)
- African Americans and Native Americans (CDC 1998)
- The poorest Americans (Istre 2001)
- Persons living in rural areas (Ahrens 2003)
- Persons living in manufactured homes or substandard housing (Runyan 1992; Parker 1993)

Risk Factors

Approximately half of home fire deaths occur in homes without smoke alarms (Ahrens 2004).

Most residential fires occur during the winter months (CDC 1998).

Alcohol use contributes to an estimated 40 percent of residential fire deaths (Smith 1999).

References

Ahrens M. *The U.S. fire problem overview report: leading causes and other patterns and trends*. Quincy (MA): National Fire Protection Association; 2003.

Ahrens M. *U.S. experience with smoke alarms and other fire alarms*. Quincy (MA): National Fire Protection Association; 2004.

Centers for Disease Control and Prevention. Deaths resulting from residential fires and the prevalence of smoke alarms—United States 1991–1995. *Morbidity and Mortality Weekly Report* 1998; 47(38): 803–6.

Centers for Disease Control and Prevention, National Center for Health Statistics (NCHS). National vital statistics system. Hyattsville (MD): U.S. Department of Health and Human Services, CDC, National Center for Health Statistics; 1998.

Centers for Disease Control and Prevention. Web-based Injury Statistics Query and Reporting System (WISQARS) [Online]. (2005). National Center for Injury Prevention and Control, Centers for Disease Control and Prevention (producer). Available from: URL: www.cdc.gov/ncipc/wisqars. [Cited 2006 Aug 21].

Finkelstein EA, Corso PS, Miller TR, Associates. *Incidence and Economic Burden of Injuries in the United States.* New York: Oxford University Press; 2006.

Hall JR. *Burns, toxic gases, and other hazards associated with fires: Deaths and injuries in fire and non-fire situations*. Quincy (MA): National Fire Protection Association, Fire Analysis and Research Division; 2001.

International Association for the Study of Insurance Economics. *World fire statistics: information bulletin of the world fire statistics*. Geneva (Switzerland): The Geneva Association; 2003.

Istre GR, McCoy MA, Osborn L, Barnard JJ, Bolton A. Deaths and injuries from house fires. *New England Journal of Medicine* 2001; 344:1911–16.

Karter MJ. *Fire loss in the United States during 2006*. Quincy (MA): National Fire Protection Association, Fire Analysis and Research Division; 2007.

Parker DJ, Sklar DP, Tandberg D, Hauswald M, Zumwalt RE. Fire fatalities among New Mexico children. *Annals of Emergency Medicine* 1993;22(3):517–22.

Runyan CW, Bangdiwala SI, Linzer MA, Sacks JJ, Butts J. Risk factors for fatal residential fires. *New England Journal of Medicine* 1992;327(12):859–63.

Runyan SW, Casteel C (Eds.). *The state of home safety in America: Facts about unintentional injuries in the home*, 2nd edition. Washington, D.C.: Home Safety Council, 2004.

Smith GS, Branas C, Miller TR. Fatal nontraffic injuries involving alcohol: a meta-analysis. *Annals of Emergency Medicine* 1999;33(6): 659–68.

Fire Prevention Tips

According to the Home Safety Council's State of Home Safety in America™ Report, fires and burns are the third leading cause of unintentional home injury and related deaths. Fire safety and survival begin with everyone in your household being prepared. Follow these safety measures from the Home Safety Council to reduce the chance of fire in your home:

- Prevent fires caused by cooking:
  - Always stay in the kitchen while cooking.
  - Keep things that can burn, such as dishtowels, paper or plastic bags, and curtains at least three feet away from the range top.
  - Before cooking, roll up sleeves and use oven mitts. Loose-fitting clothes can touch a hot burner and catch on fire.
  - Never leave barbecue grills unattended while in use.
  - Keep grills at least ten feet away from other objects, including the house and any shrubs or bushes.
  - Always stay by the grill when cooking.
- Prevent fires caused by heating:
  - Store matches and lighters in a locked cabinet.
  - Keep space heaters at least three feet away from things that can burn, such as curtains or stacks of newspaper. Always turn off heaters when leaving the room or going to bed.
  - Have a service person inspect chimneys, fireplaces, wood and coal stoves, and central furnaces once a year. Have them cleaned when necessary.

    - Keep things that can burn away from your fireplace and keep a glass or metal screen in front of your fireplace.
- Prevent fires caused by smoking:
    - Use "fire-safe" cigarettes and smoke outside.
    - Use large, deep ashtrays on sturdy surfaces like a table.
    - Douse cigarette and cigar butts with water before dumping them in the trash.
- Prevent fires caused by candles:
    - Never leave burning candles unattended. Do not allow children to keep candles or incense in their rooms.
    - Always use stable candle holders made of material that won't catch fire, such as metal, glass, etc.
    - Blow out candles when adults leave the room.
- Prevent fires caused by gasoline and other products:
    - Store gasoline in a garage or shed in a container approved for gasoline storage.
    - Never bring or use gasoline indoors; and use it as a motor fuel only.
    - Close the lid on all dangerous products and put them away after using them.
    - Store them away from the home and in a safe place with a lock.
    - Don't plug in too many appliances at once.
- Keep your family safe at home:
    - Make a fire escape plan for your family. Find two exits out of every room. Pick a meeting place outside. Practice makes perfect—hold a family fire drill at least twice each year.
    - Install smoke alarms on every level of your home. For the best detection and notification protection, install both ionization- and photoelectric-type smoke alarms. Some models provide dual coverage. The type will be printed on the box or package. Put them inside or near every bedroom. Test them monthly to make sure they work. Put in new batteries once a year.
    - Know how to put out a small pan fire by sliding a lid over the flames.

- Teach every family member to "Stop, Drop, and Roll" if clothes catch fire.
- Consider having a home fire sprinkler system installed in your new home, or when you remodel.
- Learn how and when to use a fire extinguisher.
- If you have a fire in your home, once you get out, stay out.
- Do not go back inside for any reason.

Section 19.3

Preventing Motor Vehicle Accidents

"Older Drivers" is reprinted from the National Institute on Aging, February 16, 2008. "Impaired Driving" is reprinted from the Centers for Disease Control and Prevention, June 2, 2008. Permission to reprint "Driving Defensively" is granted by the National Safety Council, a membership organization dedicated to protecting life and promoting health.

Older Drivers

How Does Age Affect Driving?

More and more older drivers are on the roads these days. It's important to know that getting older doesn't automatically turn people into bad drivers. Many of us continue to be good, safe drivers as we age. But there are changes that can affect driving skills as we age.

Changes to our bodies: Over time your joints may get stiff and your muscles weaken. It can be harder to move your head to look back, quickly turn the steering wheel, or safely hit the brakes.

Your eyesight and hearing may change, too. As you get older, you need more light to see things. Also, glare from the sun, oncoming headlights, or other street lights may trouble you more than before. The area you can see around you (called peripheral vision) may become narrower. The vision problems from eye diseases such as cataracts, macular degeneration, or glaucoma can also affect your driving ability.

You may also find that your reflexes are getting slower. Or, your attention span may shorten. Maybe it's harder for you to do two things at once. These are all normal changes, but they can affect your driving skills.

Some older people have conditions like Alzheimer disease (AD) that change their thinking and behavior. People with AD may forget familiar routes or even how to drive safely. They become more likely to make driving mistakes, and they have more "close calls" than other drivers. However, people in the early stages of AD may be able to keep driving for a while. Caregivers should watch their driving over time. As the disease worsens, it will affect driving ability. Doctors can help you decide whether it's safe for the person with AD to keep driving.

Other health changes: While health problems can affect driving at any age, some occur more often as we get older. For example, arthritis, Parkinson disease, and diabetes may make it harder to drive. People who are depressed may become distracted while driving. The effects of a stroke or even lack of sleep can also cause driving problems. Devices such as an automatic defibrillator or pacemaker might cause an irregular heartbeat or dizziness, which can make driving dangerous.

Medicine side effects: Some medicines can make it harder for you to drive safely. These medicines include sleep aids, anti-depression drugs, antihistamines for allergies and colds, strong painkillers, and diabetes medications. If you take one or more of these or other medicines, talk to your doctor about how they might affect your driving.

Smart Driving Tips

Planning before you leave:

- Plan to drive on streets you know.
- Limit your trips to places that are easy to get to and close to home.
- Take routes that let you avoid risky spots like ramps and left turns.
- Add extra time for travel if driving conditions are bad.
- Don't drive when you are stressed or tired.

While you are driving:

- Always wear your seatbelt.

- Stay off the cell phone.
- Avoid distractions such as listening to the radio or having conversations.
- Leave a big space, at least two car lengths, between your car and the one in front of you. If you are driving at higher speeds or if the weather is bad, leave even more space between you and the next car.
- Make sure there is enough space behind you. (Hint: if someone follows you too closely, slow down so that the person will pass you.)
- Use your rear window defroster to keep the back window clear at all times.
- Keep your headlights on at all times.

Car safety:

- Drive a car with features that make driving easier, such as power steering, power brakes, automatic transmission, and large mirrors.
- Drive a car with airbags.
- Check your windshield wiper blades often and replace them when needed.
- Keep your headlights clean and aligned.
- Think about getting hand controls for the accelerator and brakes if you have leg problems.

Driving skills:

- Take a driving refresher class every few years. (Hint: Some car insurance companies lower your bill when you pass this type of class. Check with the American Association of Retired Persons [AARP], the American Automobile Association [AAA], or local private driving schools to find a class near you.)

Am I a Safe Driver?

Maybe you already know of some driving situations that are hard for you—nights, highways, rush hours, or bad weather. If so, try to change your driving habits to avoid them. Other hints? Older drivers are most at risk when yielding the right of way, turning (especially making left turns), changing lanes, passing, and using expressway ramps. Pay special attention at those times.

Is It Time to Give Up Driving?

We all age differently. For this reason, there is no way to say what age should be the upper limit for driving. So, how do you know if you should stop driving? To help you decide, ask yourself the following questions:

- Do other drivers often honk at me?
- Have I had some accidents, even "fender benders"?
- Do I get lost, even on roads I know?
- Do cars or people walking seem to appear out of nowhere?
- Have family, friends, or my doctor said they are worried about my driving?
- Am I driving less these days because I am not as sure about my driving as I used to be?

If you answered yes to any of these questions, you should think seriously about whether or not you are still a safe driver. If you answered no to all these questions, don't forget to have your eyes and ears checked regularly. Talk to your doctor about any changes to your health that could affect your ability to drive safely.

How Will I Get Around?

You can stay active and do the things you like to do, even if you decide to give up driving. There may be more options for getting around than you think. Some areas offer low-cost bus or taxi service for older people. Some also have carpools or other transportation on request. Religious and civic groups sometimes have volunteers who take seniors where they want to go. Your local Agency on Aging has information about transportation services in your area.

If you do not have these services where you live, look into taking taxis. Too expensive, you think? Well, think about this: the AAA now estimates that the average cost of owning and running a car is about $6,420 a year. So, by giving up your car, you might have as much as $123 a week to use for taxis, buses, or to buy gas for friends and relatives who can drive you!

Impaired Driving

Alcohol-related motor vehicle crashes kill someone every thirty-one minutes and nonfatally injure someone every two minutes (NHTSA 2006). But there are effective measures that can be taken to prevent injuries and deaths from impaired driving.

Occurrence and Consequences

- During 2005, 16,885 people in the U.S. died in alcohol-related motor vehicle crashes, representing 39 percent of all traffic-related deaths (NHTSA 2006).
- In 2005, nearly 1.4 million drivers were arrested for driving under the influence of alcohol or narcotics (Department of Justice 2005). That's less than 1 percent of the 159 million self-reported episodes of alcohol–impaired driving among U.S. adults each year (Quinlan et al. 2005).
- Drugs other than alcohol (e.g., marijuana and cocaine) are involved in about 18 percent of motor vehicle driver deaths. These other drugs are generally used in combination with alcohol (Jones et al. 2003).
- More than half of the 414 child passengers ages fourteen and younger who died in alcohol-related crashes during 2005 were riding with the drinking driver (NHTSA 2006).
- In 2005, 48 children age fourteen years and younger who were killed as pedestrians or pedal cyclists were struck by impaired drivers (NHTSA 2006).

Cost

Each year, alcohol-related crashes in the United States cost about $51 billion (Blincoe et al. 2002).

Groups at Risk

- Male drivers involved in fatal motor vehicle crashes are almost twice as likely as female drivers to be intoxicated with a blood alcohol concentration (BAC) of 0.08 percent or greater (NHTSA 2006). It is illegal to drive with a BAC of 0.08 percent or higher in all fifty states, the District of Columbia, and Puerto Rico.

- At all levels of blood alcohol concentration, the risk of being involved in a crash is greater for young people than for older people (Zador et al. 2000). In 2005, 16 percent of drivers ages sixteen to twenty who died in motor vehicle crashes had been drinking alcohol (NHTSA 2006).
- Young men ages eighteen to twenty (under the legal drinking age) reported driving while impaired more frequently than any other age group (Shults et al. 2002, Quinlan et al. 2005).
- Among motorcycle drivers killed in fatal crashes, 30 percent have BACs of 0.08 percent or greater (Paulozzi et al. 2004).
- Nearly half of the alcohol-impaired motorcyclists killed each year are age forty or older, and motorcyclists ages forty to forty-four years have the highest percentage of fatalities with BACs of 0.08 percent or greater (Paulozzi et al. 2004).
- Of the 1,946 traffic fatalities among children ages zero to fourteen years in 2005, 21 percent involved alcohol (NHTSA 2006b).
- Among drivers involved in fatal crashes, those with BAC levels of 0.08 percent or higher were nine times more likely to have a prior conviction for driving while impaired (DWI) than were drivers who had not consumed alcohol (NHTSA 2006).

Prevention Strategies

Effective measures to prevent injuries and deaths from impaired driving include the following:

- Aggressively enforcing existing 0.08 percent BAC laws, minimum legal drinking age laws, and zero tolerance laws for drivers younger than twenty-one years old in all states (Shults et al. 2002, Quinlan et al. 2005).
- Promptly suspending the driver's licenses of people who drive while intoxicated (DeJong et al. 1998).
- Sobriety checkpoints (Elder et al. 2002).
- Health promotion efforts that use an ecological framework to influence economic, organizational, policy, and school/community action (Howat et al. 2004; Hingson et al. 2006).
- Multifaceted community-based approaches to alcohol control and DWI prevention (Holder et al. 2000, DeJong et al. 1998).

- Mandatory substance abuse assessment and treatment for driving-under-the-influence offenders (Wells-Parker et al. 1995).

Other suggested measures include the following:

- Reducing the legal limit for blood alcohol concentration (BAC) to 0.05 percent (Howat et al. 1991; National Committee on Injury Prevention and Control 1989).
- Raising state and federal alcohol excise taxes (National Committee on Injury Prevention and Control 1989).
- Implementing compulsory blood alcohol testing when traffic crashes result in injury (National Committee on Injury Prevention and Control 1989).

References

Blincoe L, Seay A, Zaloshnja E, Miller T, Romano E, Luchter S, et al. The Economic Impact of Motor Vehicle Crashes, 2000. Washington (DC): Dept of Transportation (US), National Highway Traffic Safety Administration (NHTSA); 2002. Available from URL: http://www.nhtsa.dot.gov/people/economic/econimpact2000/index.htm.

DeJong W. Hingson R. Strategies to reduce driving under the influence of alcohol. *Annual Review of Public Health* 1998;19:359–78.

Department of Justice (US), Federal Bureau of Investigation (FBI). Crime in the United States 2005: Uniform Crime Reports. Washington (DC): FBI; 2005 [cited 2006 Nov 3]. Available from URL: http://www.fbi.gov/ucr/05cius/index.html.

Dept of Transportation (US), National Highway Traffic Safety Administration (NHTSA). Traffic safety facts 2005: alcohol. Washington (DC): NHTSA; 2006 [cited 2006 Oct 3]. Available from URL: http://www-nrd.nhtsa.dot.gov/pdf/nrd-30/NCSA/TSF2005/AlcoholTSF05.pdf.

Dept of Transportation (US), National Highway Traffic Safety Administration (NHTSA). Traffic safety facts 2005: children. Washington (DC): NHTSA; 2006b [cited 2006 Oct 3]. Available from URL: http://www-nrd.nhtsa.dot.gov/pdf/nrd-30/NCSA/TSF2005/ChildrenTSF05.pdf.

Elder RW, Shults RA, Sleet DA, et al. Effectiveness of sobriety checkpoints for reducing alcohol-involved crashes. *Traffic Injury Prevention* 2002;3:266-74.

Hingson, R, Sleet, DA. Modifying alcohol use to reduce motor vehicle injury. In Gielen, Ac, Sleet, DA, DiClemente, R (Eds). *Injury and Violence Prevention: Behavior change Theories, Methods, and Applications.* San Francisco, CA: Jossey-Bass, 2006.

Holder HD, Gruenewald PJ, Ponicki WR, Treno AJ, Grube JW, Saltz RF, et al. Effect of community-based interventions on high-risk drinking and alcohol-related injuries. *Journal of the American Medical Association* 2000;284:2341–47.

Howat P, Sleet D, Smith I. Alcohol and driving: is the .05% blood alcohol concentration limit justified? *Drug and Alcohol Review* 1991; 10(1):151–66.

Howat, P, Sleet, D, Elder, R, Maycock, B. Preventing Alcohol-related traffic injury: a health promotion approach. *Traffic Injury Prevention* 2004;5:208–19.

Jones RK, Shinar D, Walsh JM. State of knowledge of drug-impaired driving. Dept of Transportation (US), National Highway Traffic Safety Administration (NHTSA); 2003. Report DOT HS 809 642.

National Committee on Injury Prevention and Control. Injury prevention: meeting the challenge. *American Journal of Preventive Medicine* 1989;5(3 Suppl):123–27.

Paulozzi LJ, Patel R. Changes in motorcycle crash mortality rates by blood alcohol concentration and age—United States, 1983–2003. *MMWR* 2004;53(47):1103–6.

Quinlan KP, Brewer RD, Siegel P, Sleet DA, Mokdad AH, Shults RA, Flowers N. Alcohol-impaired driving among U.S. adults, 1993–2002. *American Journal of Preventive Medicine* 2005;28(4):345–50.

Shults RA, Sleet DA, Elder RW, Ryan GW, Sehgal M. Association between state-level drinking and driving countermeasures and self-reported alcohol-impaired driving. *Inj Prev* 2002;8:106–10.

Wells-Parker E, Bangert-Drowns R, McMillen R, Williams M. Final results from a meta-analysis of remedial interventions with drink/drive offenders. *Addiction* 1995;90:907–26.

Zador PL, Krawchuk SA, Voas RB. Alcohol-related relative risk of driver fatalities and driver involvement in fatal crashes in relation to driver age and gender: an update using 1996 data. *Journal of Studies on Alcohol* 2000;61:387–95.

Driving Defensively

More than forty-one thousand people lose their lives in motor vehicle crashes each year and over two million more suffer disabling injuries, according to the National Safety Council. The triple threat of high speeds, impaired or careless driving, and not using occupant restraints threatens every driver—regardless of how careful or how skilled.

Driving defensively means not only taking responsibility for yourself and your actions but also keeping an eye on "the other guy." The National Safety Council suggests the following guidelines to help reduce your risks on the road:

- Don't start the engine without securing each passenger in the car, including children and pets. Safety belts save thousands of lives each year! Lock all doors.
- Remember that driving too fast or too slow can increase the likelihood of collisions.
- Don't kid yourself. If you plan to drink, designate a driver who won't drink. Alcohol is a factor in almost half of all fatal motor vehicle crashes.
- Be alert! If you notice that a car is straddling the center line, weaving, making wide turns, stopping abruptly or responding slowly to traffic signals, the driver may be impaired.
- Avoid an impaired driver by turning right at the nearest corner or exiting at the nearest exit. If it appears that an oncoming car is crossing into your lane, pull over to the roadside, sound the horn, and flash your lights.
- Notify the police immediately after seeing a motorist who is driving suspiciously.
- Follow the rules of the road. Don't contest the "right of way" or try to race another car during a merge. Be respectful of other motorists.
- Don't follow too closely. Always use a "three-second following distance" or a "three-second plus following distance."
- While driving, be cautious, aware, and responsible.

Section 19.4

Occupational Injuries

Excerpted from "National Census of Fatal Occupational Injuries in 2007," Bureau of Labor Statistics, August 20, 2008.

A total of 5,488 fatal work injuries were recorded in the United States in 2007, a decrease of 6 percent from the revised total of 5,840 fatal work injuries reported for 2006. While these results are considered preliminary, this figure represents the smallest annual preliminary total since the Census of Fatal Occupational Injuries (CFOI) program was first conducted in 1992. Final results for 2007 will be released in April 2009.

Based on these preliminary counts, the rate of fatal injury for U.S. workers in 2007 was 3.7 fatal work injuries per 100,000 workers, down from the final rate of 4.0 per 100,000 workers in 2006, and the lowest annual fatality rate ever reported by the fatality census.

Key Findings of the 2007 Census of Fatal Occupational Injuries

- The number of fatal falls in 2007 rose to a series high of 835—a 39 percent increase since 1992 when the CFOI program was first conducted.
- Transportation incidents, which typically account for two-fifths of all workplace fatalities, fell to a series low of 2,234 cases in 2007.
- Workplace homicides rose 13 percent to 610 in 2007 after reaching a series low of 540 in 2006.
- The number of fatal workplace injuries among protective service occupations rose 19 percent in 2007 to 337, led by an increase in the number of police officers fatally injured on the job.
- Fatal occupational injuries incurred by non-Hispanic black or African American workers were at the highest level since 1999, but fatal work injuries among Hispanic workers were lower by 8 percent in 2007.

Profile of 2007 Fatal Work Injuries by Type of Incident

Nearly all types of transportation fatalities saw sizable decreases in 2007 relative to 2006, including non-highway incidents (down 15 percent); workers struck by vehicle, mobile equipment (down 10 percent); water vehicle incidents (down 28 percent); railway incidents (down 26 percent); and aircraft incidents (down 23 percent). Highway incidents also decreased, but only by 3 percent.

The 835 fatal falls in 2007 represented a series high for the fatality census. The increase for falls overall was driven primarily by increases in falls on same level (up 21 percent from 2006) and falls from nonmoving vehicles (up 17 percent). Falls from roofs, however, were down 13 percent from the number in 2006.

Table 19.1. Number of Work-Related Fatal Events in Four Most Common Categories, 1992–2007

	Highway Incidents	Homicides	Falls	Struck by Object
1992	1,158	1,044	600	557
1993	1,242	1,074	618	565
1994	1,343	1,080	665	591
1995	1,346	1,036	651	547
1996	1,346	927	691	582
1997	1,393	860	716	579
1998	1,442	714	706	520
1999	1,496	651	721	585
2000	1,365	677	734	571
2001	1,409	643	810	553
2002	1,373	609	719	505
2003	1,353	632	696	531
2004	1,398	599	822	602
2005	1,437	567	770	607
2006	1,356	540	827	589
2007	1,311	610	835	504

Note: Data from 2001 exclude fatalities resulting from the September 11 terrorist attacks.

Source: U.S. Bureau of Labor Statistics, U.S. Department of Labor, 2008.

Workplace homicides increased by 13 percent in 2007. Even with the increase, workplace homicides have declined 44 percent from the high of 1,080 reported in 1994. Workplace homicides involving police officers and supervisors of retail sales workers both saw substantial increases in 2007.

Profile of Fatal Work Injuries by Industry

Overall, 90 percent of the fatal work injuries involved workers in private industry. Service-providing industries in the private sector recorded 48 percent of all fatal work injuries in 2007, while goods-producing industries recorded 42 percent. Another 10 percent of the fatal work injury cases in 2007 involved government workers. The number of fatal work injuries in the private sector decreased 7 percent in 2007, while fatalities among government workers, including resident military personnel, increased 2 percent.

Fatalities declined in the construction industry, but construction continued to incur the most fatalities of any industry in the private sector, as it has for the five years since the CFOI program began using the North American Industry Classification System (NAICS) to categorize industry. The percentage decrease in fatalities from 2006 (1,239 to 1,178, a 5 percent drop) was about the same as the decrease for all fatal work injuries in 2007. Of the three major subsectors within construction, fatalities among workers in construction of buildings actually rose 11 percent from 2006, with most of the increase in non-residential construction industries. The largest construction subsector, specialty trade contractors, had 6 percent fewer fatalities in 2007 as compared to 2006.

Fatalities among private sector workers in transportation and warehousing sector, which had the second largest number of fatalities, decreased 3 percent from the number reported in 2006. Truck transportation, the largest subsector in transportation and warehousing, also had a 3 percent decrease in 2007. The number of fatal injuries in air, rail, and water transportation were also lower.

Fatalities were down 13 percent among private sector workers in the agriculture, forestry, fishing, and hunting industry sector in 2007. Non-highway incidents in agriculture, forestry, fishing, and hunting decreased 17 percent, and incidents of being struck by an object decreased 12 percent, each of which accounts for about one-fifth of fatalities in the agriculture, forestry, fishing, and hunting industry. Fatalities to workers in crop production fell 19 percent while fatalities to workers in animal production rose 7 percent. Fishing and logging, two of the industries with the highest fatality rates, had lower numbers of fatalities in 2007.

In the trade industry (wholesale and retail), fatal work injuries were down 8 percent from their 2006 level. While most wholesale trade subsectors declined, fatal work injuries in retail grocery stores were up 26 percent (from 57 in 2006 to 72 in 2007), due largely to an increase in workplace homicides in that industry.

The preliminary total of 392 fatal work injuries in manufacturing represents the lowest total recorded in the five years since the CFOI program began using the North American Industry Classification System (NAICS). The 2007 total for manufacturing represents a 14 percent decrease from the 2006 count.

Fatalities among government workers were up 2 percent from 2006, primarily due to a 14 percent increase in workplace fatalities among local government workers. The increase among local government workers was primarily attributable to higher numbers of fatalities in police protection and fire protection (up 32 and 43 percent, respectively). Fatal work injury rates were lower for federal and state workers.

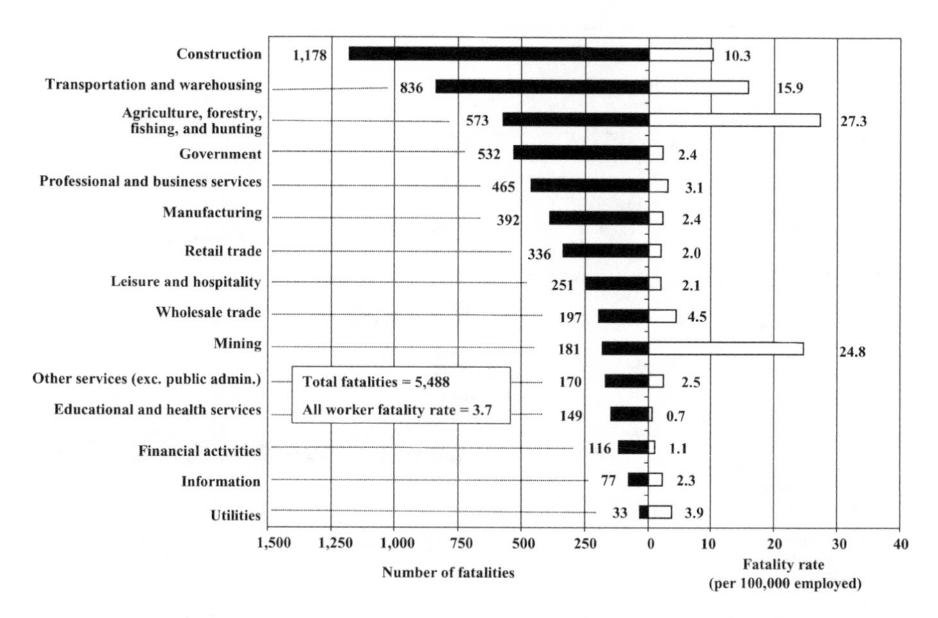

Figure 19.1. *Number and Rate of Fatal Occupational Injuries, by Industry Sector, 2007 (Source: U.S. Bureau of Labor Statistics, U.S. Department of Labor, 2008).*

Profile of Fatal Work Injuries by Occupation

About one-fourth of all occupational fatalities in 2007 involved workers in transportation and material moving occupations, though fatalities among these workers declined by 5 percent in 2007. This decline was largely the result of a 6 percent decline in highway incidents, which account for about 50 percent of the fatalities in this occupation. Construction and extraction occupations, which accounted for 21 percent of all fatalities, decreased by 10 percent from 2006 to 2007 after increasing the previous three years. Operating engineers and other construction equipment operators; painters, construction and maintenance; and electricians all saw decreases of 20 percent or more.

Fatalities among workers employed in protective service occupations rose 19 percent from 2006 to 2007, including police officers (up 30 percent), firefighters (up 17 percent), and security guards (up 11 percent). Among other occupation groups, fatalities incurred by workers in sales and related occupations decreased 2 percent although fatalities incurred by supervisors of sales workers increased by 10 percent. Office and administrative support occupations had 50 percent more workplace fatalities in 2007 (from 88 in 2006 to 132 in 2007), due in part to an increase in fatal transportation incidents.

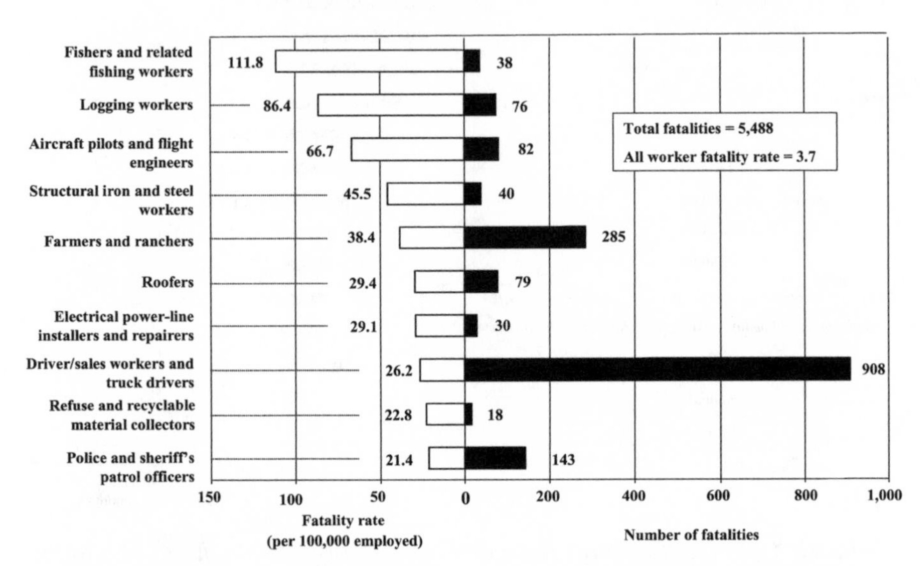

Figure 19.2. *Selected Occupations with High Fatality Rates, 2007 (Source: U.S. Bureau of Labor Statistics, U.S. Department of Labor, 2008).*

The four occupations with the highest fatality rates were fishers and related fishing workers with a fatality rate of 111.8 per 100,000 workers, logging workers (86.4), aircraft pilots and flight engineers (66.7), and structural iron and steel workers (45.5).

Profile of Fatal Work Injuries by Demographic Characteristics

While fatal work injuries in general fell 6 percent, those incurred by non-Hispanic black or African American workers increased by 5 percent to 591 in 2007. This is the highest number reported for black or African American workers since 1999. A tripling in the number of fatalities involving black or African American police officers in local government (from 6 to 18) was one of the reasons for the higher number of fatalities. Fatalities among Hispanic or Latino workers decreased 8 percent from 2006 and among white, non-Hispanic workers by 6 percent.

While fatalities incurred by workers age sixty-five and older decreased 7 percent, these workers were about three times more likely than all workers to be killed on the job. Self-employed workers had a 2 percent drop in fatalities, while their wage and salary counterparts fell by 7 percent. Workplace fatalities incurred by both male and female workers decreased 6 percent.

Of the 5,488 fatal occupational injuries in 2007, 959 were incurred by workers who were born outside of the United States. Of the foreign-born workers who were fatally injured in the United States in 2007, the largest share were born in Mexico (44 percent).

Section 19.5

Water-Related Injuries and Water Safety

Reprinted from "Water-Related Injuries Fact Sheet," Centers for Disease Control and Prevention, June 12, 2008.

How big is the problem?

In 2005, there were 3,582 fatal unintentional drownings in the United States, averaging ten deaths per day. An additional 710 people died, from drowning and other causes, in boating-related incidents.[1, 2]

More than one in four fatal drowning victims are children fourteen and younger.[1] For every child who dies from drowning, another four received emergency department care for nonfatal submersion injuries.[1]

Nonfatal drownings can cause brain damage that may result in long-term disabilities including memory problems, learning disabilities, and permanent loss of basic functioning (i.e., permanent vegetative state).

Who is most at risk?

Males: In 2005, males were four times more likely than females to die from unintentional drownings in the United States.[1]

Children: In 2005, of all children one to four years old who died, almost 30 percent died from drowning.[1] Although drowning rates have slowly declined,[1, 3] fatal drowning remains the second-leading cause of unintentional injury-related death for children ages one to fourteen years.[4]

Minorities: Between 2000 and 2005, the fatal unintentional drowning rate for African Americans across all ages was 1.3 times that of whites. For American Indians and Alaskan Natives, this rate was 1.8 times that of whites.[1]

Rates of fatal drowning are notably higher among these populations in certain age groups. The fatal drowning rate of African American children ages five to fourteen is 3.2 times that of white children in the same age range. For American Indian and Alaskan Native children, the fatal drowning rate is 2.4 times higher than for white children.[1]

Factors such as the physical environment (e.g., access to swimming pools) and a combination of social and cultural issues (e.g., valuing swimming skills and choosing recreational water-related activities) may contribute to the racial differences in drowning rates. If minorities participate less in water-related activities than whites, their drowning rates (per exposure) may be higher than currently reported.[5]

What are the major risk factors?

Lack of barriers and supervision: Children under one year most often drown in bathtubs, buckets, or toilets.[6] Among children ages one to four years, most drownings occur in residential swimming pools.[6] Most young children who drowned in pools were last seen in the home, had been out of sight less than five minutes, and were in the care of one or both parents at the time.[7] Barriers, such as pool fencing, can help prevent children from gaining access to the pool area without caregivers' awareness.[8]

Age and recreation in natural water settings (such as lakes, rivers, or the ocean): The percent of drownings in natural water settings increases with age. Most drownings in those over fifteen years of age occur in natural water settings.[9]

Lack of appropriate choices in recreational boating: In 2006, the U.S. Coast Guard received reports for 4,967 boating incidents; 3,474 boaters were reported injured, and 710 died. Among those who drowned, nine out of ten were not wearing life jackets. Most boating fatalities from 2006 (70 percent) were caused by drowning; the remainder were due to trauma, hypothermia, carbon monoxide poisoning, or other causes. Open motor boats were involved in 45 percent of all reported incidents, and personal watercraft were involved in another 24 percent.[2]

Alcohol use: Alcohol use is involved in up to half of adolescent and adult deaths associated with water recreation and about one in five reported boating fatalities.[10, 11] Alcohol influences balance, coordination, and judgment, and its effects are heightened by sun exposure and heat.[12]

Seizure disorders: For persons with seizure disorders, drowning is the most common cause of unintentional injury death, with the bathtub as the site of highest drowning risk.[13]

What has Centers for Disease Control and Prevention (CDC) research found?

A CDC study about self-reported swimming ability[14] found that:

- younger respondents reported greater swimming ability than older respondents;
- self-reported ability increased with level of education (i.e., high school graduate, college graduate, etc.);
- among racial groups, African Americans reported the most limited swimming ability; and
- men of all ages, races, and educational levels consistently reported greater swimming ability than women.

How can water-related injuries be prevented?

To help prevent water-related injuries:[1, 8, 9, 12, 13]

- Designate a responsible adult to watch young children while in the bath and all children swimming or playing in or around water. Adults should not be involved in any other distracting activity (such as reading, playing cards, talking on the phone, or mowing the lawn) while supervising children.
- Always swim with a buddy. Select swimming sites that have lifeguards whenever possible.
- Avoid drinking alcohol before or during swimming, boating, or water skiing. Do not drink alcohol while supervising children.
- Learn to swim. Be aware that the American Academy of Pediatrics does not recommend swimming classes as the primary means of drowning prevention for children younger than four. Constant, careful supervision and barriers such as pool fencing are necessary even when children have completed swimming classes.
- Learn cardiopulmonary resuscitation (CPR). In the time it might take for paramedics to arrive, your CPR skills could make a difference in someone's life. CPR performed by bystanders has been shown to improve outcomes in drowning victims.

- Do not use air-filled or foam toys, such as "water wings," "noodles," or inner-tubes, in place of life jackets (personal flotation devices). These toys are not designed to keep swimmers safe.

If you have a swimming pool at home:

- Install a four-sided, isolation pool fence that completely separates the house and play area of the yard from the pool area. The fence should be at least four feet high. Use self-closing and self-latching gates that open outward with latches that are out of reach of children. Also, consider additional barriers such as automatic door locks or alarms to prevent access or notify you if someone enters the pool area.
- Remove floats, balls, and other toys from the pool and surrounding area immediately after use. The presence of these toys may encourage children to enter the pool area or lean over the pool and potentially fall in.

If you are in or around natural bodies of water:

- Know the local weather conditions and forecast before swimming or boating. Strong winds and thunderstorms with lightning strikes are dangerous.
- Use U.S. Coast Guard approved life jackets when boating, regardless of distance to be traveled, size of boat, or swimming ability of boaters.
- Know the meaning of and obey warnings represented by colored beach flags.
- Watch for dangerous waves and signs of rip currents (e.g., water that is discolored and choppy, foamy, or filled with debris and moving in a channel away from shore). If you are caught in a rip current, swim parallel to shore; once free of the current, swim toward shore.

References

1. Centers for Disease Control and Prevention, National Center for Injury Prevention and Control. Web-based Injury Statistics Query and Reporting System (WISQARS) [online]. (2008) [cited 2008 March 23]. Available from: URL: www.cdc.gov/ncipc/wisqars.

2. U.S. Coast Guard, Department of Homeland Security (US). Boating Statistics—2006 [online]. 2008. [cited 2008 March 26]. Available from URL: www.uscgboating.org/statistics/Boating_Statistics_2006.pdf.

3. Branche CM. What is happening with drowning rates in the United States? In: Fletemeyer JR and Freas SJ, editors. *Drowning: New perspectives on intervention and prevention*. Boca Raton (FL): CRC Press LLC; 1999.

4. Centers for Disease Control and Prevention. Swimming and Recreational Water Safety. In: *Health Information for International Travel 2005–2006*. Atlanta: US Department of Health and Human Services, Public Health Service, 2005.

5. Branche CM, Dellinger AM, Sleet DA, Gilchrist J, Olson SJ. Unintentional injuries: the burden, risks and preventive strategies to address diversity. In: Livingston IL, editor. *Praeger handbook of Black American health (2nd edition): Policies and issues behind disparities in health*. Westport (CT): Praeger Publishers; 2004. p. 317–27.

6. Brenner RA, Trumble AC, Smith GS, Kessler EP, Overpeck MD. Where children drown, United States, 1995. *Pediatrics* 2001;108(1):85–89.

7. Present P. *Child drowning study. A report on the epidemiology of drowning in residential pools to children under age five*. Washington (DC): Consumer Product Safety Commission (US); 1987.

8. U. S. Consumer Product Safety Commission. Safety barrier guidelines for home pools [online]. [cited 2007 Mar 21]. Available from URL: www.cpsc.gov/cpscpub/pubs/pool.pdf.

9. Gilchrist J, Gotsch K, Ryan GW. Nonfatal and Fatal Drownings in Recreational Water Settings—United States, 2001 and 2002. *MMWR* 2004;53(21):447–52.

10. Howland J, Mangione T, Hingson R, Smith G, Bell N. Alcohol as a risk factor for drowning and other aquatic injuries. In: Watson RR, editor. *Alcohol and accidents. Drug and alcohol abuse reviews*. Vol 7. Totowa (NJ): Humana Press, Inc.; 1995.

11. Howland J, Hingson R. Alcohol as a risk factor for drownings: A review of the literature (1950–1985). *Accident Analysis and Prevention* 1988;20(1):19–25.

12. Smith GS, Kraus JF. Alcohol and residential, recreational, and occupational injuries: A review of the epidemiologic evidence. *Annual Rev of Public Health* 1988;9:99–121.

13. Quan L, Bennett E, Branche C. Interventions to prevent drowning. In Doll L, Bonzo S, Mercy J, Sleet D (Eds). *Handbook of injury and violence prevention*. New York: Springer, 2007.

14. Gilchrist J, Sacks JJ, Branche CM. Self-reported swimming ability in U.S. adults, 1994. *Public Health Reports* 2000;115(2–3):110–11.

Chapter 20

Stroke

Stroke Facts and Statistics

Stroke is the third leading cause of death in the United States. Over 160,000 people die each year from stroke in the United States.

Stroke is a leading cause of serious long–term disability.

About 700,000 strokes occur in the United States each year. About 500,000 of these are first or new strokes. About 200,000 occur in people who have already had a stroke before.

Nearly three-quarters of all strokes occur in people over the age of sixty-five. The risk of having a stroke more than doubles each decade after the age of fifty-five.

Strokes can—and do—occur at *any* age. Nearly one quarter of strokes occur in people under the age of sixty-five.

Stroke death rates are higher for African Americans than for whites, even at younger ages.

According to the American Heart Association, stroke cost almost $57 billion in both direct and indirect costs in 2005.

It has been noted for several decades that the southeastern United States has the highest stroke mortality rates in the country. It is not

---

Reprinted from the following documents from the Centers for Disease Control and Prevention: "Stroke Facts," October 10, 2007; "Stroke," October 10, 2007; "Types of Stroke," October 10, 2007; "Outcomes from Stroke," October 10, 2007; "Treatment," October 10, 2007; "Risk Factors," October 10, 2007; and "Signs and Symptoms of Stroke," May 12, 2008.

completely clear what factors might contribute to the higher incidence of and mortality from stroke in this region.

About Stroke

A stroke occurs either when the blood supply to part of the brain is blocked or when a blood vessel in the brain bursts, causing damage to a part of the brain. A stroke is also sometimes called a brain attack.

Stroke is the third leading cause of death in the United States. Among survivors, stroke can cause significant disability including paralysis as well as speech and emotional problems. New treatments are available that can reduce the damage caused by a stroke for some victims. But these treatments need to be given soon after the symptoms start.

Knowing the symptoms of stroke, calling 911 right away, and getting to a hospital are crucial to the most beneficial outcomes after having a stroke. The best treatment is to try to prevent a stroke by taking steps to lower your risk for stroke.

Types of Stroke

Ischemic stroke: An ischemic stroke occurs when an artery that supplies blood and oxygen to the brain becomes blocked. Most strokes are of this type. Blood clots are the most common cause of artery blockage. Ischemic strokes can also be caused by a narrowing of the arteries (called stenosis). The most common condition that causes stenosis is atherosclerosis. In atherosclerosis, plaque (a mixture of fatty substances including cholesterol and other lipids) and blood clots build up inside the artery walls, causing thickening, hardening, and loss of elasticity. These lead to decreased blood flow.

Hemorrhagic stroke: A hemorrhagic stroke occurs when an artery in the brain bursts. Hemorrhage can occur in several ways. One cause is an aneurysm, a weak or thin spot on an artery wall that can expand like a balloon. The thin walls of the stretched artery can rupture or break. Hemorrhage also occurs when arterial walls lose their elasticity and become brittle and thin. They can then crack and bleed. This can happen with atherosclerosis. High blood pressure increases the risk of a hemorrhagic stroke.

There are two main types of hemorrhagic stroke. An intracerebral hemorrhage occurs when a blood vessel in the brain leaks blood into the brain itself. A subarachnoid hemorrhage is bleeding under the outer membranes of the brain and into the thin, fluid-filled space that surrounds the brain.

Transient ischemic attacks: A transient ischemic attack (TIA) is sometimes called a mini-stroke. It starts just like a stroke but then clears up within twenty-four hours, leaving no apparent symptoms or deficits. A TIA is a warning that the person is at risk for a more serious stroke. Having other risk factors increases a person's chances of a recurrent stroke if they have had a TIA. For most TIAs the symptoms go away within an hour. However, there is no way to tell whether symptoms will be a TIA or a more serious stroke that can lead to death or disability. The sudden onset of the symptoms of a stroke should signal an emergency. Patients and witnesses should not wait to see if the symptoms go away.

Outcomes from Stroke

Stroke is the third leading cause of death in the United States. It is also a leading cause of serious long-term disability. While most strokes occur in people over the age of sixty-five, strokes can occur at any age.

Among people who survive, strokes can affect the entire body. Stroke can leave victims with physical, mental, and emotional deficits. The amount of disability is related to the severity of the stroke. People who survive a stroke are also at risk for having another stroke.

Physical: Persons who have had a stroke can have weakness or even complete paralysis on one side of the body. The paralysis or weakness may affect only the face, an arm, or a leg or may affect one entire side of the body and face. Some stroke patients may have trouble with swallowing. Slurred speech due to weakness of the muscles used in speaking may also occur.

Activity and balance: A stroke victim may have problems performing daily activities, such as walking, dressing, eating, and using the bathroom. Balance and coordination may also be a problem.

Cognitive deficits: Stroke may cause problems with thinking, awareness, attention, learning, judgment, and memory.

Language: Stroke victims may find it hard to understand or form speech. This is called aphasia. Aphasia usually occurs along with problems in reading or writing.

Emotional: Stroke patients may find it difficult to control their emotions or may express inappropriate emotions in certain situations. One common emotional problem with many stroke patients is depression. Post-stroke depression may be more than a general sadness resulting from the stroke. Medications and therapy might be needed to treat the depression.

Pain: Stroke patients may experience pain, uncomfortable numbness, or strange sensations after a stroke. These sensations may be due to many factors including damage to the sensory regions of the brain, stiff joints, or a disabled limb.

Recurrent stroke: Recurrent stroke is a major contributor to stroke disability and death, with the risk of severe disability or death from stroke increasing with each stroke. The risk of a recurrent stroke is greatest right after a stroke.

Treatment

Medical treatments can help to control the risk factors that put people at higher risk for stroke. These include treating high blood pressure, heart disease, and diabetes. Lifestyle changes such as quitting smoking can also lower the risk of stroke.

Acute stroke therapies try to stop a stroke while it is happening. These treatments try to dissolve the blood clot causing an ischemic stroke or to stop the bleeding of a hemorrhagic stroke. These therapies are most effective when given very soon after the onset of a stroke.

Post-stroke treatment and rehabilitation are used to lower the risk of another stroke and to help patients overcome disabilities that result from stroke. People who have had a stroke can do things to lower their risk of having another stroke. These include controlling their underlying risk factors.

Rehabilitation helps stroke victims relearn skills that may be lost when the brain is damaged. Rehabilitation may include the following:

- Physical therapy to help restore movement, balance, and coordination.
- Occupational therapy to help the patient relearn everyday activities such as eating, drinking, dressing, bathing, cooking, reading, and writing.

- Speech therapy to help stroke patients relearn language and speaking skills, including swallowing, or learn other forms of communication.
- Psychological or psychiatric help after a stroke. Psychological problems, such as depression, anxiety, frustration, and anger, can be common after a stroke.

The best treatment for stroke is the take steps to lower the risk for stroke.

Risk Factors

Some conditions as well as some lifestyle factors can put people at a higher risk for stroke. The most important risk factors for stroke are high blood pressure, heart disease, diabetes, and cigarette smoking. Persons who have already had a stroke need to control the risk factors in order to lower their risk of having another stroke. All persons can take steps to lower their risk for stroke.

High blood pressure: High blood pressure, or hypertension, is a major risk factor for stroke. It is a condition where the pressure of the blood in the arteries is too high. There are often no symptoms to signal high blood pressure. About sixty million people in the United States have high blood pressure. Lowering blood pressure can lower the risk of stroke. Medicines to lower blood pressure can decrease the risk of stroke among those with high blood pressure.

Heart disease: Common heart disorders such as coronary artery disease can also increase a person's risk for stroke. Coronary artery disease (CAD) occurs when the arteries that supply blood to the heart muscle become hardened and narrowed due to the buildup of plaque. Plaque (a mixture of fatty substances, including cholesterol and other lipids) and blood clots can build up inside the artery walls, causing thickening, hardening, and loss of elasticity. They can result in decreased or blocked blood flow and lead to a heart attack. Also, heart problems such as valve defects, irregular heartbeat, and enlargement of one of the heart's chambers can result in blood clots that may break loose and cause a stroke. Persons with heart disease may be given medicines such as aspirin to help prevent clots from forming.

Atrial fibrillation: A heart condition known as atrial fibrillation is a major concern. Atrial fibrillation is irregular beating of the upper chambers, or atria, of the heart. When the atria quivers instead of beating in a regular pattern, blood is not fully pumped out of them and may pool and clot. The clots can then leave the heart and travel to the brain, causing a stroke. Atrial fibrillation affects as many as 2.2 million Americans. About 15 percent of stroke patients have had atrial fibrillation before they experience a stroke.

Diabetes: Diabetes is another disease that increases a person's risk for stroke. With diabetes, the body does not make enough insulin, cannot use its own insulin as well as it should, or both. This causes sugars to be unavailable to the body tissues and to build up in the blood. People with diabetes have two to four times the risk of stroke compared to people without diabetes. Further, having diabetes can worsen the outcome of stroke.

Tobacco use: Smoking almost doubles a person's risk for ischemic stroke, independently of other risk factors. Cigarette smoking increases the risk of stroke by promoting atherosclerosis and increasing the levels of blood clotting factors, such as fibrinogen. Also, nicotine raises blood pressure, and carbon monoxide reduces the amount of oxygen that blood can carry to the brain.

Other Factors

Blood cholesterol levels: Some strokes can be caused by a narrowing of the arteries through the buildup of plaque, a mixture of fatty substances, including cholesterol and other lipids. This is called atherosclerosis. Plaque and blood clots build up inside the artery walls, causing thickening, hardening, and loss of elasticity. These can lead to decreased blood flow and to stroke if they occur in the arteries to the brain.

Cholesterol is a waxy substance produced by the liver. It is needed by the body, and the liver makes enough cholesterol for the body's needs. Excess cholesterol—usually from eating foods that contain high levels of cholesterol and saturated fats—contributes to atherosclerosis.

There are two major kinds of cholesterol, one that is good, and one that is bad when there is too much of it. A higher level of high-density lipoprotein cholesterol, or HDL, is considered good. However, higher levels of low-density lipoprotein, or LDL, can lead to atherosclerosis and stroke. A lipoprotein profile can be done to measure several different kinds of cholesterol as well as triglycerides (another kind of fat found in the blood).

Alcohol: Generally, excessive alcohol use can lead to an increase in blood pressure, which increases the risk for stroke.

Genetic risk factors: Stroke can run in families. Genes play a role in stroke risk factors such as high blood pressure, heart disease, diabetes, and vascular conditions. It is also possible that an increased risk for stroke within a family is due to factors such as a common sedentary lifestyle or poor eating habits, rather than hereditary factors.

Signs and Symptoms of Stroke

A stroke, or cerebrovascular accident, occurs when the blood supply to the brain is cut off (an ischemic stroke) or when a blood vessel bursts (a hemorrhagic stroke). Without oxygen, brain cells begin to die. Death or permanent disability can result. High blood pressure, smoking, and having had a previous stroke or heart attack increase a person's chances of having a stroke. With timely treatment, the risk of death and disability from stroke can be lowered. It is very important to know the symptoms of a stroke and act right away.

The National Institute of Neurological Disorders and Stroke notes these five major signs of stroke:

- Sudden numbness or weakness of the face, arms, or legs
- Sudden confusion or trouble speaking or understanding others
- Sudden trouble seeing in one or both eyes
- Sudden trouble walking, dizziness, or loss of balance or coordination
- Sudden severe headache with no known cause

All of the major symptoms of stroke appear suddenly, and often there is more than one symptom at the same time.

If you think someone is having a stroke, you should call 9–1–1 or emergency medical services immediately. Receiving immediate treatment is critical in lowering the risk of disability and even death.

Chapter 21

Chronic Obstructive Pulmonary Disease (COPD)

What Is COPD?

Chronic obstructive pulmonary disease (COPD) is a serious lung disease that, over time, makes it hard to breathe. You may also have heard COPD called other names, like emphysema or chronic bronchitis. In people who have COPD, the airways—tubes that carry air in and out of your lungs—are partially blocked, which makes it hard to get air in and out.

When COPD is severe, shortness of breath and other symptoms of COPD can get in the way of even the most basic tasks, such as doing light housework, taking a walk, even washing and dressing.

Did You Know?

- COPD is the 4th leading cause of death in the United States and causes serious, long-term disability.
- COPD kills more than 120,000 Americans each year. That's one death every four minutes.
- More than twelve million people have been diagnosed with COPD.
- An additional twelve million likely have COPD and don't even know it.

Reprinted from "What Is COPD?" "How Does COPD Affect Breathing?" "Symptoms," "Getting Tested," "Taking Action," "Am I at Risk?" and "Treatment Options," National Heart, Lung, and Blood Institute, National Institutes of Health, 2007.

How Does COPD Affect Breathing?

The "airways" are the tubes that carry air in and out of the lungs through the nose and mouth. Healthy airways and air sacs in the lungs are elastic—they try to bounce back to their original shape after being stretched or filled with air, just the way a new rubber band or balloon does. This elastic quality helps retain the normal structure of the lung and helps to move the air quickly in and out.

In people with COPD, the air sacs no longer bounce back to their original shape. The airways can also become swollen or thicker than normal, and mucus production might increase. The floppy airways are blocked, or obstructed, making it even harder to get air out of the lungs.

Symptoms

Many people with COPD avoid activities that they used to enjoy because they become short of breath more easily.

Symptoms of COPD include the following:

- Constant coughing, sometimes called "smoker's cough"
- Shortness of breath while doing activities you used to be able to do
- Excess sputum production
- Feeling like you can't breathe
- Not being able to take a deep breath
- Wheezing

When COPD is severe, shortness of breath and other symptoms can get in the way of doing even the most basic tasks, such as doing light housework, taking a walk, even bathing and getting dressed.

COPD develops slowly, and can worsen over time, so be sure to report any symptoms you might have to your doctor as soon as possible, no matter how mild they may seem.

Getting Tested

Everyone at risk for COPD who has cough, sputum production, or shortness of breath should be tested for the disease. The test for COPD is called spirometry.

Spirometry can detect COPD before symptoms become severe. It is a simple, non-invasive breathing test that measures the amount of air a person can blow out of the lungs (volume) and how fast he or she can blow it out (flow). Based on this test, your doctor can tell if you have COPD, and if so, how severe it is. The spirometry reading can help your doctor determine the best course of treatment.

How Spirometry Works

Spirometry is one of the best and most common lung function tests. The test is done with a spirometer, a machine that measures how well your lungs function, records the results, and displays them on a graph for your doctor. You will be asked to take a deep breath, then blow out as hard and as fast as you can using a mouthpiece connected to the machine with tubing. The spirometer then measures the total amount exhaled, called the forced vital capacity or FVC, and how much you exhaled in the first second, called the forced expiratory volume in one second or FEV1. Your doctor will read the results to assess how well your lungs are working and whether or not you have COPD.

Taking Action

There are many things people at risk for COPD can do.

Quit smoking: If you smoke, the best thing you can to do prevent more damage to your lungs is to quit. To help you quit, there are many online resources and several new aids available from your doctor.

Avoid exposure to pollutants: Try to stay away from other things that could irritate your lungs, like dust and strong fumes. Stay indoors when the outside air quality is poor. You should also stay away from places where there might be cigarette smoke.

Visit your doctor on a regular basis: See your doctor regularly even if you are feeling fine. Make a list of your breathing symptoms and think about any activities that you can no longer do because of shortness of breath. Be sure to bring a list of all the medicines you are taking to each doctor's visit.

Take precautions against the flu: Do your best to avoid crowds during flu season. It is also a good idea to get a flu shot every year, since the flu can cause serious problems for people with COPD. You should also ask your doctor about the pneumonia vaccine.

Am I At Risk?

Most people who are at risk for getting COPD have never even heard of it and, in many cases, don't even realize that the condition has a name. Some of the things that put you at risk for COPD include smoking, environmental exposure, and genetic factors.

Smoking: COPD most often occurs in people age forty and over with a history of smoking (either current or former smokers), although as many as one out of six people with COPD never smoked. Smoking is the most common cause of COPD—it accounts for as many as nine out of ten COPD-related deaths.

Environmental exposure: COPD can also occur in people who have had long-term exposure to things that can irritate your lungs, like certain chemicals, dust, or fumes in the workplace. Heavy or long-term exposure to secondhand smoke or other air pollutants may also contribute to COPD.

Genetic factors: In some people, COPD is caused by a genetic condition known as alpha-1 antitrypsin, or AAT, deficiency. While very few people know they have AAT deficiency, it is estimated that close to one hundred thousand Americans have it. People with AAT deficiency can get COPD even if they have never smoked or had long-term exposure to harmful pollutants.

Treatment Options

Once you have been diagnosed with COPD, there are many ways that you and your doctor can work together to manage the symptoms of the disease and improve your quality of life. Your doctor may suggest one or more of the following options.

Medications (such as bronchodilators and inhaled steroids): Bronchodilators are medicines that usually come in the form of an inhaler. They work to relax the muscles around your airways, to help open them and make it easier to breathe. Inhaled steroids help prevent the airways from getting inflamed. Each patient is different—your doctor may suggest other types of medications that might work better for you.

Pulmonary rehabilitation: Your doctor may recommend that you participate in pulmonary rehabilitation, or "rehab." This is a program that helps you learn to exercise and manage your disease with physical activity and counseling. It can help you stay active and carry out your day-to-day tasks.

Physical activity training: Your doctor or a pulmonary therapist recommended by your doctor might teach you some activities to help your arms and legs get stronger and/or breathing exercises that strengthen the muscles needed for breathing.

Lifestyle changes: Lifestyle changes such as quitting smoking can help you manage the effects of COPD.

Oxygen treatment: If your COPD is severe, your doctor might suggest oxygen therapy to help with shortness of breath. You might need oxygen all of the time or just some of the time—your doctor will work with you to learn which treatment will be most helpful.

Surgery: COPD patients with very severe symptoms may have a hard time breathing all the time. In some of these cases, doctors may suggest lung surgery to improve breathing and help lessen some of the most severe symptoms.

Managing complications: Symptoms of COPD can get worse all of a sudden. When this happens, it is much harder to catch your breath. You might also have chest tightness, more coughing or a change in your cough (becomes more productive, more mucus is expelled), and a fever.

When symptoms get worse quickly, it could be a sign of a lung infection. There could be other causes for symptoms getting worse, such as heart disease related to severe lung damage. The best thing to do is call your doctor right away so he or she can find out what the cause of the problem is and take steps to treat it.

When to Get Emergency Help

Seek emergency help if your usual medications aren't working and one or more of the following is true:

- You find that it is unusually hard to walk or talk (such as difficulty completing a sentence).
- Your heart is beating very fast or irregularly.
- Your lips or fingernails are gray or blue.

- Your breathing is fast and hard, even when you are using your medication.

Be prepared and have information on hand that you or others would need in a medical emergency, such as a list of medicines you are taking, the name of your doctor and his or her contact information, directions to the hospital or your doctor's office, and people to contact if you are unable to speak or drive yourself to the doctor or hospital.

Chapter 22

Diabetes

Basics about Diabetes

What is diabetes?

Diabetes is a disease in which blood glucose levels are above normal. Most of the food we eat is turned into glucose, or sugar, for our bodies to use for energy. The pancreas, an organ that lies near the stomach, makes a hormone called insulin to help glucose get into the cells of our bodies. When you have diabetes, your body either doesn't make enough insulin or can't use its own insulin as well as it should. This causes sugar to build up in your blood.

Diabetes can cause serious health complications including heart disease, blindness, kidney failure, and lower-extremity amputations. Diabetes is the sixth leading cause of death in the United States.

What are the symptoms of diabetes?

People who think they might have diabetes must visit a physician for diagnosis. They might have some or none of the following symptoms:

- Frequent urination

"Basics about Diabetes" is excerpted from "Frequently Asked Questions: Basics about Diabetes" and "Preventing Diabetes" is reprinted from "Frequently Asked Questions: Preventing Diabetes," Centers for Disease Control and Prevention, July 12, 2007.

- Excessive thirst
- Unexplained weight loss
- Extreme hunger
- Sudden vision changes
- Tingling or numbness in hands or feet
- Feeling very tired much of the time
- Very dry skin
- Sores that are slow to heal
- More infections than usual.

Nausea, vomiting, or stomach pains may accompany some of these symptoms in the abrupt onset of insulin-dependent diabetes, now called type 1 diabetes.

What are the types of diabetes?

Type 1 diabetes, which was previously called insulin-dependent diabetes mellitus (IDDM) or juvenile-onset diabetes, may account for 5 to 10 percent of all diagnosed cases of diabetes. Type 2 diabetes, which was previously called non-insulin-dependent diabetes mellitus (NIDDM) or adult-onset diabetes, may account for about 90 to 95 percent of all diagnosed cases of diabetes. Gestational diabetes is a type of diabetes that only pregnant women get. If not treated, it can cause problems for mothers and babies. Gestational diabetes develops in 2 to 5 percent of all pregnancies but usually disappears when a pregnancy is over. Other specific types of diabetes resulting from specific genetic syndromes, surgery, drugs, malnutrition, infections, and other illnesses may account for 1 to 2 percent of all diagnosed cases of diabetes.

What are the risk factors for diabetes?

Risk factors for type 2 diabetes include older age, obesity, family history of diabetes, prior history of gestational diabetes, impaired glucose tolerance, physical inactivity, and race/ethnicity. African Americans, Hispanic/Latino Americans, American Indians, and some Asian Americans and Pacific Islanders are at particularly high risk for type 2 diabetes.

Risk factors are less well defined for type 1 diabetes than for type 2 diabetes, but autoimmune, genetic, and environmental factors are involved in developing this type of diabetes.

Gestational diabetes occurs more frequently in African Americans, Hispanic/Latino Americans, American Indians, and people with a family history of diabetes than in other groups. Obesity is also associated with higher risk. Women who have had gestational diabetes are at increased risk for later developing type 2 diabetes. In some studies, nearly 40 percent of women with a history of gestational diabetes developed diabetes in the future.

Other specific types of diabetes, which may account for 1 to 2 percent of all diagnosed cases, result from specific genetic syndromes, surgery, drugs, malnutrition, infections, and other illnesses.

What is the treatment for diabetes?

Healthy eating, physical activity, and insulin injections are the basic therapies for type 1 diabetes. The amount of insulin taken must be balanced with food intake and daily activities. Blood glucose levels must be closely monitored through frequent blood glucose testing.

Healthy eating, physical activity, and blood glucose testing are the basic therapies for type 2 diabetes. In addition, many people with type 2 diabetes require oral medication, insulin, or both to control their blood glucose levels.

People with diabetes must take responsibility for their day-to-day care, and keep blood glucose levels from going too low or too high.

People with diabetes should see a health care provider who will monitor their diabetes control and help them learn to manage their diabetes. In addition, people with diabetes may see endocrinologists, who may specialize in diabetes care; ophthalmologists for eye examinations; podiatrists for routine foot care; and dietitians and diabetes educators who teach the skills needed for daily diabetes management.

What causes type 1 diabetes?

The causes of type 1 diabetes appear to be much different than those for type 2 diabetes, though the exact mechanisms for developing both diseases are unknown. The appearance of type 1 diabetes is suspected to follow exposure to an "environmental trigger," such as an unidentified virus, stimulating an immune attack against the beta cells of the pancreas (that produce insulin) in some genetically predisposed people.

Is there a cure for diabetes?

In response to the growing health burden of diabetes, the diabetes community has three choices: prevent diabetes; cure diabetes; and improve the quality of care of people with diabetes to prevent devastating complications. All three approaches are actively being pursued by the U.S. Department of Health and Human Services.

Both the National Institutes of Health (NIH) and the Centers for Disease Control and Prevention (CDC) are involved in prevention activities. The NIH is involved in research to cure both type 1 and type 2 diabetes, especially type 1. CDC focuses most of its programs on being sure that the proven science is put into daily practice for people with diabetes. The basic idea is that if all the important research and science are not applied meaningfully in the daily lives of people with diabetes, then the research is, in essence, wasted.

Several approaches to "cure" diabetes are being pursued:

- Pancreas transplantation
- Islet cell transplantation (islet cells produce insulin)
- Artificial pancreas development
- Genetic manipulation (fat or muscle cells that don't normally make insulin have a human insulin gene inserted—then these "pseudo" islet cells are transplanted into people with type 1 diabetes)

Each of these approaches still has a lot of challenges, such as preventing immune rejection; finding an adequate number of insulin cells; keeping cells alive; and others. But progress is being made in all areas.

Preventing Diabetes

What are the most important things to do to prevent diabetes?

The Diabetes Prevention Program (DPP), a major federally funded study of 3,234 people at high risk for diabetes, showed that people can delay and possibly prevent the disease by losing a small amount of weight (5 to 7 percent of total body weight) through thirty minutes of physical activity five days a week and healthier eating.

When should I be tested for diabetes?

Anyone aged forty-five years or older should consider getting tested for diabetes, especially if you are overweight. If you are younger than forty-five, but are overweight and have one or more additional risk factors (see below), you should consider testing.

What are the risk factors that increase the likelihood of developing diabetes?

- Being overweight or obese
- A parent, brother, or sister with diabetes
- African American, American Indian, Asian American, Pacific Islander, or Hispanic American/Latino heritage
- Prior history of gestational diabetes or birth of at least one baby weighing more than nine pounds
- High blood pressure measuring 140/90 or higher
- Abnormal cholesterol with HDL ("good") cholesterol is 35 or lower, or triglyceride level is 250 or higher
- Physical inactivity—exercising fewer than three times a week

How does body weight affect the likelihood of developing diabetes?

Being overweight or obese is a leading risk factor for type 2 diabetes. Being overweight can keep your body from making and using insulin properly, and can also cause high blood pressure. The Diabetes Prevention Program (DPP), a major federally funded study of 3,234 people at high risk for diabetes, showed that moderate diet and exercise of about thirty minutes or more, five or more days per week, or of 150 or more minutes per week, resulting in a 5 to 7 percent weight loss can delay and possibly prevent type 2 diabetes.

What is pre-diabetes?

People with blood glucose levels that are higher than normal but not yet in the diabetic range have "pre-diabetes." Doctors sometimes call this condition impaired fasting glucose (IFG) or impaired glucose tolerance (IGT), depending on the test used to diagnose it. Insulin resistance and pre-diabetes usually have no symptoms. You may have one or both conditions for several years without noticing anything.

If you have pre-diabetes, you have a higher risk of developing type 2 diabetes. Studies have shown that most people with pre-diabetes go on to develop type 2 diabetes within ten years, unless they lose weight through modest changes in diet and physical activity. People with pre-diabetes also have a higher risk of heart disease.

Can vaccines cause diabetes?

No. Carefully performed scientific studies show that vaccines do not cause diabetes or increase a person's risk of developing diabetes. In 2002, the Institute of Medicine reviewed the existing studies and released a report concluding that the scientific evidence favors rejection of the theory that immunizations cause diabetes. The only evidence suggesting a relationship between vaccination and diabetes comes from Dr. John B. Classen, who has suggested that certain vaccines if given at birth may decrease the occurrence of diabetes, whereas if initial vaccination is performed after two months of age the occurrence of diabetes increases. Dr. Classen's studies have a number of limitations and have not been verified by other researchers.

Chapter 23

Influenza and Pneumonia

Chapter Contents

Section 23.1

Influenza

Reprinted from "Key Facts about Seasonal Influenza (Flu)," Centers for Disease Control and Prevention, July 16, 2008.

What Is Influenza (Also Called Flu)?

The flu is a contagious respiratory illness caused by influenza viruses. It can cause mild to severe illness, and at times can lead to death. The best way to prevent the flu is by getting a flu vaccination each year.

Every year in the United States, on average, 5 to 20 percent of the population gets the flu, more than 200,000 people are hospitalized from flu complications, and about 36,000 people die from flu. Some people, such as older people, young children, and people with certain health conditions (such as asthma, diabetes, or heart disease), are at high risk for serious flu complications.

Symptoms of Flu

Symptoms of flu include the following:

- Fever (usually high)
- Headache
- Extreme tiredness
- Dry cough
- Sore throat
- Runny or stuffy nose
- Muscle aches

Stomach symptoms, such as nausea, vomiting, and diarrhea, also can occur but are more common in children than adults

Complications of Flu

Complications of flu can include bacterial pneumonia, ear infections, sinus infections, dehydration, and worsening of chronic medical conditions, such as congestive heart failure, asthma, or diabetes.

How Flu Spreads

Flu viruses spread mainly from person to person through coughing or sneezing of people with influenza. Sometimes people may become infected by touching something with flu viruses on it and then touching their mouth or nose. Most healthy adults may be able to infect others beginning one day before symptoms develop and up to five days after becoming sick. That means that you may be able to pass on the flu to someone else before you know you are sick, as well as while you are sick.

Preventing Seasonal Flu: Get Vaccinated

The single best way to prevent the flu is to get a flu vaccination each year. There are two types of vaccines:

- **The "flu shot":** An inactivated vaccine (containing killed virus) that is given with a needle. The flu shot is approved for use in people six months of age and older, including healthy people and people with chronic medical conditions.
- **The nasal-spray flu vaccine:** A vaccine made with live, weakened flu viruses that do not cause the flu (sometimes called LAIV for "live attenuated influenza vaccine"). LAIV is approved for use in healthy people two to forty-nine years of age who are not pregnant.

About two weeks after vaccination, antibodies develop that protect against influenza virus infection. Flu vaccines will not protect against flu-like illnesses caused by non-influenza viruses.

When to Get Vaccinated

Yearly flu vaccination should begin in September or as soon as vaccine is available and continue throughout the influenza season, into December, January, and beyond. This is because the timing and duration of influenza seasons vary. While influenza outbreaks can happen as early as October, most of the time influenza activity peaks in January or later.

Who Should Get Vaccinated?

In general, anyone who wants to reduce their chances of getting the flu can get vaccinated. However, certain people should get vaccinated each year either because they are at high risk of having serious flu-related complications or because they live with or care for high-risk persons. During flu seasons when vaccine supplies are limited or delayed, the Advisory Committee on Immunization Practices (ACIP) makes recommendations regarding priority groups for vaccination.

People who should get vaccinated each year are as follows:

- Children aged six months up to their nineteenth birthday.
- Pregnant women.
- People fifty years of age and older.
- People of any age with certain chronic medical conditions.
- People who live in nursing homes and other long-term care facilities.
- People who live with or care for those at high risk for complications from flu, including health care workers, household contacts of persons at high risk for complications from the flu, and household contacts and out of home caregivers of children less than six months of age (these children are too young to be vaccinated).

Use of the Nasal Spray Flu Vaccine

Vaccination with the nasal-spray flu vaccine is an option for healthy people two to forty-nine years of age who are not pregnant, even healthy persons who live with or care for those in a high-risk group. The one exception is healthy persons who care for persons with severely weakened immune systems who require a protected environment; these healthy persons should get the inactivated vaccine.

Who Should Not Be Vaccinated?

Some people should not be vaccinated without first consulting a physician. They include the following:

- People who have a severe allergy to chicken eggs
- People who have had a severe reaction to an influenza vaccination in the past
- People who developed Guillain-Barré syndrome (GBS) within six weeks of getting an influenza vaccine previously

- Children less than six months of age (influenza vaccine is not approved for use in this age group)

People who have a moderate or severe illness with a fever should wait to get vaccinated until their symptoms lessen.

If you have questions about whether you should get a flu vaccine, consult your health-care provider.

Section 23.2

Pneumonia

What Is Pneumonia?

Pneumonia is a serious infection and/or inflammation of your lungs. The air sacs in the lungs fill with pus and other liquid. Oxygen has trouble reaching your blood. If there is too little oxygen in your blood, your body cells can't work properly. Because of this and spreading infection through the body pneumonia can cause death.

Until 1936, pneumonia was the number one cause of death in the United States. Since then, the use of antibiotics brought it under control. In 2004, pneumonia and influenza combined ranked as the eighth leading cause of death.[1]

Pneumonia affects your lungs in two ways. Lobar pneumonia affects a section (lobe) of a lung. Bronchial pneumonia (or bronchopneumonia) affects patches throughout both lungs.

Causes of Pneumonia

Pneumonia is not a single disease. It can have over thirty different causes. There are five main causes of pneumonia:

- Bacteria
- Viruses
- Mycoplasmas
- Other infectious agents, such as fungi—including Pneumocystis
- Various chemicals

Bacterial Pneumonia

Bacterial pneumonia can attack anyone from infants through the elderly. Alcoholics, the debilitated, postoperative patients, people with respiratory diseases or viral infections, and people who have weakened immune systems are at greater risk.

Pneumonia bacteria are present in some healthy throats. When body defenses are weakened in some way, by illness, old age, malnutrition, general debility, or impaired immunity, the bacteria can multiply and cause serious damage. Usually, when a person's resistance is lowered, bacteria work their way into the lungs and inflame the air sacs.

The tissue of part of a lobe of the lung, an entire lobe, or even most of the lung's five lobes becomes completely filled with liquid (this is called "consolidation"). The infection quickly spreads through the bloodstream and the whole body is invaded.

The organism *Streptococcus pneumoniae* is the most common cause of bacterial pneumonia. It is one form of pneumonia for which a vaccine is available.

Symptoms: The onset of bacterial pneumonia can vary from gradual to sudden. In the most severe cases, the patient may experience shaking chills, chattering teeth, severe chest pain, and a cough that produces rust-colored or greenish mucus.

A person's temperature may rise as high as 105 degrees F. The patient sweats profusely, and breathing and pulse rate increase rapidly. Lips and nail beds may have a bluish color due to lack of oxygen in the blood. A patient's mental state may be confused or delirious.

Viral Pneumonia

Half of all pneumonias are believed to be caused by viruses. More and more viruses are being identified as the cause of respiratory infection, and though most attack the upper respiratory tract, some produce pneumonia, especially in children. Most of these pneumonias are not serious and last a short time but some may be.

Infection with the influenza virus may be severe and occasionally fatal. The virus invades the lungs and multiplies, but there are almost no physical signs of lung tissue becoming filled with fluid. It finds many of its victims among those who have preexisting heart or lung disease or are pregnant.

Symptoms: The initial symptoms of viral pneumonia are the same as influenza symptoms: fever, a dry cough, headache, muscle pain, and weakness. Within twelve to thirty-six hours, there is increasing breathlessness; the cough becomes worse and produces a small amount of mucus. There is a high fever and there may be blueness of the lips.

In extreme cases, the patient has a desperate need for air and extreme breathlessness. Viral pneumonias may be complicated by an invasion of bacteria, with all the typical symptoms of bacterial pneumonia.

Mycoplasma Pneumonia

Because of its somewhat different symptoms and physical signs, and because the course of the illness differed from classical pneumococcal pneumonia, mycoplasma pneumonia was once believed to be caused by one or more undiscovered viruses and was called "primary atypical pneumonia."

Identified during World War II, mycoplasmas are the smallest free-living agents of disease in humankind, unclassified as to whether bacteria or viruses, but having characteristics of both. They generally cause a mild and widespread pneumonia. They affect all age groups, occurring most frequently in older children and young adults. The death rate is low, even in untreated cases.

Symptoms: The most prominent symptom of mycoplasma pneumonia is a cough that tends to come in violent attacks, but produces only sparse whitish mucus. Chills and fever are early symptoms, and some patients experience nausea or vomiting. Patients may experience profound weakness that lasts for a long time.

Other Kinds of Pneumonia

Pneumocystis carinii pneumonia (PCP) is caused by an organism believed to be a fungus. PCP may be the first sign of illness in many persons with acquired immunodeficiency syndrome (AIDS).

PCP can be successfully treated in many cases. It may recur a few months later, but treatment can help to prevent or delay its recurrence.

Other less common pneumonias may be quite serious and are occurring more often. Various special pneumonias are caused by the inhalation of food, liquid, gases, or dust, and by fungi. Foreign bodies or a bronchial obstruction such as a tumor may promote the occurrence of pneumonia, although they are not causes of pneumonia.

Rickettsia (also considered an organism somewhere between viruses and bacteria) cause Rocky Mountain spotted fever, Q fever, typhus, and psittacosis, diseases that may have mild or severe effects on the lungs. Tuberculosis pneumonia is a very serious lung infection and extremely dangerous unless treated early.

Treating Pneumonia

If you develop pneumonia, your chances of a fast recovery are greatest under certain conditions: if you're young, if your pneumonia is caught early, if your defenses against disease are working well, if the infection hasn't spread, and if you're not suffering from other illnesses.

In the young and healthy, early treatment with antibiotics can cure bacterial pneumonia and speed recovery from mycoplasma pneumonia and a certain percentage of rickettsia cases. There is not yet a general treatment for viral pneumonia, although antiviral drugs are used for certain kinds. Most people can be treated at home.

The drugs used to fight pneumonia are determined by the germ causing the pneumonia and the judgment of the doctor. After a patient's temperature returns to normal, medication must be continued according to the doctor's instructions, otherwise the pneumonia may recur. Relapses can be far more serious than the first attack.

Besides antibiotics, patients are given supportive treatment: proper diet, and oxygen to increase oxygen in the blood when needed. In some patients, medication to ease chest pain and to provide relief from violent cough may be necessary.

The vigorous young person may lead a normal life within a week of recovery from pneumonia. For the middle-aged, however, weeks may elapse before they regain their accustomed strength, vigor, and feeling of well-being. A person recovering from mycoplasma pneumonia may be weak for an extended period of time.

Adequate rest is important to maintain progress toward full recovery and to avoid relapse. Remember, don't rush recovery!

Preventing Pneumonia Is Possible

Because pneumonia is a common complication of influenza (flu), getting a flu shot every fall is good pneumonia prevention.

A vaccine is also available to help fight pneumococcal pneumonia, one type of bacterial pneumonia. Your doctor can help you decide if you, or a member of your family, need the vaccine against pneumococcal pneumonia. It is usually given only to people at high risk of getting the disease and its life-threatening complications.

The greatest risk of pneumococcal pneumonia is usually among people who:

- have chronic illnesses such as lung disease, heart disease, kidney disorders, sickle cell anemia, or diabetes;
- are recovering from severe illness;
- are in nursing homes or other chronic care facilities;
- are age sixty-five or older.

If you are at risk, ask your doctor for the vaccine.

Ask your doctor about any revaccination recommendations. The vaccine is not recommended for pregnant women or children under age two.

Since pneumonia often follows ordinary respiratory infections, the most important preventive measure is to be alert to any symptoms of respiratory trouble that linger more than a few days. Good health habits, proper diet and hygiene, rest, regular exercise, etc., increase resistance to all respiratory illnesses. They also help promote fast recovery when illness does occur.

If You Have Symptoms of Pneumonia

Call your doctor immediately. Even with the many effective antibiotics, early diagnosis and treatment are important.

Follow your doctor's advice. In serious cases, your doctor may advise a hospital stay. Or recovery at home may be possible.

Continue to take the medicine your doctor prescribes until told you may stop. This will help prevent recurrence of pneumonia and relapse.

Remember, even though pneumonia can be treated, it is an extremely serious illness. Don't wait, get treatment early.

Sources

1. National Center for Health Statistics. *National Vital Statistics Report. Deaths: Preliminary Data for 2004*. Vol. 54, 19 June 2006.

Chapter 24

Suicide

Suicide is a major, preventable public health problem. In 2004, it was the eleventh leading cause of death in the United States, accounting for 32,439 deaths.[1] The overall rate was 10.9 suicide deaths per 100,000 people.[1] An estimated eight to twenty-five attempted suicides occur per every suicide death.[2]

Suicidal behavior is complex. Some risk factors vary with age, gender, or ethnic group and may occur in combination or change over time.

If you are in a crisis and need help right away, call this toll-free number, available twenty-four hours a day, every day: 800-273-TALK (8255). You will reach the National Suicide Prevention Lifeline, a service available to anyone. You may call for yourself or for someone you care about. All calls are confidential.

What Are the Risk Factors for Suicide?

Research shows that risk factors for suicide include the following:

- Depression and other mental disorders, or a substance-abuse disorder (often in combination with other mental disorders). More than 90 percent of people who die by suicide have these risk factors.[2]

The first part of this chapter is reprinted from "Suicide in the U.S.: Statistics and Prevention," National Institute of Mental Health, National Institutes of Health, June 26, 2008. "Suicide Warning Signs" is reprinted from the U.S. Department of Health and Human Services Substance Abuse and Mental Health Services Administration, September 2005.

- Stressful life events, in combination with other risk factors, such as depression. However, suicide and suicidal behavior are not normal responses to stress; many people have these risk factors but are not suicidal.
- Prior suicide attempt.
- Family history of mental disorder or substance abuse.
- Family history of suicide.
- Family violence, including physical or sexual abuse.
- Firearms in the home,[3] the method used in more than half of suicides.
- Incarceration.
- Exposure to the suicidal behavior of others, such as family members, peers, or media figures.[2]

Research also shows that the risk for suicide is associated with changes in brain chemicals called neurotransmitters, including serotonin. Decreased levels of serotonin have been found in people with depression, impulsive disorders, and a history of suicide attempts, and in the brains of suicide victims.[4]

Are Women or Men at Higher Risk?

Suicide was the eighth leading cause of death for males and the sixteenth leading cause of death for females in 2004.[1]

Almost four times as many males as females die by suicide.[1]

Firearms, suffocation, and poison are by far the most common methods of suicide, overall. However, men and women differ in the method used, as shown in Table 24.1.[1]

Is Suicide Common among Children and Young People?

In 2004, suicide was the third leading cause of death in each of the following age groups.[1] Of every 100,000 young people in each age group, the following number died by suicide:[1]

- Children ages 10 to 14—1.3 per 100,000
- Adolescents ages 15 to 19—8.2 per 100,000
- Young adults ages 20 to 24—12.5 per 100,000

Table 24.1. Methods of Suicide

Suicide by:	Males (%)	Females (%)
Firearms	57	32
Suffocation	23	20
Poisoning	13	38

As in the general population, young people were much more likely to use firearms, suffocation, and poisoning than other methods of suicide, overall. However, while adolescents and young adults were more likely to use firearms than suffocation, children were dramatically more likely to use suffocation.[1]

There were also gender differences in suicide among young people, as follows:

- Almost four times as many males as females ages fifteen to nineteen died by suicide.[1]
- More than six times as many males as females ages twenty to twenty-four died by suicide.[1]

Are Older Adults at Risk?

Older Americans are disproportionately likely to die by suicide:

- Of every 100,000 people ages sixty-five and older, 14.3 died by suicide in 2004. This figure is higher than the national average of 10.9 suicides per 100,000 people in the general population.[1]
- Non-Hispanic white men age eighty-five or older had an even higher rate, with 17.8 suicide deaths per 100,000.[1]

Are Some Ethnic Groups or Races at Higher Risk?

Of every 100,000 people in each of the following ethnic/racial groups below, the following number died by suicide in 2004.[1]

- Highest rates:
    - Non-Hispanic Whites—12.9 per 100,000
    - American Indian and Alaska Natives—12.4 per 100,000
- Lowest rates:
    - Non-Hispanic Blacks—5.3 per 100,000

- Asian and Pacific Islanders—5.8 per 100,000
- Hispanics—5.9 per 100,000

What Are Some Risk Factors for Nonfatal Suicide Attempts?

As noted, an estimated eight to twenty-five nonfatal suicide attempts occur per every suicide death. Men and the elderly are more likely to have fatal attempts than are women and youth.[2]

Risk factors for nonfatal suicide attempts by adults include depression and other mental disorders, alcohol abuse, cocaine use, and separation or divorce.[5,6]

Risk factors for attempted suicide by youth include depression, alcohol or other drug-use disorder, physical or sexual abuse, and disruptive behavior.[6,7]

Most suicide attempts are expressions of extreme distress, not harmless bids for attention. A person who appears suicidal should not be left alone and needs immediate mental health treatment.

What Can Be Done to Prevent Suicide?

Research helps determine which factors can be modified to help prevent suicide and which interventions are appropriate for specific groups of people. Before being put into practice, prevention programs should be tested through research to determine their safety and effectiveness.[8] For example, because research has shown that mental and substance-abuse disorders are major risk factors for suicide, many programs also focus on treating these disorders.

Studies showed that a type of psychotherapy called cognitive therapy reduced the rate of repeated suicide attempts by 50 percent during a year of follow-up. A previous suicide attempt is among the strongest predictors of subsequent suicide, and cognitive therapy helps suicide attempters consider alternative actions when thoughts of self-harm arise.[9]

Specific kinds of psychotherapy may be helpful for specific groups of people. For example, a recent study showed that a treatment called dialectical behavior therapy reduced suicide attempts by half, compared with other kinds of therapy, in people with borderline personality disorder (a serious disorder of emotion regulation).[10]

The medication clozapine is approved by the Food and Drug Administration for suicide prevention in people with schizophrenia.[11]

Other promising medications and psychosocial treatments for suicidal people are being tested.

Since research shows that older adults and women who die by suicide are likely to have seen a primary care provider in the year before death, improving primary-care providers' ability to recognize and treat risk factors may help prevent suicide among these groups.[12] Improving outreach to men at risk is a major challenge in need of investigation.

What Should I Do If I Think Someone Is Suicidal?

If you think someone is suicidal, do not leave him or her alone. Try to get the person to seek immediate help from his or her doctor or the nearest hospital emergency room, or call 911. Eliminate access to firearms or other potential tools for suicide, including unsupervised access to medications.

References

1. Centers for Disease Control and Prevention, National Center for Injury Prevention and Control. Web-based Injury Statistics Query and Reporting System (WISQARS): www.cdc.gov/ncipc/wisqars

2. Moscicki EK. Epidemiology of completed and attempted suicide: toward a framework for prevention. *Clinical Neuroscience Research*, 2001; 1: 310–23.

3. Miller M, Azrael D, Hepburn L, Hemenway D, Lippmann SJ. The association between changes in household firearm ownership and rates of suicide in the United States, 1981–2002. *Injury Prevention* 2006;12:178–82; doi:10.1136/ip.2005.010850

4. Arango V, Huang YY, Underwood MD, Mann JJ. Genetics of the serotonergic system in suicidal behavior. *Journal of Psychiatric Research*. Vol. 37: 375–86. 2003.

5. Kessler RC, Borges G, Walters EE. Prevalence of and risk factors for lifetime suicide attempts in the National Comorbidity Survey. *Archives of General Psychiatry*, 1999; 56(7): 617–26.

6. Petronis KR, Samuels JF, Moscicki EK, Anthony JC. An epidemiologic investigation of potential risk factors for suicide

attempts. *Social Psychiatry and Psychiatric Epidemiology*, 1990; 25(4): 193–99.

7. U.S. Public Health Service. National strategy for suicide prevention: goals and objectives for action. Rockville, MD: USDHHS, 2001.

8. Gould MS, Greenberg T, Velting DM, Shaffer D. Youth suicide risk and preventive interventions: a review of the past 10 years. *Journal of the American Academy of Child and Adolescent Psychiatry*, 2003; 42(4): 386–405.

9. Brown GK, Ten Have T, Henriques GR, Xie SX, Hollander JE, Beck AT. Cognitive therapy for the prevention of suicide attempts: a randomized controlled trial. *Journal of the American Medical Association*. 2005 Aug 3;294(5):563–70.

10. Linehan MM, Comtois KA, Murray AM, Brown MZ, Gallop RJ, Heard HL, Korslund KE, Tutek DA, Reynolds SK, Lindenboim N. Two-Year Randomized Controlled Trial and Follow-up of Dialectical Behavior Therapy vs Therapy by Experts for Suicidal Behaviors and Borderline Personality Disorder. *Archives of General Psychiatry*, 2006 Jul;63(7):757–66.

11. Meltzer HY, Alphs L, Green AI, Altamura AC, Anand R, Bertoldi A, Bourgeois M, Chouinard G, Islam MZ, Kane J, Krishnan R, Lindenmayer JP, Potkin S; International Suicide Prevention Trial Study Group. Clozapine treatment for suicidality in schizophrenia: International Suicide Prevention Trial (InterSePT). *Archives of General Psychiatry*, 2003; 60(1): 82–91.

12. Luoma JB, Pearson JL, Martin CE. Contact with mental health and primary care prior to suicide: a review of the evidence. *American Journal of Psychiatry*, 2002; 159: 909–16.

Suicide Warning Signs

Seek help as soon as possible by contacting a mental health professional or by calling the National Suicide Prevention Lifeline at 800-273-TALK if you or someone you know exhibits any of the following signs:

- Threatening to hurt or kill oneself or talking about wanting to hurt or kill oneself

- Looking for ways to kill oneself by seeking access to firearms, pills, or other means
- Talking or writing about death, dying, or suicide when these actions are out of the ordinary for the person
- Feeling hopeless
- Feeling rage or uncontrolled anger or seeking revenge
- Acting reckless or engaging in risky activities—seemingly without thinking
- Feeling trapped—like there's no way out
- Increasing alcohol or drug use
- Withdrawing from friends, family, and society
- Feeling anxious, agitated, or unable to sleep or sleeping all the time
- Experiencing dramatic mood changes
- Seeing no reason for living or having no sense of purpose in life

Chapter 25

Alzheimer Disease

Introduction

Dementia is a brain disorder that seriously affects a person's ability to carry out daily activities. The most common form of dementia among older people is Alzheimer disease (AD), which initially involves the parts of the brain that control thought, memory, and language. Although scientists are learning more every day, right now they still do not know what causes AD, and there is no cure.

Scientists think that as many as 4.5 million Americans suffer from AD. The disease usually begins after age sixty, and risk goes up with age. While younger people also may get AD, it is much less common. About 5 percent of men and women ages sixty-five to seventy-four have AD, and nearly half of those age eighty-five and older may have the disease. It is important to note, however, that AD is not a normal part of aging.

AD is named after Dr. Alois Alzheimer, a German doctor. In 1906, Dr. Alzheimer noticed changes in the brain tissue of a woman who had died of an unusual mental illness. He found abnormal clumps (now called amyloid plaques) and tangled bundles of fibers (now called neurofibrillary tangles). Today, these plaques and tangles in the brain are considered signs of AD.

Excerpted from "Alzheimer's Disease Fact Sheet," National Institute on Aging, July 24, 2008.

Scientists also have found other brain changes in people with AD. Nerve cells die in areas of the brain that are vital to memory and other mental abilities, and connections between nerve cells are disrupted. There also are lower levels of some of the chemicals in the brain that carry messages back and forth between nerve cells. AD may impair thinking and memory by disrupting these messages.

What Causes AD?

Scientists do not yet fully understand what causes AD. There probably is not one single cause, but several factors that affect each person differently. Age is the most important known risk factor for AD. The number of people with the disease doubles every five years beyond age sixty-five.

Family history is another risk factor. Scientists believe that genetics may play a role in many AD cases. For example, early-onset familial AD, a rare form of AD that usually occurs between the ages of thirty and sixty, is inherited. The more common form of AD is known as late-onset. It occurs later in life, and no obvious inheritance pattern is seen in most families. However, several risk factor genes may interact with each other and with nongenetic factors to cause the disease. The only risk factor gene identified so far for late-onset AD is a gene that makes one form of a protein called apolipoprotein E (ApoE). Everyone has ApoE, which helps carry cholesterol in the blood. Only about 15 percent of people have the form that increases the risk of AD. It is likely that other genes also may increase the risk of AD or protect against AD, but they remain to be discovered.

Scientists still need to learn a lot more about what causes AD. In addition to genetics and ApoE, they are studying education, diet, and environment to learn what role they might play in the development of this disease. Scientists are finding increasing evidence that some of the risk factors for heart disease and stroke, such as high blood pressure, high cholesterol, and low levels of the vitamin folate, may also increase the risk of AD. Evidence for physical, mental, and social activities as protective factors against AD is also increasing.

What Are the Symptoms of AD?

AD begins slowly. At first, the only symptom may be mild forgetfulness, which can be confused with age-related memory change. Most people with mild forgetfulness do not have AD. In the early stage of AD, people may have trouble remembering recent events, activities, or the names of familiar people or things. They may not be able to solve simple math problems. Such difficulties may be a bother, but usually they are not serious enough to cause alarm.

However, as the disease goes on, symptoms are more easily noticed and become serious enough to cause people with AD or their family members to seek medical help. Forgetfulness begins to interfere with daily activities. People in the middle stages of AD may forget how to do simple tasks like brushing their teeth or combing their hair. They can no longer think clearly. They can fail to recognize familiar people and places. They begin to have problems speaking, understanding, reading, or writing. Later on, people with AD may become anxious or aggressive, or wander away from home. Eventually, patients need total care.

How Is AD Diagnosed?

An early, accurate diagnosis of AD helps patients and their families plan for the future. It gives them time to discuss care while the patient can still take part in making decisions. Early diagnosis will also offer the best chance to treat the symptoms of the disease.

Today, the only definite way to diagnose AD is to find out whether there are plaques and tangles in brain tissue. To look at brain tissue, however, doctors usually must wait until they do an autopsy, which is an examination of the body done after a person dies. Therefore, doctors can only make a diagnosis of "possible" or "probable" AD while the person is still alive.

At specialized centers, doctors can diagnose AD correctly up to 90 percent of the time. Doctors use several tools to diagnose "probable" AD, including the following:

- Questions about the person's general health, past medical problems, and ability to carry out daily activities
- Tests of memory, problem solving, attention, counting, and language
- Medical tests—such as tests of blood, urine, or spinal fluid, and brain scans

Sometimes these test results help the doctor find other possible causes of the person's symptoms. For example, thyroid problems, drug reactions, depression, brain tumors, and blood vessel disease in the brain can cause AD-like symptoms. Some of these other conditions can be treated successfully.

How Is AD Treated?

AD is a slow disease, starting with mild memory problems and ending with severe brain damage. The course the disease takes and how fast changes occur vary from person to person. On average, AD patients live from eight to ten years after they are diagnosed, though some people may live with AD for as many as twenty years.

No treatment can stop AD. However, for some people in the early and middle stages of the disease, the drugs tacrine (Cognex®, which is still available but no longer actively marketed by the manufacturer), donepezil (Aricept®), rivastigmine (Exelon®), or galantamine (Razadyne®, previously known as Reminyl®) may help prevent some symptoms from becoming worse for a limited time. Another drug, memantine (Namenda®), has been approved to treat moderate to severe AD, although it also is limited in its effects. Also, some medicines may help control behavioral symptoms of AD such as sleeplessness, agitation, wandering, anxiety, and depression. Treating these symptoms often makes patients more comfortable and makes their care easier for caregivers.

New Areas of Research

Neuroimaging: Scientists are finding that damage to parts of the brain involved in memory, such as the hippocampus, can sometimes be seen on brain scans before symptoms of the disease occur. An NIA public-private partnership—the AD Neuroimaging Initiative (ADNI)—is a large study that will determine whether magnetic resonance imaging (MRI) and positron emission tomography (PET) scans, or other imaging or biological markers, can see early AD changes or measure disease progression. The project is designed to help speed clinical trials and find new ways to determine the effectiveness of treatments.

AD genetics: The NIA is sponsoring the AD Genetics Study to learn more about risk factor genes for late-onset AD.

Mild cognitive impairment: During the past several years, scientists have focused on a type of memory change called mild cognitive impairment (MCI), which is different from both AD and normal age-related memory change. People with MCI have ongoing memory problems, but they do not have other losses such as confusion, attention problems, and difficulty with language. The NIA-funded Memory Impairment Study compared donepezil, vitamin E, or placebo in participants with MCI to see whether the drugs might delay or prevent progression to AD. The study found that the group with MCI taking donepezil were at reduced risk of progressing to AD for the first eighteen months of a three-year study, when compared with their counterparts on placebo. The reduced risk of progressing from MCI to a diagnosis of AD among participants on donepezil disappeared after eighteen months, and by the end of the study, the probability of progressing to AD was the same in the two groups. Vitamin E had no effect at any time point in the study when compared with placebo.

Inflammation: There is evidence that inflammation in the brain may contribute to AD damage. Some studies have suggested that drugs such as nonsteroidal anti-inflammatory drugs (NSAIDs) might help slow the progression of AD, but clinical trials thus far have not demonstrated a benefit from these drugs. A clinical trial studying two of these drugs, rofecoxib (Vioxx®) and naproxen (Aleve®) showed that they did not delay the progression of AD in people who already have the disease. Another trial, testing whether the NSAIDs celecoxib (Celebrex®) and naproxen could prevent AD in healthy older people at risk of the disease, was suspended due to concerns over possible cardiovascular risk. Researchers are continuing to look for ways to test how other anti-inflammatory drugs might affect the development or progression of AD.

Antioxidants: Several years ago, a clinical trial showed that vitamin E slowed the progress of some consequences of AD by about seven months. Additional studies are investigating whether antioxidants—vitamins E and C—can slow AD. Another clinical trial is examining whether vitamin E and/or selenium supplements can prevent AD or cognitive decline, and additional studies on other antioxidants are ongoing or being planned, including a study of the antioxidant treatments—vitamins E, C, alpha-lipoic acid, and coenzyme Q—in patients with mild to moderate AD.

Ginkgo biloba: Early studies suggested that extracts from the leaves of the ginkgo biloba tree may be of some help in treating AD symptoms. There is no evidence yet that ginkgo biloba will cure or prevent AD, but scientists now are trying to find out in a clinical trial whether ginkgo biloba can delay cognitive decline or prevent dementia in older people.

Estrogen: Some studies have suggested that estrogen used by women to treat the symptoms of menopause also protects the brain.

Experts also wondered whether using estrogen could reduce the risk of AD or slow the disease. Clinical trials to test estrogen, however, have not shown that estrogen can slow the progression of already diagnosed AD. And one study found that women over the age of sixty-five who used estrogen with a progestin were at greater risk of dementia, including AD, and that older women using only estrogen could also increase their chance of developing dementia.

Scientists believe that more research is needed to find out if estrogen may play some role in AD. They would like to know whether starting estrogen therapy around the time of menopause, rather than at age sixty-five or older, will protect memory or prevent AD.

Chapter 26

Kidney Disease

What do my kidneys do?

Your kidneys are bean-shaped organs, each about the size of your fist. They are located near the middle of your back, just below the ribcage.

Your kidneys filter blood. The filtering occurs in tiny units inside your kidneys called nephrons. One kidney has about a million nephrons. They remove waste products and extra water, which become urine. The urine flows through tubes called ureters to your bladder, which stores the urine until you go to the bathroom.

The wastes in your blood come from the normal breakdown of active tissues and from food you eat. After your body has taken what it needs from the food, waste is sent to the blood. If your kidneys did not remove these wastes, the wastes would build up in the blood and damage your body.

What is kidney disease?

Kidney disease results from damage to the nephrons, the tiny structures inside your kidneys that filter blood.

Usually the damage occurs very gradually over years. It happens in both kidneys. There aren't any obvious symptoms, so you don't know it's happening.

Reprinted from "Kidney Disease Information," National Kidney Disease Education Program, National Institutes of Health, March 2005.

Common causes of kidney disease are as follows:

- **Diabetes:** In diabetes, the body doesn't use glucose (sugar) very well. The glucose stays in your blood and acts like a poison. If you have diabetes, you can prevent kidney disease by controlling your blood sugar levels.
- **High blood pressure:** High blood pressure can damage the small blood vessels in your kidneys. When this happens your kidneys cannot filter wastes from your blood very well. If you have high blood pressure (hypertension) be sure to take any medicines your doctor prescribes.
- **Heredity:** Some kidney diseases result from hereditary factors, and can run in families. If your family has a history of any kind of kidney problems, you may be at risk for kidney disease and should talk to your doctor.

Am I at risk for kidney disease?

- Do you have diabetes (problems with your blood sugar)?
- Do you have high blood pressure?
- Did your mother, father, sister, or brother ever have kidney failure? Kidney disease runs in families.

If you answered "yes" to any of these questions, you are at risk for kidney disease. Now is the time to talk to your doctor or health care professional about getting tested. It could save your life.

How can my doctor tell if I have kidney disease?

Early kidney disease is a silent problem, like high blood pressure, and does not have any symptoms. You may have it, but not know it, because you don't feel sick.

To detect the disease doctors can do very simple tests that include the following:

- Measure the level of serum creatinine in your blood to estimate your glomerular filtration rate (GFR)
- Measure the level of protein in your urine (increased levels of protein show your kidneys are not working right)
- Check your blood pressure

If I have kidney disease, how can it be treated?

Unfortunately, kidney disease often cannot be cured. But if you are in the early stages of a kidney disease, you may be able to make your kidneys last longer by taking certain steps. You will also want to be sure that risks for heart attack and stroke are minimized, since kidney patients are susceptible to these problems.

If you have diabetes, watch your blood glucose closely to keep it under control. Consult your doctor for the latest in treatment.

People with reduced kidney function should have their blood pressure controlled, and an angiotensin-converting enzyme (ACE) inhibitor or an angiotensin II receptor blocker (ARB) should be one of their medications. Many people will require two or more types of medication to keep the blood pressure below 130/80 mm Hg. A diuretic is an important addition to the ACE inhibitor or ARB.

What happens if my kidneys fail completely?

Complete and irreversible kidney failure is sometimes called end-stage renal disease, or ESRD. If your kidneys stop working completely, your body fills with extra water and waste products. This condition is called uremia. Your hands or feet may swell. You will feel tired and weak because your body needs clean blood to function properly.

Untreated uremia may lead to seizures or coma and will ultimately result in death. If your kidneys stop working completely, you will need to undergo dialysis or kidney transplantation.

Dialysis: There are two major forms of dialysis. In hemodialysis, your blood is sent through a machine that filters away waste products. The clean blood is returned to your body. Hemodialysis is usually performed at a dialysis center three times per week for three to four hours. In peritoneal dialysis, a fluid is put into your abdomen. This fluid, called dialysate, captures the waste products from your blood. After a few hours, the dialysate containing your body's wastes is drained away. Then, a fresh bag of dialysate is dripped into the abdomen. Patients can perform peritoneal dialysis themselves. Patients using continuous ambulatory peritoneal dialysis (CAPD), the most common form of peritoneal dialysis, change dialysate four times a day.

Transplantation: A donated kidney may come from an anonymous donor who has recently died or from a living person, usually a relative. The kidney that you receive must be a good match for your body. The more the new kidney is like you, the less likely your immune system is to reject it. You will take special drugs to help trick your immune system so it does not reject the transplanted kidney.

Chapter 27

Chronic Liver Disease and Cirrhosis

Viral Hepatitis

What Is Viral Hepatitis?

Viral hepatitis is inflammation of the liver caused by a virus. Several different viruses, named the hepatitis A, B, C, D, and E viruses, cause viral hepatitis.

All of these viruses cause acute, or short-term, viral hepatitis. The hepatitis B, C, and D viruses can also cause chronic hepatitis, in which the infection is prolonged, sometimes lifelong. Chronic hepatitis can lead to cirrhosis, liver failure, and liver cancer.

Researchers are looking for other viruses that may cause hepatitis, but none have been identified with certainty. Other viruses that less often affect the liver include cytomegalovirus; Epstein-Barr virus, also called infectious mononucleosis; herpesvirus; parvovirus; and adenovirus.

"Viral Hepatitis" is excerpted from "Viral Hepatitis: A through E and Beyond," National Institute of Diabetes and Digestive and Kidney Diseases, National Institutes of Health, NIH Publication No. 08-4762, February 2008. "Cirrhosis of the Liver" is excerpted from "What I Need to Know about Cirrhosis of the Liver," National Institute of Diabetes and Digestive and Kidney Diseases, National Institutes of Health, NIH Publication No. 06-5166, October 2005.

What Are the Symptoms of Viral Hepatitis?

Symptoms include the following:

- Jaundice, which causes a yellowing of the skin and eyes
- Fatigue
- Abdominal pain
- Loss of appetite
- Nausea
- Vomiting
- Diarrhea
- Low-grade fever
- Headache

However, some people do not have symptoms.

Hepatitis A

Disease spread: Hepatitis A is spread primarily through food or water contaminated by feces from an infected person. Rarely, it spreads through contact with infected blood.

People at risk: People most likely to get hepatitis A are: international travelers, particularly those traveling to developing countries; people who live with or have sex with an infected person ; people living in areas where children are not routinely vaccinated against hepatitis A, where outbreaks are more likely; day care children and employees, during outbreaks; men who have sex with men; and users of illicit drugs.

Prevention: The hepatitis A vaccine offers immunity to adults and children older than age one. The Centers for Disease Control and Prevention recommends routine hepatitis A vaccination for children aged twelve to twenty-three months and for adults who are at high risk for infection. Treatment with immune globulin can provide short-term immunity to hepatitis A when given before exposure or within two weeks of exposure to the virus. Avoiding tap water when traveling internationally and practicing good hygiene and sanitation also help prevent hepatitis A.

Treatment: Hepatitis A usually resolves on its own over several weeks.

Hepatitis B

Disease spread: Hepatitis B is spread through contact with infected blood, through sex with an infected person, and from mother to child during childbirth, whether the delivery is vaginal or via cesarean section.

People at risk: People most likely to get hepatitis B are: people who live with or have sexual contact with an infected person; men who have sex with men; people who have multiple sex partners; injection drug users; immigrants and children of immigrants from areas with high rates of hepatitis B; infants born to infected mothers; health care workers; hemodialysis patients; people who received a transfusion of blood or blood products before 1987, when better tests to screen blood donors were developed; and international travelers.

Prevention: The hepatitis B vaccine offers the best protection. All infants and unvaccinated children, adolescents, and at-risk adults should be vaccinated. For people who have not been vaccinated, reducing exposure to the virus can help prevent hepatitis B. Reducing exposure means using latex condoms, which may lower the risk of transmission; not sharing drug needles; and not sharing personal items such as toothbrushes, razors, and nail clippers with an infected person.

Treatment: Drugs approved for the treatment of chronic hepatitis B include alpha interferon and peginterferon, which slow the replication of the virus in the body and also boost the immune system, and the antiviral drugs lamivudine, adefovir dipivoxil, entecavir, and telbivudine. Other drugs are also being evaluated. Infants born to infected mothers should receive hepatitis B immune globulin and the hepatitis B vaccine within twelve hours of birth to help prevent infection.

People who develop acute hepatitis B are generally not treated with antiviral drugs because, depending on their age at infection, the disease often resolves on its own. Infected newborns are most likely to progress to chronic hepatitis B, but by young adulthood, most people with acute infection recover spontaneously. Severe acute hepatitis B can be treated with an antiviral drug such as lamivudine.

Hepatitis C

Disease spread: Hepatitis C is spread primarily through contact with infected blood. Less commonly, it can spread through sexual contact and childbirth.

People at risk: People most likely to be exposed to the hepatitis C virus are: injection drug users; people who have sex with an infected person; people who have multiple sex partners; health care workers; infants born to infected women; hemodialysis patients; people who received a transfusion of blood or blood products before July 1992, when sensitive tests to screen blood donors for hepatitis C were introduced; and people who received clotting factors made before 1987, when methods to manufacture these products were improved.

Prevention: There is no vaccine for hepatitis C. The only way to prevent the disease is to reduce the risk of exposure to the virus. Reducing exposure means avoiding behaviors like sharing drug needles or personal items such as toothbrushes, razors, and nail clippers with an infected person.

Treatment: Chronic hepatitis C is treated with peginterferon together with the antiviral drug ribavirin.

If acute hepatitis C does not resolve on its own within two to three months, drug treatment is recommended.

Hepatitis D

Disease spread: Hepatitis D is spread through contact with infected blood. This disease occurs only at the same time as infection with hepatitis B or in people who are already infected with hepatitis B.

People at risk: Anyone infected with hepatitis B is at risk for hepatitis D. Injection drug users have the highest risk. Others at risk include people who live with or have sex with a person infected with hepatitis D and people who received a transfusion of blood or blood products before 1987.

Prevention: People not already infected with hepatitis B should receive the hepatitis B vaccine. Other preventive measures include avoiding exposure to infected blood, contaminated needles, and an infected person's personal items such as toothbrushes, razors, and nail clippers.

Treatment: Chronic hepatitis D is usually treated with pegylated interferon, although other potential treatments are under study.

Hepatitis E

Disease spread: Hepatitis E is spread through food or water contaminated by feces from an infected person. This disease is uncommon in the United States.

People at risk: People most likely to be exposed to the hepatitis E virus are: international travelers, particularly those traveling to developing countries; people living in areas where hepatitis E outbreaks are common; and people who live with or have sex with an infected person.

Prevention: There is no U.S. Food and Drug Administration (FDA)-approved vaccine for hepatitis E. The only way to prevent the disease is to reduce the risk of exposure to the virus. Reducing risk of exposure means avoiding tap water when traveling internationally and practicing good hygiene and sanitation.

Treatment: Hepatitis E usually resolves on its own over several weeks to months.

Other Causes of Viral Hepatitis

Some cases of viral hepatitis cannot be attributed to the hepatitis A, B, C, D, or E viruses, or even the less common viruses that can infect the liver, such as cytomegalovirus, Epstein-Barr virus, herpesvirus, parvovirus, and adenovirus. These cases are called non-A–E hepatitis. Scientists continue to study the causes of non-A–E hepatitis.

Cirrhosis of the Liver

What is cirrhosis of the liver?

Cirrhosis refers to scarring of the liver. Scar tissue forms because of injury or long-term disease. It replaces healthy tissue.

Scar tissue cannot do what healthy liver tissue does—make protein, help fight infections, clean the blood, help digest food, and store energy for when you need it. Scar tissue also blocks the normal flow of blood through the liver. Too much scar tissue means that your liver cannot work properly. To live, you need a liver that works.

Cirrhosis can be life threatening, but it can also be controlled if treated early.

What are the symptoms of cirrhosis?

You may have no symptoms at all in the early stages. As cirrhosis progresses you may:

- feel tired or weak;
- lose your appetite;
- feel sick to your stomach;
- lose weight.

Cirrhosis can also lead to other problems:

- You may bruise or bleed easily, or have nosebleeds.
- Bloating or swelling may occur as fluid builds up in the abdomen or legs. Fluid buildup in the abdomen is called ascites and in the legs is called edema.
- Medications may have a stronger effect on you because your liver does not break them down as quickly.
- Waste materials from food may build up in the blood or brain and may cause confusion or difficulty thinking. For example, protein that you eat breaks down into chemicals like ammonia. When red blood cells get old, they break down and leave a substance called bilirubin. A healthy liver removes these byproducts, but a diseased liver leaves them in the body.
- Blood pressure may increase in the vein entering the liver, a condition called portal hypertension.
- Enlarged veins, called varices, may develop in the esophagus and stomach. Varices can bleed suddenly, causing vomiting of blood or passing of blood in a bowel movement.
- The kidneys may not work properly or may fail.

As cirrhosis progresses, your skin and the whites of your eyes may turn yellow, a condition called jaundice. You may also develop severe itching or gallstones.

In the early stages, cirrhosis causes your liver to swell. Then, as more scar tissue replaces normal tissue, the liver shrinks.

About 5 percent of patients with cirrhosis also get cancer of the liver.

What causes cirrhosis?

Cirrhosis has many causes, including the following:

- Alcohol abuse (alcoholic liver disease)
- Chronic viral hepatitis (hepatitis B, C, or D)
- Autoimmune hepatitis, which is destruction of liver cells by the body's immune system
- Nonalcoholic fatty liver disease or nonalcoholic steatohepatitis (NASH), which is fat deposits and inflammation in the liver
- Some drugs, toxins, and infections
- Blocked bile ducts, the tubes that carry bile from the liver
- Some inherited diseases such as hemochromatosis, a disease that occurs when the body absorbs too much iron and stores the excess iron in the liver, pancreas, and other organs; Wilson disease, which is caused by the buildup of too much copper in the liver; or protoporphyria, a disorder that affects the skin, bone marrow, and liver

Sometimes the cause of cirrhosis remains unknown even after a thorough medical examination.

How is cirrhosis diagnosed?

Your symptoms, a physical examination, and certain tests can help your doctor diagnose cirrhosis. Some tests are as follows:

- Blood tests to see whether your liver is working properly. Routine blood tests may be normal in cirrhosis. However, with advanced cirrhosis, blood tests may reveal abnormal levels of bilirubin and other substances.
- X-rays, magnetic resonance imaging, or ultrasound images (pictures developed from sound waves), which may show an enlarged or shrunken liver.
- Liver biopsy, an examination of a piece of your liver under a microscope, to look for scar tissue. This is the most accurate way to diagnose cirrhosis.

How is cirrhosis treated?

Once you have cirrhosis, nothing can make the scar tissue go away completely. However, treating the cause will keep cirrhosis from getting worse. For example, if cirrhosis is due to alcoholic liver disease, the treatment is to completely stop drinking alcohol. If cirrhosis is caused by hepatitis C, then that disease may be treated with medication.

Your doctor will suggest treatment based on the cause of your cirrhosis and your symptoms. Early diagnosis and carefully following an appropriate treatment plan can help many people with cirrhosis. In very advanced cirrhosis, however, certain treatments may not be possible. In that situation, your doctors will work with you to prevent or manage the complications that cirrhosis can cause.

How can I prevent cirrhosis if I already have liver disease?

- See your doctor for treatment of your liver disease. Many of the causes of cirrhosis are treatable, and early treatment may prevent cirrhosis.
- Follow a healthy lifestyle, eat a healthy diet, and stay active.
- Try to keep your weight in the normal range. Being overweight can make several liver diseases worse.
- Do not drink alcohol. Alcohol can harm liver cells, and chronic alcohol use is one of the major causes of cirrhosis.
- Stay away from illegal (street) drugs, which can increase your chances of getting hepatitis B or hepatitis C.
- See your doctor if you have chronic viral hepatitis. Effective treatments for both hepatitis B and hepatitis C are available. If you are on treatment, follow your treatment directions exactly.
- If you have autoimmune hepatitis, take medications and have regular check-ups as recommended by your doctor or a liver specialist (hepatologist).

What can I do to keep cirrhosis from getting worse?

- Stop drinking alcohol completely.
- Do not take any medications, including those you can buy without a prescription such as vitamins and herbal supplements,

without discussing them with your doctor. Cirrhosis makes your liver sensitive to certain medications.

- Get vaccinated against hepatitis A and hepatitis B. These forms of liver disease are preventable. Also, ask your doctor about getting a flu shot and being vaccinated against pneumonia.
- Avoid eating raw oysters or other raw shellfish. Raw shellfish can harbor bacteria (*Vibrio vulnificus*) that cause severe infections in people with cirrhosis.

Part Three

Reproductive and Sexual Concerns

Chapter 28

Male Reproductive System

All living things reproduce. Reproduction—the process by which organisms make more organisms like themselves—is one of the things that sets living things apart from nonliving matter. But even though the reproductive system is essential to keeping a species alive, unlike other body systems it's not essential to keeping an individual alive.

In the human reproductive process, two kinds of sex cells, or gametes (pronounced: gah-meetz), are involved. The male gamete, or sperm, and the female gamete, the egg or ovum, meet in the female's reproductive system to create a new individual. Both the male and female reproductive systems are essential for reproduction.

Humans, like other organisms, pass certain characteristics of themselves to the next generation through their genes, the special carriers of human traits. The genes parents pass along to their children are what make children similar to others in their family, but they are also what make each child unique. These genes come from the father's sperm and the mother's egg, which are produced by the male and female reproductive systems.

"Male Reproductive System," November 2007, reprinted with permission from www.kidshealth.org. This information was provided by KidsHealth, one of the largest resources online for medically reviewed health information written for parents, kids, and teens. For more articles like this one, visit www.KidsHealth.org, or www.TeensHealth.org.

What Is the Male Reproductive System?

Most species have two sexes: male and female. Each sex has its own unique reproductive system. They are different in shape and structure, but both are specifically designed to produce, nourish, and transport either the egg or sperm.

Unlike the female, whose sex organs are located entirely within the pelvis, the male has reproductive organs, or genitals (pronounced: jen-ih-tulz), that are both inside and outside the pelvis. The male genitals include:

- the testicles;
- the duct system, which is made up of the epididymis and the vas deferens;
- the accessory glands, which include the seminal vesicles and prostate gland;
- the penis.

In a guy who's reached sexual maturity, the two testicles (pronounced: tes-tih-kulz), or testes (pronounced: tes-teez) produce and store millions of tiny sperm cells. The testicles are oval-shaped and grow to be about two inches (five centimeters) in length and one inch (three centimeters) in diameter. The testicles are also part of the endocrine system because they produce hormones, including testosterone (pronounced: tes-tos-tuh-rone). Testosterone is a major part of puberty in guys, and as a guy makes his way through puberty, his testicles produce more and more of it. Testosterone is the hormone that causes guys to develop deeper voices, bigger muscles, and body and facial hair, and it also stimulates the production of sperm.

Alongside the testicles are the epididymis (pronounced: ep-ih-did-uh-mus) and the vas deferens (pronounced: vas def-uh-runz), which make up the duct system of the male reproductive organs. The vas deferens is a muscular tube that passes upward alongside the testicles and transports the sperm-containing fluid called semen (pronounced: see-mun). The epididymis is a set of coiled tubes (one for each testicle) that connects to the vas deferens.

The epididymis and the testicles hang in a pouch-like structure outside the pelvis called the scrotum. This bag of skin helps to regulate the temperature of testicles, which need to be kept cooler than body temperature to produce sperm. The scrotum changes size to maintain the right temperature. When the body is cold, the scrotum shrinks and becomes tighter to hold in body heat. When it's warm, the scrotum becomes larger and more floppy to get rid of extra heat. This happens without a guy ever having to think about it. The brain and the nervous system give the scrotum the cue to change size.

The accessory glands, including the seminal vesicles and the prostate gland, provide fluids that lubricate the duct system and nourish the sperm. The seminal vesicles (pronounced: sem-uh-nul ves-ih-kulz) are sac-like structures attached to the vas deferens to the side of the bladder. The prostate gland, which produces some of the parts of semen, surrounds the ejaculatory ducts at the base of the urethra (pronounced: yoo-ree-thruh), just below the bladder. The urethra is the channel that carries the semen to the outside of the body through the penis. The urethra is also part of the urinary system because it is also the channel through which urine passes as it leaves the bladder and exits the body.

The penis is actually made up of two parts: the shaft and the glans (pronounced: glanz). The shaft is the main part of the penis and the glans is the tip (sometimes called the head). At the end of the glans is a small slit or opening, which is where semen and urine exit the body through the urethra. The inside of the penis is made of a spongy tissue that can expand and contract.

All boys are born with a foreskin, a fold of skin at the end of the penis covering the glans. Some boys have a circumcision (pronounced: sur-kum-sih-zhun), which means that a doctor or clergy member cuts away the foreskin. Circumcision is usually performed during a baby boy's first few days of life. Although circumcision is not medically necessary, parents who choose to have their children circumcised often do so based on religious beliefs, concerns about hygiene, or cultural or social reasons. Boys who have circumcised penises and those who don't are no different: All penises work and feel the same, regardless of whether the foreskin has been removed.

What Does the Male Reproductive System Do?

The male sex organs work together to produce and release semen into the reproductive system of the female during sexual intercourse. The male reproductive system also produces sex hormones, which help a boy develop into a sexually mature man during puberty (pronounced: pyoo-bur-tee).

When a baby boy is born, he has all the parts of his reproductive system in place, but it isn't until puberty that he is able to reproduce. When puberty begins, usually between the ages of ten and fourteen, the pituitary (pronounced: pih-too-uh-ter-ee) gland—which is located near the brain—secretes hormones that stimulate the testicles to produce testosterone. The production of testosterone brings about many physical changes. Although the timing of these changes is different for every guy, the stages of puberty generally follow a set sequence:

- During the first stage of male puberty, the scrotum and testes grow larger.
- Next, the penis becomes longer, and the seminal vesicles and prostate gland grow.
- Hair begins to appear in the pubic area and later it grows on the face and underarms. During this time, a male's voice also deepens.
- Boys also undergo a growth spurt during puberty as they reach their adult height and weight.

Once a guy has reached puberty, he will produce millions of sperm cells every day. Each sperm is extremely small: only 1/600 of an inch (0.05 millimeters long). Sperm develop in the testicles within a system of tiny tubes called the seminiferous tubules (pronounced: sem-uh-nih-fuh-rus too-byoolz). At birth, these tubules contain simple round cells, but during puberty, testosterone and other hormones cause these cells to transform into sperm cells. The cells divide and change until they have a head and short tail, like tadpoles. The head contains genetic material (genes). The sperm use their tails to push themselves into the epididymis, where they complete their development. It takes sperm about four to six weeks to travel through the epididymis.

The sperm then move to the vas deferens, or sperm duct. The seminal vesicles and prostate gland produce a whitish fluid called seminal fluid, which mixes with sperm to form semen when a male is sexually stimulated. The penis, which usually hangs limp, becomes hard when a male is sexually excited. Tissues in the penis fill with blood and it becomes stiff and erect (an erection). The rigidity of the erect penis makes it easier to insert into the female's vagina during sexual intercourse. When the erect penis is stimulated, muscles around the reproductive organs contract and force the semen through the duct system and urethra. Semen is pushed out of the male's body through his urethra—this process is called ejaculation (pronounced: ih-jak-yuh-lay-shun). Each time a guy ejaculates, it can contain up to five hundred million sperm.

When the male ejaculates during intercourse, semen is deposited into the female's vagina. From the vagina the sperm make their way up through the cervix and move through the uterus with help from uterine contractions. If a mature egg is in one of the female's fallopian tubes, a single sperm may penetrate it, and fertilization, or conception, occurs.

This fertilized egg is now called a zygote (pronounced: zy-goat) and contains forty-six chromosomes—half from the egg and half from the sperm. The genetic material from the male and female has combined so that a new individual can be created. The zygote divides again and again as it grows in the female's uterus, maturing over the course of the pregnancy into an embryo, a fetus, and finally a newborn baby.

Things That Can Go Wrong with the Male Reproductive System

Guys may sometimes experience reproductive system problems. Below are some examples of disorders that affect the male reproductive system.

Disorders of the Scrotum, Testicles, or Epididymis

Conditions affecting the scrotal contents may involve the testicles, epididymis, or the scrotum itself.

Testicular injury: Even a mild injury to the testicles can cause severe pain, bruising, or swelling. Most testicular injuries occur when the testicles are struck, hit, kicked, or crushed, usually during sports or due to other trauma. Testicular torsion (pronounced: tor-zhun), when one of the testicles twists around, cutting off its blood supply, is also a problem that some teen guys experience—although it's not common.

Varicocele (pronounced: var-uh-koh-seal): This is a varicose vein (an abnormally swollen vein) in the network of veins that run from the testicles. Varicoceles commonly develop while a guy is going through puberty. A varicocele is usually not harmful, although in some people it may damage the testicle or decrease sperm production, so it helps for a guy to see his doctor if he's concerned about changes in his testicles.

Testicular cancer: This is one of the most common cancers in men younger than forty. It occurs when cells in the testicle divide abnormally and form a tumor. Testicular cancer can spread to other parts of the body, but if it's detected early, the cure rate is excellent. All guys should perform testicular self-examinations regularly to help with early detection.

Epididymitis (pronounced: ep-uh-did-ih-my-tus): This is inflammation of the epididymis, the coiled tubes that connect the testes with the vas deferens. It is usually caused by an infection, such as the sexually transmitted disease chlamydia, and results in pain and swelling next to one of the testicles.

Hydrocele: A hydrocele (pronounced: high-druh-seel) occurs when fluid collects in the membranes surrounding the testes. Hydroceles may cause swelling in the scrotum around the testicle but are generally painless. In some cases, surgery may be needed to correct the condition.

Inguinal hernia: When a portion of the intestines pushes through an abnormal opening or weakening of the abdominal wall and into the groin or scrotum, it is known as an inguinal hernia (pronounced: in-gwuh-nul her-nee-uh). The hernia may look like a bulge or swelling in the groin area. It can be corrected with surgery.

Disorders of the Penis

Disorders affecting the penis include the following.

Inflammation of the penis: Symptoms of penile inflammation include redness, itching, swelling, and pain. Balanitis occurs when the glans (the head of the penis) becomes inflamed. Posthitis is foreskin inflammation, which is usually due to a yeast or bacterial infection.

Hypospadias: This is a disorder in which the urethra opens on the underside of the penis, not at the tip.

If you think you have symptoms of a problem with your reproductive system or if you have questions about your growth and development, talk to your doctor—many problems with the male reproductive system can be treated.

Chapter 29

Circumcision

Alternative Names

Foreskin removal; removal of foreskin

Definition

Circumcision is the surgical removal of the foreskin of the penis.

Description

The healthcare provider will usually numb the penis with local anesthesia before the procedure starts. The numbing medicine may be injected at the base of the penis, in the shaft, or applied as a cream.

There are a variety of ways to perform a circumcision. Most commonly, the foreskin is pushed from the head of the penis and clamped with a metal or plastic ring-like device.

If the ring is metal, the foreskin is cut off and the metal device is removed. The wound heals in five to seven days.

If the ring is plastic, a piece of suture is tied tightly around the foreskin. This pushes the tissue into a groove in the plastic over the head of the penis. Within five to seven days, the plastic covering the penis falls free, leaving a completely healed circumcision.

The baby may be given a sweetened pacifier or lollipop during the procedure. Tylenol (acetaminophen) may be given afterward.

In older and adolescent boys, circumcision is usually done under general anesthesia while the child is completely asleep. The foreskin is removed and stitched onto the remaining skin of the penis. Stitches that dissolve are used to close the wound. They will be absorbed by the body within seven to ten days. The wound may take up to three weeks to heal.

Why the Procedure Is Performed

Circumcision is often performed in healthy boys for cultural or religious reasons. In the United States, a newborn boy is usually circumcised before he leaves the hospital. Jewish boys, however, are circumcised when they are eight days old.

In other parts of the world, including Europe, Asia, and South and Central America, circumcision is rare in the general population.

The merits of circumcision have been debated. Opinions about the need for circumcision in healthy boys vary among healthcare providers. Some believe there is great value to having an intact foreskin, such as allowing for a more natural sexual response during adulthood.

Rather than routinely recommending circumcision for healthy boys, many healthcare providers allow the parents to make the decision after presenting them with the pros and cons.

There is no compelling medical rationale for the procedure in healthy boys, although some boys have a medical condition requiring circumcision.

In 1999 the American Academy of Pediatrics revised their policy statement on circumcision, and this policy is supported by the American Medical Association. A summary of the policy is below:

> "Existing scientific evidence demonstrates potential medical benefits of newborn male circumcision; however, these data are not sufficient to recommend routine neonatal circumcision. In circumstances in which there are potential benefits and risks, yet the procedure is not essential to the child's current well-being, parents should determine what is in the best interest of the child. To make an informed choice, parents of all male infants should be given accurate and unbiased information and be provided the opportunity to discuss this decision. If a decision for circumcision is made, procedural analgesia should be provided."

Risks

Risks related to circumcision:

- Bleeding
- Infection
- Redness around the surgery site
- Injury to the penis

Some research has suggested that uncircumcised male infants have an increased risk of certain conditions, including:

- cancer of the penis;
- certain sexually transmitted diseases including human immunodeficiency virus (HIV);
- infections of the penis;
- phimosis (tightness of the foreskin that prevents it from retracting);
- urinary tract infections.

The overall increased risk for these conditions is thought to be relatively small.

Proper hygiene of the penis and safe sexual practices can help prevent many of these conditions. Proper hygiene is always important, but is thought to be especially important for uncircumcised males.

Outlook (Prognosis)

Circumcision is considered a very safe procedure for both newborns and older children.

Recovery

Healing time for newborns after circumcision usually is about one week. Place petroleum jelly (Vaseline) onto the area after changing the diaper. This helps protect the healing area. Some swelling and yellow crust formation around the site is normal.

For older children and adolescents, healing may take up to three weeks. In most cases, the child will be released from the hospital on the day of the surgery.

At home, older children should avoiding vigorous exercise while the wound heals. If bleeding occurs during the first twenty-four hours after surgery, use a clean cloth to apply pressure to the wound for ten minutes. Place an ice pack on the area (twenty minutes on, twenty minutes off) for the first twenty-four hours after surgery. This helps reduce swelling and pain.

Bathing or showering is usually allowed. The surgical cut may be gently washed with mild, unscented soap.

Change the dressing at least once a day and apply an antibiotic ointment. If the dressing gets wet, change it promptly.

Use prescribed pain medicine as directed. Pain medicines should not be needed longer than four to seven days. In infants, use only acetaminophen (Tylenol), if needed.

Call your pediatrician or surgeon if:

- new bleeding occurs;
- pus drains from the area of the surgical cut;
- pain becomes severe or lasts for longer than expected;
- the entire penis looks red and swollen.

Chapter 30

Preventing Pregnancy

Chapter Contents

Section 30.1

Birth Control Methods: How Well Do They Work?

"Birth Control Methods: How Well Do They Work?," March 2007, reprinted with permission from www.kidshealth.org. Copyright © 2007 The Nemours Foundation. This information was provided by KidsHealth, one of the largest resources online for medically reviewed health information written for parents, kids, and teens. For more articles like this one, visit www.KidsHealth.org, or www.TeensHealth.org.

Some birth control methods work better than others. Table 30.1 below compares how well different birth control methods work.

The most effective way to prevent pregnancy is abstinence. However, within the first year of committing to abstinence, many couples become pregnant because they have sex anyway but don't use protection. So it's a good idea even for people who don't plan to have sex to be informed about birth control.

Couples who do have sex need to use birth control properly and every time to prevent pregnancy. For example, Table 30.1 below shows that the birth control pill can be effective in preventing pregnancy. But if a girl forgets to take her birth control pills, then this is not an effective method for her. Condoms can be an effective way to prevent pregnancy, too. But if a guy forgets to use a condom or doesn't use it correctly, then it's not an effective way for him to prevent pregnancy.

For every one hundred couples using each type of birth control, Table 30.1 shows how many of these couples will get pregnant within a year. The information shown is for *all* couples, not just teenage couples. Some birth control methods may be less effective for teen users. For example, teenage girls who use fertility awareness (also called the rhythm method) may have an even greater chance of getting pregnant than adult women because their bodies have not yet settled into a regular menstrual cycle.

We list the effectiveness of different birth control methods based on their typical use rates. Typical use refers to how the average person uses that method of birth control (compared to "perfect" use, which means no mistakes are made in using that method).

For us to consider a birth control method completely effective, no couples will become pregnant while using that method. Very effective means that between 1 and 2 out of 100 couples become pregnant while using that method. Effective means that 2 to 12 out of 100 couples become pregnant while using that method. Moderately effective means that 13 to 20 out of 100 couples become pregnant while using that method. Less effective means that 21 to 40 out of 100 couples become

Table 30.1. Effectiveness of Birth Control Methods

Method of Birth Control	How Many Couples Using This Method Will Get Pregnant in a Year?	How Well Does This Method Work in Preventing Pregnancy?	Can This Method Also Protect Against STDs?
Consistent Abstinence	None	Completely effective	Yes
Birth Control Patch ("The Patch")	5 to 8 out of 100	Effective	No
Birth Control Pill ("The Pill")	5 to 8 out of 100	Effective	No
Birth Control Ring ("The Ring")	5 to 8 out of 100	Effective	No
Female Condom	21 out of 100	Less effective	Yes
Male Condom	15 out of 100	Moderately effective	Yes
Birth Control Shot	3 out of 100	Effective	No
Diaphragm	16 out of 100	Moderately effective	No
Emergency Contraception	1 to 2 out of 100	Very effective	No
Intrauterine Device (IUD)	Fewer than 1 out of 100	Very effective	No
Fertility Awareness	25 out of 100	Less effective	No
Spermicide	29 out of 100	Less effective	No
Withdrawal ("Pulling Out")	27 out of 100	Less effective	No
Not Using Any Birth Control	85 out of 100	Not effective	No

pregnant while using that method. And not effective means that more than 40 out of 100 couples become pregnant while using that method.

In addition to preventing pregnancy, abstinence and condoms provide some protection against sexually transmitted diseases (STDs). However, most birth control methods do not provide much protection against STDs.

Choosing a birth control method based on how well it works is important, but there are other things to keep in mind when choosing a form of birth control. These include:

- how easy a particular birth control method is to use;
- how much a particular birth control method costs;
- whether a person has a health condition or is taking medication that will interfere; with how well a particular birth control method works.

Section 30.2

Condoms: Basic Facts

"Birth Control: Condom," February 2007, reprinted with permission from www.kidshealth.org. Copyright © 2007 The Nemours Foundation. This information was provided by KidsHealth, one of the largest resources online for medically reviewed health information written for parents, kids, and teens. For more articles like this one, visit www.KidsHealth.org, or www.TeensHealth.org.

What Is It?

Condoms are considered a barrier method of contraception. There are male condoms and female condoms. A male condom is a thin latex (a type of rubber) sheath that is worn on the penis. A female condom is a polyurethane sheath with a flexible ring at either end. One end is closed and is inserted into the vagina, the other end is open and the ring sits outside the opening of the vagina. The male condom is far more widely used and is sometimes called a "rubber" or "prophylactic."

How Does It Work?

The condom works by keeping semen (the fluid that contains sperm) from entering the vagina. The male condom is placed on a guy's penis when it becomes erect. It is unrolled all the way to the base of the penis while holding the tip of the condom to leave some extra rubber. This creates a space for semen after ejaculation and makes it less likely that the condom will break.

After the guy ejaculates, he should hold the condom at the base of the penis as he pulls out of the vagina. He must do this while the penis is still erect to prevent the condom from slipping off when he gets soft. If this happens, sperm could enter the vagina.

The female condom is inserted into the vagina using the closed-end ring. The other ring creates the open end of the condom. The sheath then lines the walls of the vagina creating a barrier between the sperm and the cervix. The male and female condoms should not be used at the same time because they can get stuck together and cause one or the other to slip during intercourse, making them ineffective. The female condom can be inserted up to eight hours prior to intercourse. It should be removed immediately after sex.

A used condom should be thrown in the garbage, not down the toilet. Once a condom is used, it cannot be reused. A new condom should be used each time you have sex and it must be used from start to finish every time you have sex to prevent pregnancy and sexually transmitted diseases (STDs). Never use oil-based lubricants such as mineral oil, petroleum jelly, or baby oil with condoms because these substances can break down the rubber.

And if a condom ever seems dry, sticky, or stiff when it comes out of the package, or if it is past its expiration date, throw it away and use a new one. It's a good idea to have several condoms on hand in case there is a problem with one. It's best to store unused condoms in a cool, dry place.

How Well Does It Work?

Over the course of one year, fifteen out of one hundred typical couples who rely on male condoms alone to prevent pregnancy will have an accidental pregnancy. The use of the female condom is a little less reliable and twenty-one out of one hundred couples will have an unintended pregnancy.

Of course, these are average figures and the chance of getting pregnant depends on whether you use this method correctly and every time you have sex. In fact studies show that, although it's possible for condoms to break or slip during intercourse, the most common reason that condoms "fail" is that the couple fails to use one at all.

Experts used to think that using spermicide with a condom would decrease the pregnancy rate as well as help fight against STDs. However, more recent information indicates that this is not necessarily true and spermicide does not help make condoms more effective.

In general, how well each type of birth control method works depends on a lot of things. One factor is whether the method chosen is convenient—and whether the person remembers to use it correctly all the time.

Abstinence (not having sex) is the only method that always prevents pregnancy and STDs.

Protection Against STDs

Most male condoms are made of latex. Those made of lambskin may offer less protection against some STDs, including human immunodeficiency virus (HIV), so use of latex condoms is recommended. For people who may have an allergic skin reaction to latex, both male and female condoms made of polyurethane are available.

When properly used, latex and polyurethane condoms are effective against most STDs. Condoms do not protect against infections spread from sores on the skin not covered by a condom (such as the base of the penis or scrotum). For those having sex, condoms must always be used to protect against STDs even when using another method of birth control.

Possible Side Effects

Most men and women have no problems using condoms. Side effects that can occasionally occur include:

- allergy to latex condoms;
- irritation of the penis or the vagina from spermicides or lubricants that some condoms are treated with.

Who Uses It?

Couples who are responsible enough to stop and put a condom on each time before sex and people who want protection against STDs use condoms. Because condoms are the only method of birth control currently available for men, they allow the guy to take responsibility for birth control and STD protection. Condoms are also a good choice for people who do not have a lot of money to spend on birth control.

How Do You Get It?

Condoms are available without a prescription and are sold in drugstores, supermarkets, and even vending machines (in some stores, they're in the "Family Planning" aisle). Condoms come in different sizes, textures, and colors.

How Much Does It Cost?

Condoms are the least expensive and most available method of birth control—other than abstinence, of course. Male condoms cost about $0.50 to $1 each and are less expensive when they are bought in boxes that contain several condoms.

In addition, many health centers and family planning clinics (such as Planned Parenthood) and some schools distribute them free of charge. Female condoms are a little more expensive and cost about $2 to $3 per condom.

Section 30.3

Vasectomy

Excerpted from "Facts about Vasectomy Safety," National Institute of Child Health and Human Development, August 17, 2006.

Vasectomy is a simple operation designed to make a man sterile, or unable to father a child. It is used as a means of contraception in many parts of the world. A total of about fifty million men have had a vasectomy—a number that corresponds to roughly 5 percent of all married couples of reproductive age. In comparison, about 15 percent of couples rely on female sterilization for birth control.

Approximately half a million vasectomies are performed in the United States each year. About one out of six men over age thirty-five has been vasectomized, the prevalence increasing along with education and income. Among married couples in this country, only female sterilization and oral contraception are relied upon more often for family planning.

Vasectomy involves blocking the tubes through which sperm pass into the semen. Sperm are produced in a man's testis and stored in an adjacent structure known as the epididymis. During sexual climax, the sperm move from the epididymis through a tube called the vas deferens and mix with other components of semen to form the ejaculate. All vasectomy techniques involve cutting or otherwise blocking both the left and right vas deferens, so the man's ejaculate will no longer contain sperm, and he will not be able to make a woman pregnant.

Vasectomy Techniques

In the conventional approach, a physician makes one or two small incisions, or cuts, in the skin of the scrotum, which has been numbed with a local anesthetic. The vas is cut, and a small piece may be removed. Next, the doctor ties the cut ends and sews up the scrotal incision. The entire procedure is then repeated on the other side.

An improved method, devised by a Chinese surgeon, has been widely used in China since 1974. This so-called nonsurgical or no-scalpel vasectomy was introduced into the United States in 1988, and many doctors are now using the technique here.

In a no-scalpel vasectomy, the doctor feels for the vas under the skin of the scrotum and holds it in place with a small clamp. Then a special instrument is used to make a tiny puncture in the skin and stretch the opening so the vas can be cut and tied. This approach produces very little bleeding, and no stitches are needed to close the punctures, which heal quickly by themselves. The newer method also produces less pain and fewer complications than conventional vasectomy.

Post-Vasectomy

Regardless of how it is performed, vasectomy offers many advantages as a method of birth control. Like female sterilization, it is a highly effective one-time procedure that provides permanent contraception. But vasectomy is medically much simpler than female sterilization, has a lower incidence of complications, and is much less expensive.

After vasectomy, the patient will probably feel sore for a few days, and he should rest for at least one day. However, he can expect to recover completely in less than a week. Many men have the procedure on a Friday and return to work on Monday. Although complications such as swelling, bruising, inflammation, and infection may occur, they are relatively uncommon and almost never serious. Nevertheless, men who develop these symptoms at any time should inform their physician.

A man can resume sexual activity within a few days after vasectomy, but precautions should be taken against pregnancy until a test shows that his semen is free of sperm. Generally, this test is performed after the patient has had ten to twenty post-vasectomy ejaculations. If sperm are still present in the semen, the patient is told to return later for a repeat test.

A major study of vasectomy side effects occurring within eight to ten years after the procedure was published in the *British Medical Journal* in 1992. This study—the Health Status of American Men, or HSAM—was sponsored by the National Institute of Child Health and Human Development (NICHD). Investigators questioned 10,590 vasectomized men, and an equal number of nonvasectomized men, to see if they had developed any of ninety-nine different disorders. After a total of 182,000 person-years of follow-up, only one condition, epididymitis/orchitis (defined as painful, swollen, and tender epididymis or testis)—was found to be more common after vasectomy. This local inflammation most often occurs during the first year after surgery. Treated with heat, it usually clears up within a week.

Disadvantages of Vasectomy

The chief advantage of vasectomy—its permanence—is also its chief disadvantage. The procedure itself is simple, but reversing it is difficult, expensive, and often unsuccessful. Researchers are studying new methods of blocking the vas that may produce less tissue damage and scarring and might thus permit more successful reversal. But these methods are all experimental, and their effectiveness has not yet been confirmed. It is possible to store semen in a sperm bank to preserve the possibility of producing a pregnancy at some future date. However, doing this is costly, and the sperm in stored semen do not always remain viable (able to cause pregnancy). For all of these reasons, doctors advise that vasectomy be undertaken only by men who are prepared to accept the fact that they will no longer be able to father a child. The decision should be considered along with other contraceptive options and discussed with a professional counselor. Men who are married or in a serious relationship should also discuss the issue with their partners.

Although it is extremely effective for preventing pregnancy, vasectomy does not offer protection against acquired immunodeficiency syndrome (AIDS) or other sexually transmitted diseases. Consequently, it is important that vasectomized men continue to use condoms, preferably latex, which offer considerable protection against the spread of disease, in any sexual encounter that carries the risk of contracting or transmitting infection.

Masculinity and Sexuality

Vasectomy does not affect production or release of testosterone, the male hormone responsible for a man's sex drive, beard, deep voice, and other masculine traits. The operation also has no effect on sexuality. Erections, climaxes, and the amount of ejaculate remain the same.

Occasionally, a man may experience sexual difficulties after vasectomy, but these almost always have an emotional basis and can usually be alleviated with counseling. More often, men who have undergone the procedure, and their partners, find that sex is more spontaneous and enjoyable once they are freed from concerns about contraception and accidental pregnancy.

Immune Reactions to Sperm

After vasectomy, the testes continue to make sperm. When the sperm cells die, they are absorbed by the body, much like unused sperm in a nonvasectomized man. Nevertheless, many vasectomized men develop immune reactions to sperm, although current evidence indicates that these reactions do not cause any harm.

Ordinarily, sperm do not come in contact with immune cells, so they do not elicit an immune response. But vasectomy breaches the barriers that separate immune cells from sperm, and many men develop anti-sperm antibodies after undergoing the procedure. This has given rise to concern on the part of doctors and researchers, because immune reactions against parts of one's own body sometimes cause disease. Rheumatoid arthritis, juvenile diabetes, and multiple sclerosis are just some of the illnesses suspected or known to be caused by immune reactions of this type.

Immune reactions can also contribute to the development of atherosclerosis, the clogging of arteries that leads to heart attacks. In the late 1970s, after a study of ten monkeys showed an increased risk of atherosclerosis in vasectomized animals, doctors became concerned that vasectomy might increase the risk of heart disease in men.

Other, more persuasive research results, however, indicated that these concerns were not warranted. In particular, the HSAM study provided a high level of reassurance. Researchers conducting this study found no evidence that vasectomized men were more likely than others to develop heart disease or any other immune illnesses.

Vasectomy has been used for about a century as a means of sterilization. It has a long track record as a safe and effective method of contraception and is relied upon by millions of people throughout the world. On the basis of much evidence, experts believe that vasectomy can safely continue to be used as it has been in the past, while further research is carried out.

Chapter 31

Vasectomy Reversal

Vasectomies can be reversed even after very long periods of time, sometimes after more than twenty-five years. Sperm are constantly being produced in men and even after time, there should be viable sperm. However, the success of the reversal, in terms of achieving a pregnancy, is dependent upon the experience of the surgeon, the age and fertility status of the female partner, and the length of time since the vasectomy.

The surgeon noted that he both cauterized and tied the vas during surgery. Would that reduce the positive outcome of an operation?

No. The outcome of the surgery is more dependent upon what is found at the time of the reversal as well as the experience of the surgeon performing the reversal surgery. During the reversal, the surgeon will check for sperm within the vas. If sperm is present, then the two ends of the vas deferens can be put back together, and the success rate should be fairly high. However, if there is no sperm at the end of the vas, there is likely a blockage closer to the testicle. Then, a more complicated surgery may be performed, but this procedure has a lower success rate.

"Vasectomy Reversals: Frequently Asked Questions," by Moshe Wald, M.D. Reprinted with permission of the University of Iowa Department of Urology, © 2006.

Is there ever any nerve damage when a vasectomy is performed? If reversed, will the nerves restore themselves?

It is possible but rare that significant pain from nerve damage can occur after a vasectomy. There are some cases where a reversal will help with the pain, but these are rare. A full work-up should be performed before undergoing a vasectomy reversal as the success rate in getting rid of the pain may not be very high.

How is the surgery performed? Does it require general anesthetic and how many hours? How about recovery?

Most vasectomy reversals are performed as an outpatient surgery and can be done under local, regional, or general anesthesia. It typically takes approximately three to four hours using an operating microscope to perform the surgery. Recovery is variable and can take anywhere from five to fourteen days. We recommend avoiding heavy lifting and sexual intercourse during the first four weeks after this surgery.

Does insurance pay for vasectomy reversal?

The cost of the surgery, as well as whether or not it is covered by insurance, is variable, and dependent upon where the surgery is performed and the patient's individual insurance policy.

What is the typical cost?

Cost can range anywhere from approximately $2,000 to $12,000, depending upon the surgeon, the type of practice where it is performed, and what part of the country the patient lives in.

Is there anyone who is automatically* not *a candidate for vasectomy reversal?

There are certainly some patients who are better candidates than others; time from the vasectomy is not necessarily a reason not to have a reversal. However, in the case of a couple where the woman has, for instance, had a tubal ligation, sperm aspiration combined with in-vitro fertilization is probably a better choice than performing vasectomy reversal followed by tubal ligation reversal.

Please explain the probability of any side effects . . . impotence, urinary incontinence, etc.

Side effects are typically minimal and usually would include swelling, pain, or bruising; however, the vasectomy itself and the reversal should not have any effect upon potency or urinary function.

What is the effective rate of reversal?

The success rate varies based on several factors. Time from the vasectomy certainly helps to predict how likely it would be to be able to put the two ends of the vas deferens back together; however, getting return of sperm into the ejaculate does not guarantee pregnancy, so pregnancy rates typically vary from 30 to 70 percent, whereas patency rate, that is the return of sperm, can be as high as 95 percent.

Are there other means of "fertility" that I should consider as options to reversal?

The only other option to a reversal that would allow use of a man's sperm with the woman's egg would be surgical sperm retrieval (through either extraction or aspiration) combined with in-vitro fertilization. The sperm removed from the testicle can be injected directly into the eggs that have been retrieved from the woman after she has been stimulated with hormone injections.

This is a very effective but expensive treatment with relatively good success rates. However, it is not possible to remove enough sperm from the man's testicle to inseminate the woman.

If antibodies from your immune system are present, why does this affect pregnancy rates?

There is some debate about the effects of antibodies on pregnancy rates after vasectomy reversal. Approximately 70 to 80 percent of men who have had vasectomies will have antibodies to their sperm. However, these antibodies rarely prevent the sperm from fertilizing the egg. Therefore, we counsel patients that it is unnecessary to routinely test for antibodies, as they rarely will have a bad effect upon the success rate.

What are the risks of cancer and do they increase with the reversal?

There was a report several years ago stating that men with vasectomies had a higher rate of prostate cancer. This report has since been challenged and, for the most part, disproven. There is also no evidence to show that reversal of the vasectomy would have any effect upon risk of cancer.

How many times can a reversal be done?

There is no maximum number of times that a man can have a reversal, although the success rate may decrease with increased number of reversals. However, there is good data to show that "redo-reversals" can have as high a success rate as first-time reversals. The more surgery is performed, the greater the likelihood of scarring in the scrotum, making subsequent surgeries more difficult.

What are my options if you do not find sperm in the vas at the time of surgery?

If the surgeon is experienced in doing vasectomy reversals, they should be able to find the blockage, which is likely to be in the epididymis, and perform the bypass above that point. However, if the surgeon is not able to perform this bypass, then the best thing to do is reattach the two ends of the vas and hope for the best. That is why it is important that prior to surgery, the patient question the surgeon regarding their experience in vasectomy reversals to determine if they would be able to perform both types of bypasses.

I had a reversal and checked okay at six weeks. Would scarring be a concern after this amount of time?

Scarring can occur at any time after a vasectomy reversal although it typically occurs within the first six months. Therefore, even if there was sperm in the ejaculate after six weeks, it is possible that scarring could occur later on. We typically offer sperm banking in case late scarring does occur.

How would I find a good surgeon for the procedure?

It is important to choose a surgeon who performs reversals on a regular basis, preferably someone with fellowship training or other special training in male infertility. Patients should ask the surgeon how often they perform the procedure, what their own personal success rate is, both in obtaining sperm and pregnancy rates, and if they have the ability to perform both types of reversals.

Are there any effects to the sperm quality after several years of a vasectomy and reattachment?

The sperm quality should return to normal three to six months following a reversal as it takes that long for the testicles to make new sperm. However, the count and the motility may be lower after reversal due to partial blockage or scarring.

How often should you check on scarring?

We typically recommend checking every three months, and we offer sperm banking based upon the quality of the sample. The chance of scarring is approximately 7 to 10 percent in the first one to two years following a successful reversal.

What are the statistics of men in the United States who are infertile and can that be reversed?

The incidence of male infertility is not well known, however, approximately 15 percent of U.S. couples have fertility problems and half of those are related to the male factor. Therefore, in any couple that is having fertility problems, there is a 50 percent chance that the male may be involved and therefore he should be evaluated.

Is it safe to get a boy a vasectomy for his eighteenth birthday then be able to switch it back later when he decides to have children?

No, we do not feel that is a reasonable option. Vasectomy reversals do not always work and in someone who is both young and never fathered children, it is probably not a good idea. We would counsel this patient to reconsider having a vasectomy. Prior to a vasectomy, the patient and his partner should be absolutely sure that they are done having children.

How does one prepare for the vasectomy or the reversal?

Prior to a vasectomy, the patient and his partner should be absolutely sure that they are done having children. There are no special preparations in terms of abstaining from ejaculation prior to either the vasectomy or the reversal. The patient should be aware that a vasectomy reversal is a more expensive procedure than the original vasectomy and likely will take longer to recover.

What is the recovery for a vasectomy and the reversal?

Most men will recover from a vasectomy in a couple of days. We typically recommend taking it easy for two days, using ice packs and scrotal support, and then going back to work two or three days later. However, vasectomy reversals tend to take longer, depending on the type of work that the patient does. While some men can return to a desk job in three or four days, we recommend that heavy construction and lifting should be avoided for four weeks after a vasectomy reversal.

What is the oldest age for a male to be considered for reversal?

The success of the reversal is related more to the age of the female rather than the male. Therefore, there is no age limit for a reversal.

Have any studies been done to show what the psychological/emotional problems are for a vasectomy or reversal?

A report on psychological factors prior to a vasectomy has suggested that most men are not worried about having a vasectomy, but they are a little concerned regarding the recovery of a vasectomy. Very few men have reported serious psychological or emotional problems following their vasectomy.

Chapter 32

Infertility

It is estimated that up to 15 percent of all couples encounter a problem with fertility; one-third of the cases are related to the male partner, one-third are related to the female, and one-third are a combination of both. So, in 50 percent of all infertile couples, a male fertility problem plays a role in the couple's inability to conceive. It is generally accepted that an evaluation of fertility problems should begin whenever the patients express concern and that the male and female should be evaluated simultaneously.

Why Male Infertility Occurs

There are many causes of male infertility. It is estimated that between 30 and 40 percent of men evaluated for infertility will be found to have a varicocele. It is currently believed that the number one cause of male infertility is varicocele. A varicocele is a dilation or swelling of the veins that drain the testicle. Varicocele can occur on one or both sides, but is most common on the left side. It is felt that varicoceles cause male infertility by raising the temperature of the testicles.

Abnormalities in hormone production may be a factor. Decreased testosterone levels can lead to low sperm counts. Other hormones such as follicle stimulating hormone (FSH) and leuteinizing hormone (LH) may play a role as well.

Excerpted from "Male Infertility," by Moshe Wald, M.D. and Jay I. Sandlow, M.D. Reprinted with permission of the University of Iowa Department of Urology, © 2006.

A wide range of chemical substances can affect sperm quality and/or quantity, including medications. The medications listed below all have been associated with male infertility:

- Anabolic steroids
- Antihypertensives
- Allopurinol
- Erythromycin
- Chemotherapy
- Cimetidine
- Colchicine
- Cyclosporine
- Dilantin
- Gentamicin
- Nitrofurantoin
- Tetracycline

Other drugs associated with infertility include: alcohol, tobacco, excessive caffeine, marijuana, heroin, and methadone.

Previous surgical procedures may play a role. Prior surgeries to the groin, pelvis, or abdominal area may have damaged nerves or structures necessary for ejaculation.

Testicular trauma or torsion may affect fertility. Testicular torsion is a condition in which the testicle twists on the cord that attaches it to the body. Approximately 30 to 40 percent of men with a history of testicular torsion have an abnormal semen analysis.

Diseases such as diabetes mellitus or multiple sclerosis can impair potency as well as ejaculation.

Infections of the reproductive tract also affect male fertility. Bacteria can affect semen quality and can produce an obstruction within the tract, especially at the epididymis. The most common sites of infection are the prostate gland, the epididymis, the seminal vesicles, and the testicle. The mumps virus, if contracted after puberty, can affect fertility. Testicular damage occurs in approximately 10 percent of patients who develop mumps after puberty.

What to Expect at the Initial Visit

A thorough medical history, physical examination, and a semen analysis are the cornerstones of the male fertility evaluation. The patient will be asked to abstain from ejaculation for approximately seventy-two hours prior to the doctor visit. On the day of the visit, he will be asked to provide a semen sample for analysis. The semen sample provides valuable information, and is more than just the "sperm count." Multiple parameters are examined, including the volume (amount) of the ejaculate, the sperm density (count), percent motility (the percent of sperm moving), and speed (forward progression).

Minimal Standards of Adequacy

- Volume: 1.5–5.0 milliliters
- Sperm: 20 million per milliliter
- Motility: Over 60 percent
- Speed: Grade 2 or higher
- Morphology: Greater than 60 percent are normal shape
- Fructose: Present

The sperm count is given, and it is reported in two ways. First, as the number of sperm per milliliter of ejaculate. A "normal" sperm count is typically sixty to eighty million, but could be much higher. Another very important aspect of the semen analysis is sperm motility. That is, the sperm's ability to move. Between 50 and 60 percent of the sperm cells should be motile. They are also "graded" on the quality of their movement on a scale from zero to four. The semen analysis also reports the sperm's shape or morphology. To be considered normal, a sperm must have an oval head, a normal mid-piece, and a tail. An abnormal sperm could have a tapered head or two tails. The semen analysis also reports the presence or absence of fructose. A nutrient for sperm, fructose is normally present in the semen. The volume of the ejaculate is also measured and reported. A normal amount is one and a half to five milliliters. Too little semen decreases the odds of the sperm reaching the ovum. Too much semen can dilute the sperm count and reduce the chances of impregnation.

At the initial visit, in addition to the semen analysis, a health history will be obtained. Questions regarding past infections of the urinary tract, past surgical procedures, alcohol and tobacco use, medication use, and past testicular trauma will be asked. Questions regarding conditions of the work environment, such as exposures to chemicals and high temperatures, will also be asked. The health history also includes questions regarding sexual practices, timing of intercourse, and sexual habits.

A physical examination will be performed, as well. During the physical, the patient will be evaluated for factors that may contribute to infertility, including, a varicocele.

If the physician suspects a hormone imbalance, hormone levels will be drawn.

Considerable discussion often occurs at the initial physician visit. Quite frequently, couples have questions. The physician and the patient (or couple) discuss the possible causes of the infertility, as well as decide on a treatment plan.

Treatment Options

The treatment plan begins with the physician counseling the patients regarding sexual practices. They are reminded that the optimal timing for intercourse is every forty-eight hours during the time when ovulation is most likely. They are cautioned to avoid lubricants, or use them very sparingly, as lubricants can impair sperm survival. Even saliva can impair sperm survival.

Lifestyle changes may be a part of the treatment plan. Alcohol, tobacco, and marijuana are all considered toxic to sperm. Decreasing the consumption of these drugs, or eliminating them altogether, will be recommended.

If hormonal abnormalities are found to be the cause of the infertility, hormonal replacement therapy is prescribed. This may be either in the form of an injection self-administered periodically throughout the week, or a tablet taken every day.

Treatment with antibiotics may be prescribed if a patient shows an infection or inflammation in any of the organs associated with sperm production or transportation. Such infections can lead to decreased fertility.

It is possible to correct a varicocele with a surgical procedure called varicocelectomy, or varix ligation. During this procedure, a small incision is made in the groin area and the enlarged veins are tied off. This procedure is performed on an outpatient basis.

Assisted reproductive treatments have revolutionized male infertility care. These procedures manipulate sperm in a controlled manner and have greatly facilitated pregnancy. The procedures include:

- **Intrauterine insemination (IUI):** Involves depositing a large number of specially processed sperm into the uterus at the optimal point in the menstrual cycle.
- **In vitro fertilization (IVF):** Involves harvesting eggs from the female partner and combining them with sperm in a carefully controlled laboratory procedure.
- **Gamete intrafallopian transfer (GIFT):** Involves hyperstimulation of the ovum. The ovum are not removed from the body, rather, they are mixed with processed sperm in a specialized catheter and immediately transferred to the fallopian tubes.
- **Intracytoplasmic sperm injection (ICSI):** Usually performed in a major IVF center; involves injecting a single sperm into an egg; considered a highly specialized technique.

These new technologies have added an entirely new dimension to male infertility treatment. One important consideration in the use of these "high-tech" treatments is the cost. Unfortunately, these forms of treatment may not be covered by insurance plans.

Special Populations

Men who have sustained spinal cord injuries may be unable to ejaculate. Yet it may be possible for them to father a child utilizing one of several outpatient procedures. In the first procedure, which requires approximately five minutes, a special vibrator is placed on the underside of the tip of the penis. This stimulates the ejaculatory reflex and ejaculation may occur. If it does not stimulate the reflex, other procedures such as electro-ejaculation or vasal aspiration may be performed. The sperm obtained may then be manipulated for use in any of the above-mentioned assisted reproductive treatments.

Vasectomy reversal has greatly increased over the past twenty years, owing in part to the increasing number of men who have had a vasectomy and subsequently desire more children. During the procedure, the surgeon uses an operating microscope to assist with the reconnection of the ends of the vas deferens. One factor that influences the success rate is the length of time between the vasectomy and the reversal. The longer the time interval, the lower the success rate. Another factor is surgical expertise. When researching surgeons, it is important to ask how many procedures he/she has performed, how often, and specifics regarding his/her success rate.

The diagnosis of male infertility can invoke many emotions. Frustration, fear, anger, anxiety, and depression are all common emotional responses. When approaching the diagnostic process, it is important to remember that male infertility is not uncommon, it is treatable, and that knowledgeable, expert health care professionals can assist the patients in achieving their goal.

Frequently Asked Questions

Are there any sexual positions that you recommend to increase chances of pregnancy?

Typically, the only one that has been shown to make any difference, is after ejaculation, having the woman lie with her legs elevated or propped up on a pillow for about fifteen or twenty minutes.

How can a couple tell whether their lack of ability to conceive is caused by the man or the woman?

Since approximately half of infertility problems involve the man, we typically recommend obtaining one or two semen analyses prior to the workup of the woman, unless there are obvious female problems.

Are there any over-the-counter products that increase fertility?

No. There is a dietary supplement that has been advertised but, to date, there is insufficient evidence to show that it really changes fertility.

How do tight jeans cause a low sperm count?

That is actually a myth. There is very good evidence that shows that tight jeans and tight underwear, as well as all types of clothing do not have any effect on sperm count. There is really no difference in boxers versus briefs, tight jeans versus loose pants.

Can a vasectomy be reversed?

Yes. Vasectomy reversal can be successful. It is dependent upon several factors including the time from vasectomy, the experience of the surgeon, and type of vasectomy reversal performed.

How much time do you usually let go by before testing for a fertility problem?

I leave that up to the couple. The definition of infertility is inability to get pregnant after one year of unprotected intercourse. Some couples want to know before a year, and it is not unreasonable to start with something easy such as a semen analysis.

What is retrograde ejaculation, and how can it be prevented?

Retrograde ejaculation is fairly uncommon and is typically associated with a neurologic disorder or previous abdominal surgery. It is not something that can be prevented, but it can be treated. Treatment is based on the specific underlying problem.

Quick question!! I had a tubal pregnancy; after that he had a vasectomy, what are the chances of that failing?

The chances of a vasectomy failing are dependent upon whether or not the man has undergone an adequate test to show that he truly is sterile. Once he has been confirmed to be sterile, the chances of failure are approximately 1 in 4,500.

What causes varicocele, and how does it affect fertility? What can be done to correct it?

Varicoceles are very common and tend to develop during adolescence. Fifteen percent of all men have varicoceles, but not all varicoceles affect fertility. It appears that decreased fertility is based on increased temperature within the testicles. They can be corrected by surgery or by radiologic placement of coils in the dilated veins. The success rate is fairly reasonable with improvement in sperm parameters in approximately 65 to 70 percent of patients and natural conception occurring in approximately 30 to 40 percent of patients.

What is Peyronie's disease, and can it cause infertility?

Peyronie's disease does not cause infertility, but may be associated with erectile dysfunction. It is a curvature of the penis when it is erect. It is typically seen in men between ages thirty and fifty. It tends to be self-limited, meaning, it will stop progressing by itself. It does not always need to be treated.

What are the chances of conceiving after a man has a vasectomy?

The chances of conception after a man has had a vasectomy and has been confirmed to be sterile are approximately 1 in 4,500. The chances of conception after a vasectomy reversal are related to several issues including the type of reversal, the age of the female partner, the time from vasectomy, and the sperm count after the reversal.

What chances are there if I have a spinal injury? I do ejaculate.

If you do ejaculate, then the chance of conception would be related to the ability to get an erection as well as the sperm count and motility. Assisted reproductive techniques such as artificial insemination may improve those chances.

I have heard that a new food supplement called proXeed® can help couples improve their chances for conception by improving the quality of the man's sperm. Is there any truth to this one?

This is the dietary supplement that I referred to earlier. There are very few studies that talk about the effect and none of these studies examine the chance for conception. For now, I tend to tell couples to use caution with this product, as there have not been any good studies performed to date.

What causes some men to have fertility problems?

Fertility problems can be related to many factors including varicoceles, blockages, infection, hormonal problems, as well as genetic causes. Seeking help from a male fertility specialist is a good start to determining the problem as well as the answer.

It has been a year, and no pregnancy, so should we assume he is infertile?

Although there has been no pregnancy after a year, I would not consider him sterile without a semen specimen showing no sperm.

My husband had a disease when he was a child that has led to him not producing sperm at all. Is there any way to change that?

That one is best answered by consultation with a male fertility specialist to determine if there are any reversible causes for his condition.

My boyfriend doesn't have any trouble getting an erection, but doesn't always ejaculate. Is this ok?

Yes. It is not uncommon to occasionally not ejaculate.

Do men go through any type of male menopause?

This is controversial. There are some who believe that as men age, they go through what is called "andropause." However, the evidence is conflicting, and there is no definite agreement on this condition.

What causes lack of ejaculate?

That can be due to different causes including infection, blockage, or neurologic problems. It would require evaluation by a urologist or male fertility specialist.

What are the latest treatments for infertility?

This is a fairly broad question. Much of the treatments now evolve around assisted reproductive techniques such as artificial insemination and in vitro fertilization. However, it is very important that prior to proceeding with these treatments, both partners are evaluated. There are often problems discovered, some of which are medically important when evaluating the infertile male. These should be addressed.

Can you tell us more about varicoceles?

As I mentioned, varicoceles are dilated veins around the testicles. Although they do not cause fertility problems in all men who have them, they are the most common cause of male infertility. They typically lead to increased testicular temperature, even when they are only on one side. They can cause low sperm counts, low motility, and even effect sperm function. They are typically diagnosed by physical exam and treatment is aimed at eradicating the veins. This can be either through surgery or radiographic methods.

What is the process for in-vitro?

In vitro fertilization is essentially uniting an egg and a sperm in a dish to promote fertilization. The fertilized egg is then placed back inside the woman so that implantation can occur. Typically, the woman is placed on hormonal injections so that she will make multiple eggs for fertilization.

What is the percentage of infertility being caused by psychological problems?

Male sexual problems are estimated to account for approximately 5 percent of male infertility cases. There is some evidence that psychological problems, including stress, can affect hormonal function. This, in turn, can have an effect on fertility. Other factors may also be involved.

What drugs are best for hypertension if you are trying to have a baby?

The only antihypertensives that would have an effect on the male would be those that would cause difficulties with erection. The physician monitoring hypertension can select a drug that will have minimal effects.

Does the use of marijuana cause infertility or other testicular problems?

Yes. Marijuana is a well-known cause of fertility problems. It tends to cause hormonal problems as well as having a direct effect on the testicles. This can be with long-term as well as short-term use although short-term use tends to be reversible. However, it is important to realize that it takes approximately three months for the testicles to make sperm. Therefore, even after the marijuana is no longer used, it may be several months or more before those effects have been reversed.

What other drugs cause fertility problems?

Many drugs can have an effect on sperm production. Sulfasalazine, a drug that is used in Crohn disease, is well known to do this. Most hormonal supplements, including anabolic steroids, as well as other street drugs, can have an adverse effect on fertility. Antibiotics, alcohol, and tobacco all have been shown to have some effects on fertility.

What questions should a patient ask before undergoing a vasectomy reversal?

The success rate of vasectomy reversal is dependent upon several factors. Although the time from vasectomy is important, the experience of the surgeon performing the procedure is also an important factor. A surgeon should be able to perform both a vasovasostomy as well as vasoepididymostomy. It is also important that the surgeon uses an operating microscope and performs reversals on a regular basis. Furthermore, it is important to find out that individual surgeon's success rate, not the success rate quoted in the literature. Finally, the pregnancy rates are dependent upon female factors as well. Therefore, women over forty may have a lower pregnancy rate even if the reversal is technically successful. This information should be readily shared with the patient prior to undergoing a procedure. However, it is also important not to undergo a vasectomy in the first place if you anticipate wanting to become fertile at some future time.

Do hot baths cause a low sperm count or is that just and old wives' tale?

Frequent and regular use of hot tubs can decrease a man's sperm count. Having said that, it probably should not be used as a method of birth control. Couples that are trying to conceive should probably avoid frequent hot tub use.

What other myths would you like to clear up regarding fertility and possibly men's sexual health?

One of the oldest myths is that there are no infertile men, only infertile women. This is obviously not true. Nearly 50 percent of infertility problems involve the male. Furthermore, there is much that can be done to improve male reproductive health, thus improving the couple's chances of conception.

Who should* not *get a vasectomy?

That is a difficult question—there are some physicians who will not perform a vasectomy on a young single male or on a man without children. My feeling is that the patient should be adequately counseled regarding the risks and benefits as well as the possibility of sperm banking prior to the vasectomy. There are no absolutes in terms of who should not get a vasectomy. The only other important point is that the patient's wife, or partner, is in complete agreement.

I have heard that exposure to toxic chemicals or radiation can cause infertility. Is this very common?

The number of toxic chemicals in use today that can cause infertility is becoming much smaller. However, we know that exposure to radiation can certainly have an effect on fertility.

I was here earlier, Please tell what can you do short of in-vitro? Our salaries will not allow that expense.

Options other than in vitro are dependent upon the cause of infertility, the male and the female factors involved, as well as the sperm count and motility.

Should the man be evaluated prior to in vitro fertilization?

There is good evidence that much of male factor infertility can be treated. Furthermore, a small but significant percentage of men with infertility have an underlying medical problem that is discovered during their evaluation. This can include hormonal problems as well as testicular cancer, infection, or blockages. Therefore, it is important that the urologist or male fertility specialist prior to proceeding with in vitro fertilization evaluate the male partner.

Does smoking or alcohol affect fertility?

Recently several studies have addressed the effects of smoking on male fertility. There is some very good evidence that smoking can have an adverse effect on sperm count, motility, and function. It is always a good idea to quit smoking, particularly when trying to conceive. Alcohol is slightly more controversial. Mild to moderate amounts of alcohol have not been shown to have any effects; however, moderate to heavy amounts can affect sperm count as well as hormone production.

Is infertility often an indicator of cancer?

No. It can be, but this is a rare finding. However, the most common type of cancer in men of reproductive age is testicular cancer. This would be discovered during the evaluation of the man.

I've read that bike-riders have to be careful what kind of seat they use as to not damage the testicles. True?

The best evidence regarding bicycle seats pertains to erection, not fertility. Any seat that causes numbness could potentially damage a man's erection. However, there has not been any evidence to show that fertility is affected.

I still want a baby, and I'm a paralyzed guy who can function correctly. Any advice?

If natural conception has been unsuccessful, I would seek an evaluation from an urologist including a history, physical exam, and a semen analysis. Specific treatment options can then be recommended.

Chapter 33

Sexually Transmitted Diseases (STDs)

Chapter Contents

Section 33.1

Basic Information about STDs

Reprinted from "Sexually Transmitted Diseases (STDs)," National Institute of Child Health and Human Development, May 25, 2007.

What are sexually transmitted diseases (STDs)?

STDs, also called sexually transmitted infections or STIs, are diseases that you get by having intimate sexual contact, that is, having sex (vaginal, oral, or anal intercourse), with someone who already has the disease. Every year, STDs affect more than thirteen million people.

What are the different types of STDs?

Researchers have identified more than twenty different kinds of STDs, which can fall into two main groups:

- **STDs caused by bacteria:** These diseases can be treated and often cured with antibiotics. Some bacterial STDs include: chlamydia, gonorrhea, trichomoniasis, and syphilis.
- **STDs caused by viruses:** These diseases can be controlled, but not cured. If you get a viral STD, you will always have it. Some viral STDs include: human immunodeficiency virus (HIV)/ acquired immunodeficiency syndrome (AIDS), genital herpes, genital warts, human papillomavirus (HPV), hepatitis B virus, and cytomegalovirus.

What are the symptoms of STDs?

The symptoms vary among the different types of STDs. Some examples of common symptoms include the following:

- Unusual discharge from the penis or vagina
- Sores or warts on the genital area
- Burning while urinating

- Itching and redness in the genital area
- Anal itching, soreness, or bleeding

If you are having any of these symptoms or think you might have an STD, talk to your health care provider.

How can STDs be prevented?

The only way to ensure that you won't get infected is to not have sex. This means avoiding all types of intimate sexual contact.

If you are sexually active, you can reduce your risk of getting STDs by practicing "safe sex." This means:

- using a condom for vaginal, oral, and anal intercourse—every time;
- knowing your partner and his/her STD status and health;
- having regular medical check-ups, especially if you have more than one sexual partner.

Section 33.2

Chancroid

Excerpted from "Chancroid,"

Chancroid is a bacterial disease that is spread only through sexual contact.

Causes

Chancroid is a sexually transmitted infection caused by a type of bacteria called *Haemophilus ducreyi*.

The disease is found mainly in developing and third world countries. Only a small number of cases are diagnosed in the United States each year. Most people in the United States diagnosed with chancroid have traveled outside the country to areas where the disease is known to occur frequently.

Uncircumcised men are at much higher risk than circumcised men for getting chancroid from an infected partner. Chancroid is a risk factor for the human immunodeficiency virus (HIV).

Symptoms

Within one day to two weeks after getting chancroid, a person will get a small bump in the genitals. The bump becomes an ulcer within a day of its appearance. The ulcer:

- ranges in size from one-eighth inch to two inches across;
- is painful;
- has sharply defined borders;
- has irregular or ragged borders;
- has a base that is covered with a grey or yellowish-grey material;
- has a base that bleeds easily if banged or scraped.

About half of infected men have only a single ulcer. Women often have four or more ulcers. The ulcers appear in specific locations.

Common locations in men are:

- foreskin (prepuce);
- groove behind the head of the penis (coronal sulcus);
- shaft of the penis;
- head of the penis (glans);
- opening of the penis (urethral meatus);
- scrotum.

The ulcer may look like a chancre, the typical sore of primary syphilis.

Approximately half of the people infected with a chancroid will develop enlarged inguinal lymph nodes, the nodes located in the fold between the leg and the lower abdomen.

Half of those who have swelling of the inguinal lymph nodes will progress to a point where the nodes break through the skin, producing draining abscesses. The swollen lymph nodes and abscesses are often referred to as buboes.

Exams and Tests

Chancroid is diagnosed by looking at the ulcer(s) and checking for swollen lymph nodes, as well as by getting a culture from the base of the ulcers. There are no lab tests for chancroid as there are for syphilis.

Treatment

The infection is treated with antibiotics, including azithromycin, ceftriaxone, ciprofloxacin, and erythromycin. Large lymph node swellings need to be drained, either with a needle or local surgery.

Outlook (Prognosis)

Chancroid can get better on its own. However, some people may have months of painful ulcers and draining. Antibiotic treatment usually clears up the lesions quickly with very little scarring.

Possible Complications

Complications include urethral fistulas and scars on the foreskin of the penis in uncircumcised males. Patients with chancroid should also be checked for syphilis, HIV, and genital herpes.

Chancroids in persons with HIV may take much longer to heal.

When to Contact a Medical Professional

Call for an appointment with your health care provider if you have symptoms of chancroid. Also call if you have had sexual contact with a person known to have any STD, or if you have engaged in high-risk sexual practices.

Prevention

Chancroid is a bacterial infection that is spread by sexual contact with an infected person. Although not having sex is the only sure prevention, safe sex practices are helpful for preventing the spread of chancroid.

Having sexual relations with only one partner who you know to be disease-free is the safest and most practical "safe sex" method. Condoms provide very good protection from the spread of most sexually transmitted diseases when used properly and consistently.

Section 33.3

Chlamydia

Excerpted from "Chlamydia," Centers for Disease Control and Prevention, December 20, 2007.

What is chlamydia?

Chlamydia is a common sexually transmitted disease (STD) caused by the bacterium *Chlamydia trachomatis*, which can damage a woman's reproductive organs. Even though symptoms of chlamydia are usually mild or absent, serious complications that cause irreversible damage, including infertility, can occur "silently" before a woman ever recognizes a problem. Chlamydia also can cause discharge from the penis of an infected man.

How common is chlamydia?

Chlamydia is the most frequently reported bacterial sexually transmitted disease in the United States.

How do people get chlamydia?

Chlamydia can be transmitted during vaginal, anal, or oral sex. Chlamydia can also be passed from an infected mother to her baby during vaginal childbirth.

Any sexually active person can be infected with chlamydia. The greater the number of sex partners, the greater the risk of infection. Because the cervix (opening to the uterus) of teenage girls and young women is not fully matured and is probably more susceptible to infection, they are at particularly high risk for infection if sexually active. Since chlamydia can be transmitted by oral or anal sex, men who have sex with men are also at risk for chlamydial infection.

What are the symptoms of chlamydia?

Chlamydia is known as a "silent" disease because about three quarters of infected women and about half of infected men have no symptoms. If symptoms do occur, they usually appear within one to three weeks after exposure.

Men with signs or symptoms might have a discharge from their penis or a burning sensation when urinating. Men might also have burning and itching around the opening of the penis. Pain and swelling in the testicles are uncommon.

Men or women who have receptive anal intercourse may acquire chlamydial infection in the rectum, which can cause rectal pain, discharge, or bleeding. Chlamydia can also be found in the throats of women and men having oral sex with an infected partner.

What complications can result from untreated chlamydia?

If untreated, chlamydial infections can progress to serious reproductive and other health problems with both short-term and long-term consequences. Like the disease itself, the damage that chlamydia causes is often "silent."

To help prevent the serious consequences of chlamydia, screening at least annually for chlamydia is recommended for all sexually active women age twenty-five years and younger. An annual screening test also is recommended for older women with risk factors for chlamydia (a new sex partner or multiple sex partners). All pregnant women should have a screening test for chlamydia.

Complications among men are rare. Infection sometimes spreads to the epididymis (the tube that carries sperm from the testis), causing pain, fever, and, rarely, sterility.

Rarely, genital chlamydial infection can cause arthritis that can be accompanied by skin lesions and inflammation of the eye and urethra (Reiter syndrome).

How does chlamydia affect a pregnant woman and her baby?

In pregnant women, there is some evidence that untreated chlamydial infections can lead to premature delivery. Babies who are born to infected mothers can get chlamydial infections in their eyes and respiratory tracts. Chlamydia is a leading cause of early infant pneumonia and conjunctivitis (pink eye) in newborns.

How is chlamydia diagnosed?

There are laboratory tests to diagnose chlamydia. Some can be performed on urine; other tests require that a specimen be collected from a site such as the penis or cervix.

What is the treatment for chlamydia?

Chlamydia can be easily treated and cured with antibiotics. A single dose of azithromycin or a week of doxycycline (twice daily) are the most commonly used treatments. HIV-positive persons with chlamydia should receive the same treatment as those who are HIV negative.

All sex partners should be evaluated, tested, and treated. Persons with chlamydia should abstain from sexual intercourse until they and their sex partners have completed treatment; otherwise re-infection is possible.

Women whose sex partners have not been appropriately treated are at high risk for re-infection. Having multiple infections increases a woman's risk of serious reproductive health complications, including infertility. Retesting should be encouraged for women three to four months after treatment. This is especially true if a woman does not know if her sex partner received treatment.

How can chlamydia be prevented?

The surest way to avoid transmission of STDs is to abstain from sexual contact, or to be in a long-term mutually monogamous relationship with a partner who has been tested and is known to be uninfected.

Latex male condoms, when used consistently and correctly, can reduce the risk of transmission of chlamydia.

Any genital symptoms such as an unusual sore, discharge with odor, burning during urination, or bleeding between menstrual cycles could mean an STD infection. If a woman has any of these symptoms, she should stop having sex and consult a health care provider immediately. Treating STDs early can prevent PID. Women who are told they have an STD and are treated for it should notify all of their recent sex partners (sex partners within the preceding sixty days) so they can see a health care provider and be evaluated for STDs. Sexual activity should not resume until all sex partners have been examined and, if necessary, treated.

Sources

Centers for Disease Control and Prevention. Sexually Transmitted Diseases Treatment Guidelines 2006. *MMWR* 2006;55(No. RR-11).

Centers for Disease Control and Prevention. *Sexually Transmitted Disease Surveillance, 2006*. Atlanta, GA: U.S. Department of Health and Human Services, November 2007.

SD Datta et al. Gonorrhea and chlamydia in the United States among persons 14 to 39 years of age, 1999 to 2002. *Ann Intern Med.* 2007: 147:89–96.

Stamm W E. Chlamydia trachomatis infections of the adult. In: K. Holmes, P. Sparling, P. Mardh et al (eds). *Sexually Transmitted Diseases*, 3rd edition. New York: McGraw-Hill, 1999, 407–22.

Weinstock H, Berman S, Cates W. Sexually transmitted disease among American youth: Incidence and prevalence estimates, 2000. *Perspectives on Sexual and Reproductive Health* 2004; 36: 6–10.

Section 33.4

Genital Herpes

Reprinted from "Genital Herpes," Centers for Disease Control and Prevention, January 4, 2008.

What is genital herpes?

Genital herpes is a sexually transmitted disease (STD) caused by the herpes simplex viruses type 1 (HSV-1) or type 2 (HSV-2). Most genital herpes is caused by HSV-2. Most individuals have no or only minimal signs or symptoms from HSV-1 or HSV-2 infection. When signs do occur, they typically appear as one or more blisters on or around the genitals or rectum. The blisters break, leaving tender ulcers (sores) that may take two to four weeks to heal the first time they occur. Typically, another outbreak can appear weeks or months after the first, but it almost always is less severe and shorter than the first outbreak. Although the infection can stay in the body indefinitely, the number of outbreaks tends to decrease over a period of years.

How common is genital herpes?

Results of a nationally representative study show that genital herpes infection is common in the United States. Nationwide, at least forty-five million people ages twelve and older, or one out of five adolescents and adults, have had genital HSV infection. Over the past decade, the percentage of Americans with genital herpes infection in the United States has decreased.

Genital HSV-2 infection is more common in women (approximately one out of four women) than in men (almost one out of eight). This may be due to male-to-female transmission being more likely than female-to-male transmission.

How do people get genital herpes?

HSV-1 and HSV-2 can be found in and released from the sores that the viruses cause, but they also are released between outbreaks from skin that does not appear to have a sore. Generally, a person can only get HSV-2 infection during sexual contact with someone who has a genital HSV-2 infection. Transmission can occur from an infected partner who does not have a visible sore and may not know that he or she is infected.

HSV-1 can cause genital herpes, but it more commonly causes infections of the mouth and lips, so-called fever blisters. HSV-1 infection of the genitals can be caused by oral-genital or genital-genital contact with a person who has HSV-1 infection. Genital HSV-1 outbreaks recur less regularly than genital HSV-2 outbreaks.

What are the signs and symptoms of genital herpes?

Most people infected with HSV-2 are not aware of their infection. However, if signs and symptoms occur during the first outbreak, they can be quite pronounced. The first outbreak usually occurs within two weeks after the virus is transmitted, and the sores typically heal within two to four weeks. Other signs and symptoms during the primary episode may include a second crop of sores, and flu-like symptoms, including fever and swollen glands. However, most individuals with HSV-2 infection never have sores, or they have very mild signs that they do not even notice or that they mistake for insect bites or another skin condition.

People diagnosed with a first episode of genital herpes can expect to have several (typically four or five) outbreaks (symptomatic recurrences) within a year. Over time these recurrences usually decrease in frequency. It is possible that a person becomes aware of the "first episode" years after the infection is acquired.

What are the complications of genital herpes?

Genital herpes can cause recurrent painful genital sores in many adults, and herpes infection can be severe in people with suppressed immune systems. Regardless of severity of symptoms, genital herpes frequently causes psychological distress in people who know they are infected.

In addition, genital HSV can lead to potentially fatal infections in babies. It is important that women avoid contracting herpes during pregnancy because a newly acquired infection during late pregnancy poses a greater risk of transmission to the baby. If a woman has active genital herpes at delivery, a cesarean delivery is usually performed. Fortunately, infection of a baby from a woman with herpes infection is rare.

Herpes may play a role in the spread of human immunodeficiency virus (HIV), the virus that causes acquired immunodeficiency syndrome (AIDS). Herpes can make people more susceptible to HIV infection, and it can make HIV-infected individuals more infectious.

How is genital herpes diagnosed?

The signs and symptoms associated with HSV-2 can vary greatly. Health care providers can diagnose genital herpes by visual inspection if the outbreak is typical, and by taking a sample from the sore(s) and testing it in a laboratory. HSV infections can be diagnosed between outbreaks by the use of a blood test. Blood tests, which detect antibodies to HSV-1 or HSV-2 infection, can be helpful, although the results are not always clear-cut.

Is there a treatment for herpes?

There is no treatment that can cure herpes, but antiviral medications can shorten and prevent outbreaks during the period of time the person takes the medication. In addition, daily suppressive therapy for symptomatic herpes can reduce transmission to partners.

How can herpes be prevented?

The surest way to avoid transmission of sexually transmitted diseases, including genital herpes, is to abstain from sexual contact, or to be in a long-term mutually monogamous relationship with a partner who has been tested and is known to be uninfected.

Genital ulcer diseases can occur in both male and female genital areas that are covered or protected by a latex condom, as well as in areas that are not covered. Correct and consistent use of latex condoms can reduce the risk of genital herpes.

Persons with herpes should abstain from sexual activity with uninfected partners when lesions or other symptoms of herpes are present. It is important to know that even if a person does not have any symptoms he or she can still infect sex partners. Sex partners of infected persons should be advised that they may become infected and they should use condoms to reduce the risk. Sex partners can seek testing to determine if they are infected with HSV. A positive HSV-2 blood test most likely indicates a genital herpes infection.

Sources

Centers for Disease Control and Prevention. Sexually Transmitted Diseases Treatment Guidelines 2006. *MMWR* 2006; 55(no. RR-11).

Corey L, Wald A. Genital herpes. In: Holmes KK, Sparling PF, Mardh P et al (eds). *Sexually Transmitted Disease*, 3rd Edition. New York: McGraw-Hill, 1999, p. 285–312.

Corey L, Wald A, Patel R et al. Once-daily valacyclovir to reduce the risk of transmission of genital herpes. *New England Journal of Medicine* 2004; 350:11–20.

Wald A, Langenberg AGM, Link K, et al. Effect of condoms on reducing the transmission of herpes simplex virus type 2 from men to women. *JAMA* 2001;285: 3100–3106.

Wald A, Link K. Risk of human immunodeficiency virus infection in herpes simplex virus type 2–seropositive persons: A meta-analysis. *J Infect Dis* 2002; 185: 45–52.

Weinstock H, Berman S, Cates W. Sexually transmitted diseases among American youth: Incidence and prevalence estimates, 2000. *Perspectives on Sexual and Reproductive Health* 2004; 36:6–10.

Xu F, Sternberg M, Kottiri B, McQuillan G, Lee F, Nahmias A, Berman S, Markowitz L. National trends in herpes simplex virus type 1 and type 2 in the United States: Data from the National Health and Nutrition Examination Survey (NHANES). *JAMA* 2006; Vol 296: 964–73.

Section 33.5

Gonorrhea

Excerpted from "Gonorrhea," Centers for Disease Control and Prevention, February 28, 2008.

What is gonorrhea?

Gonorrhea is a sexually transmitted disease (STD). Gonorrhea is caused by *Neisseria gonorrhoeae*, a bacterium that can grow and multiply easily in the warm, moist areas of the reproductive tract, including the cervix (opening to the womb), uterus (womb), and fallopian tubes (egg canals) in women, and in the urethra (urine canal) in women and men. The bacterium can also grow in the mouth, throat, eyes, and anus.

How common is gonorrhea?

Gonorrhea is a very common infectious disease. The Centers for Disease Control and Prevention (CDC) estimates that more than 700,000 persons in the United States get new gonorrheal infections each year.

How do people get gonorrhea?

Gonorrhea is spread through contact with the penis, vagina, mouth, or anus. Ejaculation does not have to occur for gonorrhea to be transmitted or acquired. Gonorrhea can also be spread from mother to baby during delivery.

People who have had gonorrhea and received treatment may get infected again if they have sexual contact with a person infected with gonorrhea.

Who is at risk for gonorrhea?

Any sexually active person can be infected with gonorrhea. In the United States, the highest reported rates of infection are among sexually active teenagers, young adults, and African Americans.

What are the signs and symptoms of gonorrhea?

Some men with gonorrhea may have no symptoms at all. However, some men have signs or symptoms that appear two to five days after infection; symptoms can take as long as thirty days to appear. Symptoms and signs include a burning sensation when urinating, or a white, yellow, or green discharge from the penis. Sometimes men with gonorrhea get painful or swollen testicles.

In women, the symptoms of gonorrhea are often mild, but most women who are infected have no symptoms. Even when a woman has symptoms, they can be so nonspecific as to be mistaken for a bladder or vaginal infection. The initial symptoms and signs in women include a painful or burning sensation when urinating, increased vaginal discharge, or vaginal bleeding between periods. Women with gonorrhea are at risk of developing serious complications from the infection, regardless of the presence or severity of symptoms.

Symptoms of rectal infection in both men and women may include discharge, anal itching, soreness, bleeding, or painful bowel movements. Rectal infection also may cause no symptoms. Infections in the throat may cause a sore throat but usually cause no symptoms.

What are the complications of gonorrhea?

Untreated gonorrhea can cause serious and permanent health problems in both women and men.

In women, gonorrhea is a common cause of pelvic inflammatory disease (PID). About one million women each year in the United States develop PID. The symptoms may be quite mild or can be very severe and can include abdominal pain and fever. PID can lead to internal abscesses (pus-filled "pockets" that are hard to cure) and long-lasting, chronic pelvic pain. PID can damage the fallopian tubes enough to cause infertility or increase the risk of ectopic pregnancy. Ectopic pregnancy is a life-threatening condition in which a fertilized egg grows outside the uterus, usually in a fallopian tube.

In men, gonorrhea can cause epididymitis, a painful condition of the ducts attached to the testicles that may lead to infertility if left untreated.

Gonorrhea can spread to the blood or joints. This condition can be life threatening. In addition, people with gonorrhea can more easily contract human immunodeficiency virus (HIV), the virus that causes acquired immunodeficiency syndrome (AIDS). HIV-infected people with gonorrhea can transmit HIV more easily to someone else than if they did not have gonorrhea.

How does gonorrhea affect a pregnant woman and her baby?

If a pregnant woman has gonorrhea, she may give the infection to her baby as the baby passes through the birth canal during delivery. This can cause blindness, joint infection, or a life-threatening blood infection in the baby. Treatment of gonorrhea as soon as it is detected in pregnant women will reduce the risk of these complications. Pregnant women should consult a health care provider for appropriate examination, testing, and treatment, as necessary.

How is gonorrhea diagnosed?

Several laboratory tests are available to diagnose gonorrhea. A doctor or nurse can obtain a sample for testing from the parts of the body likely to be infected (cervix, urethra, rectum, or throat) and send the sample to a laboratory for analysis. Gonorrhea that is present in the cervix or urethra can be diagnosed in a laboratory by testing a urine sample. A quick laboratory test for gonorrhea that can be done in some clinics or doctor's offices is a Gram stain. A Gram stain of a sample from a urethra or a cervix allows the doctor to see the gonorrhea bacterium under a microscope. This test works better for men than for women.

What is the treatment for gonorrhea?

Several antibiotics can successfully cure gonorrhea in adolescents and adults. However, drug-resistant strains of gonorrhea are increasing in many areas of the world, including the United States, and successful treatment of gonorrhea is becoming more difficult. Because many people with gonorrhea also have chlamydia, another STD, antibiotics for both infections are usually given together. Persons with gonorrhea should be tested for other STDs.

It is important to take all of the medication prescribed to cure gonorrhea. Although medication will stop the infection, it will not repair any permanent damage done by the disease. People who have had gonorrhea and have been treated can get the disease again if they have sexual contact with persons infected with gonorrhea. If a person's symptoms continue even after receiving treatment, he or she should return to a doctor to be reevaluated.

How can gonorrhea be prevented?

The surest way to avoid transmission of STDs is to abstain from sexual intercourse, or to be in a long-term mutually monogamous relationship with a partner who has been tested and is known to be uninfected.

Latex condoms, when used consistently and correctly, can reduce the risk of transmission of gonorrhea.

Any genital symptoms such as discharge or burning during urination or unusual sore or rash should be a signal to stop having sex and to see a doctor immediately. If a person has been diagnosed and treated for gonorrhea, he or she should notify all recent sex partners so they can see a health care provider and be treated. This will reduce the risk that the sex partners will develop serious complications from gonorrhea and will also reduce the person's risk of becoming reinfected. The person and all of his or her sex partners must avoid sex until they have completed their treatment for gonorrhea.

Sources

Centers for Disease Control and Prevention. Sexually Transmitted Diseases Treatment Guidelines, 2006. *MMWR* 2006; 55 (No. RR-11). www.cdc.gov/std/treatment

Centers for Disease Control and Prevention. *Sexually Transmitted Disease Surveillance, 2006*. Atlanta, GA: U.S. Department of Health and Human Services, November 2007.

Hook EW III and Handsfield HH. Gonococcal infections in the adult. In: K. Holmes, P. Sparling, P. Markh et al (eds). *Sexually Transmitted Diseases*, 3rd Edition. New York: McGraw-Hill, 1999, 451–66.

Weinstock H, Berman S, Cates W. Sexually transmitted disease among American youth: Incidence and prevalence estimates, 2000. *Perspectives on Sexual and Reproductive Health* 2004; 36: 6–10.

Section 33.6

Hepatitis B

"Hepatitis B," April 2007, reprinted with permission from www.kidshealth.org. Copyright © 2007 The Nemours Foundation. This information was provided by KidsHealth, one of the largest resources online for medically reviewed health information written for parents, kids, and teens. For more articles like this one, visit www.KidsHealth.org, or www.TeensHealth.org.

What is it?

Hepatitis (pronounced: hep-uh-tie-tiss) is a disease of the liver. It is usually caused by a virus, although it can also be caused by long-term overuse of alcohol or other toxins (poisons).

Although there are several different types of hepatitis, hepatitis B is a type that can move from one person to another through blood and other bodily fluids. It can be transmitted through sexual intercourse and through needles—such as those shared by intravenous drug or steroid users who have the virus, or tattoo needles that haven't been properly sterilized. A pregnant woman can also pass hepatitis B to her unborn baby. You cannot catch hepatitis B from an object, such as a toilet seat.

What are the symptoms?

Someone with hepatitis B may have symptoms similar to those caused by other viral infections, such as the flu—for example, tiredness, nausea, loss of appetite, mild fever, and vomiting—as well as abdominal pain or pain underneath the right ribcage where the liver is.

Hepatitis B can also cause jaundice, which is a yellowing of the skin and the whites of the eyes, and may cause the urine to appear brownish.

How long until symptoms appear?

Someone who has been exposed to hepatitis B may have symptoms one to four months later. Some people with hepatitis B don't notice symptoms until they become quite severe. Some have few or no symptoms, but even someone who doesn't notice any symptoms can still transmit the disease to others. Some people carry the virus in their bodies and are contagious for the rest of their lives.

What can happen?

Hepatitis B can be very dangerous to a person's health, leading to liver damage and an increased risk of liver cancer. Of babies born to women who have the hepatitis B virus, 90 percent will have the virus unless they receive a special immune injection and the first dose of hepatitis B vaccine at birth.

How is it prevented?

Because hepatitis B can easily be transmitted through blood and most body fluids, it can be prevented by:

- abstaining from sex (not having oral, vaginal, or anal sex);
- always using latex condoms for all types of sexual intercourse;
- avoiding contact with an infected person's blood;
- not using intravenous drugs or sharing any drug paraphernalia;
- not sharing things like toothbrushes or razors.

Tattoo parlors sometimes reuse needles without properly sterilizing them, so be sure to research and choose tattoo and piercing providers carefully.

To help prevent the spread of hepatitis B, health care professionals wear gloves at all times when in contact with blood or body fluids, and are usually required to be immunized against the hepatitis B virus.

There is an immunization (vaccine) against hepatitis B. The immunization is given as a series of three shots over a six-month period. Newborn babies in the United States now routinely receive this immunization series. Teens who see their health care provider for yearly exams are also likely to be given the hepatitis B immunization if they haven't had it before. Immunization programs have been responsible for a significant drop in the number of cases of hepatitis B among teens over the past ten years.

Sometimes, if someone has been recently exposed to the hepatitis B virus, a doctor may recommend a shot of immune globulin containing antibodies against the virus to try to prevent the person from coming down with the disease. For this reason, it's especially important to see a doctor quickly after any possible exposure to the virus.

How is it treated?

If you think you may have hepatitis B or if you have been intimate with someone who may have hepatitis B, you need to see your doctor or gynecologist, who will do blood tests. Let the doctor know the best way to reach you confidentially with any test results.

If your doctor diagnoses hepatitis B, you may get medicines to help fight it. Sometimes, people need to be hospitalized for a little while if they are too sick to eat or drink. Most people with hepatitis B feel better within six months.

Section 33.7

HIV and AIDS

Excerpted from "HIV and AIDS: Are You at Risk?" Centers for Disease Control and Prevention, August 1, 2007.

What is HIV and how can I get it?

HIV—the human immunodeficiency virus—is a virus that kills your body's "CD4 cells." CD4 cells (also called T-helper cells) help your body fight off infection and disease. HIV can be passed from person to person if someone with HIV infection has sex with or shares drug injection needles with another person. It also can be passed from a mother to her baby when she is pregnant, when she delivers the baby, or if she breastfeeds her baby.

What is AIDS?

AIDS—the acquired immunodeficiency syndrome—is a disease you get when HIV destroys your body's immune system. Normally, your immune system helps you fight off illness. When your immune system fails you can become very sick and can die.

What do I need to know about HIV?

The first cases of AIDS were identified in the United States in 1981, but AIDS most likely existed here and in other parts of the world for many years before that time. In 1984 scientists proved that HIV causes AIDS.

Anyone can get HIV. The most important thing to know is how you can get the virus.

You can get HIV in the following ways:

- By having unprotected sex—sex without a condom—with someone who has HIV. The virus can be in an infected person's blood, semen, or vaginal secretions and can enter your body through tiny cuts or sores in your skin, or in the lining of your vagina, penis, rectum, or mouth.
- By sharing a needle and syringe to inject drugs or sharing drug equipment used to prepare drugs for injection with someone who has HIV.
- From a blood transfusion or blood clotting factor that you got before 1985. (But today it is unlikely you could get infected that way because all blood in the United States has been tested for HIV since 1985.)

Babies born to women with HIV also can become infected during pregnancy, birth, or breastfeeding.

You cannot get HIV in the following ways:

- By working with or being around someone who has HIV
- From sweat, spit, tears, clothes, drinking fountains, phones, toilet seats, or through everyday things like sharing a meal
- From insect bites or stings
- From donating blood
- From a closed-mouth kiss (but there is a very small chance of getting it from open-mouthed or "French" kissing with an infected person because of possible blood contact)

How can I protect myself?

Don't share needles and syringes used to inject drugs, steroids, vitamins, or for tattooing or body piercing. Also, don't share equipment ("works") used to prepare drugs to be injected. Many people have been infected with HIV, hepatitis, and other germs this way. Germs from an infected person can stay in a needle and then be injected directly into the next person who uses the needle.

The surest way to avoid transmission of sexually transmitted diseases is to abstain from sexual intercourse, or to be in a long-term mutually monogamous relationship with a partner who has been tested and you know is uninfected.

For persons whose sexual behaviors place them at risk for STDs, correct and consistent use of the male latex condom can reduce the risk of STD transmission. However, no protective method is 100 percent effective, and condom use cannot guarantee absolute protection against any STD. The more sex partners you have, the greater your chances are of getting HIV or other diseases passed through sex.

Condoms used with a lubricant are less likely to break. However, condoms with the spermicide nonoxynol-9 are not recommended for STD/HIV prevention. Condoms must be used correctly and consistently to be effective and protective. Incorrect use can lead to condom slippage or breakage, thus diminishing the protective effect. Inconsistent use, e.g., failure to use condoms with every act of intercourse, can result in STD transmission because transmission can occur with a single act of intercourse.

Don't share razors or toothbrushes because they may have the blood of another person on them.

If you are pregnant or think you might be soon, talk to a doctor or your local health department about being tested for HIV. If you have HIV, drug treatments are available to help you and they can reduce the chance of passing HIV to your baby.

How do I know if I have HIV or AIDS?

You might have HIV and still feel perfectly healthy. The only way to know for sure if you are infected is to be tested. Talk with a knowledgeable health care provider or counselor both before and after you are tested. You can go to your doctor or health department for testing.

Your doctor or health care provider can give you a confidential HIV test. The information on your HIV test and test results are confidential, as is your other medical information. This means it can be shared only with people authorized to see your medical records. You can ask your doctor, health care provider, or HIV counselor at the place you are tested to explain who can obtain this information. For example, you may want to ask whether your insurance company could find out your HIV status if you make a claim for health insurance benefits or apply for life insurance or disability insurance.

The Centers for Disease Control and Prevention (CDC) recommends that everyone know their HIV status. How often you should an HIV test depends on your circumstances. If you have never been tested for HIV, you should be tested. CDC recommends being tested at least once a year if you do things that can transmit HIV infection, such as the following:

- Injecting drugs or steroids with used injection equipment
- Having sex for money or drugs
- Having sex with an HIV-infected person
- Having more than one sex partner since your HIV test
- Having a sex partner who has had other sex partners since your last HIV test

In many states, you can be tested anonymously. These tests are usually given at special places known as anonymous testing sites. When you get an anonymous HIV test, the testing site records only a number or code with the test result, not your name. A counselor gives you this number at the time your blood, saliva, or urine is taken for the test, then you return to the testing site (or perhaps call the testing site, for example with home collection kits) and give them your number or code to learn the results of your test.

If you have been tested for HIV and the result is negative and you never do things that might transmit HIV infection, then you and your health care provider can decide whether you need to get tested again.

What can I do if the test shows I have HIV?

Although HIV is a very serious infection, many people with HIV and AIDS are living longer, healthier lives today, thanks to new and effective treatments. It is very important to make sure you have a doctor who knows how to treat HIV. If you don't know which doctor to use, talk with a health care professional or trained HIV counselor. If you are pregnant or are planning to become pregnant, this is especially important.

There also are other things you can do for yourself to stay healthy. Here are a few:

- Follow your doctor's instructions. Keep your appointments. Your doctor may prescribe medicine for you. Take the medicine just the way he or she tells you to because taking only some of your medicine gives your HIV infection more chance to grow.
- Get immunizations (shots) to prevent infections such as pneumonia and flu. Your doctor will tell you when to get these shots.
- If you smoke or if you use drugs not prescribed by your doctor, quit.
- Eat healthy foods. This will help keep you strong, keep your energy and weight up, and help your body protect itself.
- Exercise regularly to stay strong and fit.
- Get enough sleep and rest.

Section 33.8

Human Papillomavirus (HPV)

Excerpted from "HPV and Men," Centers for Disease Control and Prevention, April 3, 2008.

Genital human papillomavirus (HPV) is a common virus. Most sexually active people in the United States (U.S.) will have HPV at some time in their lives. There are more than forty types of HPV that are passed on during sex. These types can infect the genital areas of men, including the skin on and around the penis or anus.

What are the health problems caused by HPV in men?

Most men who get HPV (of any type) never develop any symptoms or health problems. But some types of HPV can cause genital warts. Other types can cause penile cancer or anal cancer. The types of HPV that can cause genital warts are not the same as the types that can cause penile or anal cancer. Anal cancer is not the same as colorectal cancer. Colorectal cancer is more common than anal cancer, but it is not caused by HPV.

How common are HPV-related health problems in men?

About 1 percent of sexually active men in the United States have genital warts at any one time.

Penile cancer is rare, especially in circumcised men. In the United States, it affects about 1 in every 100,000 men. The American Cancer Society (ACS) estimated that about 1,530 men would be diagnosed with penile cancer in the United States in 2006.

Anal cancer is also uncommon—especially in men with healthy immune systems. According to the ACS, about 1,900 men will be diagnosed with anal cancer in the United States in 2007.

Some men are more likely to develop HPV-related diseases than others:

- Gay and bisexual men are seventeen times more likely to develop anal cancer than heterosexual men.
- Men with weak immune systems, including those who have human immunodeficiency virus (HIV), are more likely than other men to develop anal cancer. Men with HIV are also more likely to get severe cases of genital warts that are hard to treat.

What are the signs and symptoms?

Among men who do develop health problems, these are some of the signs to look for.

Signs of genital warts are as follows:

- One or more growths on the penis, testicles, groin, thighs, or anus.
- Warts may be raised, flat, or cauliflower-shaped. They usually do not hurt.
- Warts may appear within weeks or months after sexual contact with an infected person.

Signs and symptoms of anal cancer are as follows:

- Sometimes there are no signs or symptoms.
- Anal bleeding, pain, itching, or discharge.
- Swollen lymph nodes in the anal or groin area.
- Changes in bowel habits or the shape of your stool.

Signs of penile cancer are as follows:

- First signs: changes in color, skin thickening, or a build-up of tissue on the penis.
- Later signs: a growth or sore on the penis. It is usually painless, but in some cases, the sore may be painful and bleed.
- There may be no symptoms until the cancer is quite advanced.

How do men get HPV?

HPV is passed on through genital contact—most often during vaginal and anal sex. Since HPV usually causes no symptoms, most men and women can get HPV—and pass it on—without realizing it. People can have HPV even if years have passed since they had sex.

Is there a test for HPV in men?

Currently, there is no test designed or approved to find HPV in men. The only approved HPV test on the market is for women, for use as part of cervical cancer screening. There is no general test for men or women to check one's overall "HPV status." But HPV usually goes away on its own, without causing health problems. So an HPV infection that is found today will most likely not be there a year or two from now.

Remember, HPV is very common in men and women. Most men with HPV will never develop health problems from it. Finding out if you have HPV is not as important as finding out if you have the diseases that it can cause. Scientists are still studying how best to screen for penile and anal cancers in men who may be at highest risk for those diseases.

Is there a test to find genital warts?

Most of the time, you can see genital warts. Some doctors may use a vinegar solution to help find flat warts—but this test can sometimes wrongly identify normal skin as a wart.

Is there a test to screen for HPV-related cancers in men?

Screening tests can find early signs of disease in people who are not yet sick. Screening tests for penile or anal cancer are not widely recommended.

Some experts recommend yearly anal Pap tests for gay, bisexual, and HIV-positive men, since anal cancer is more common in these groups. This test can find abnormal cells in the anus that could turn into cancer over time. If abnormal cells are found, they can be removed. The

Centers for Disease Control and Prevention (CDC) does not recommend anal Pap tests because there is not enough research to show that removing abnormal anal cells actually prevents anal cancer from developing in the future. More studies are needed to understand if anal Pap tests and treatment of abnormal cells prevent anal cancer in men.

You can check for any abnormalities on your penis, scrotum, or around the anus. See your doctor if you find warts, blisters, sores, ulcers, white patches, or other abnormal areas on your penis—even if they do not hurt.

Is there a treatment or cure for HPV?

There is no treatment or cure for HPV. But there are ways to treat the health problems caused by HPV in men.

Genital warts can be treated with medicine, removed (surgery), or frozen off. Some of these treatments involve a visit to the doctor. Others can be treated at home by the patient himself. No one treatment is better than another. But warts often come back within a few months after treatment—so several treatments may be needed. Treating genital warts may not necessarily lower a man's chances of passing HPV on to his sex partner. Because of this, some men choose not to treat genital warts. If they are not treated, genital warts may go away on their own, stay the same, or grow (in size or number). They will not turn into cancer or threaten your health.

Penile and anal cancers can be treated with new forms of surgery, radiation therapy, and chemotherapy. Often, two or more of these treatments are used together. Patients should decide with their doctors which treatments are best for them.

Are there ways to lower my chances of getting HPV?

Because HPV is so common and usually invisible, the only sure way to prevent it is not to have sex. Even people with only one lifetime sex partner can get HPV, if their partner was infected with HPV. Condoms (used all the time and the right way) may lower your chances of passing HPV to a partner or developing HPV-related diseases. But HPV can infect areas that are not covered by a condom—so condoms may not fully protect against HPV.

I heard about a new HPV vaccine—can it help me?

The new HPV vaccine was developed to protect against most cervical cancers and genital warts. At this point, it is licensed to be used only in girls and women, ages nine to twenty-six years. Studies are now being done to find out if the vaccine is also safe in men, and if it can protect them against genital warts and certain penile and anal cancers. The U.S. Food and Drug Administration (FDA) will consider licensing the vaccine for boys and men if there is proof that it is safe and effective for them.

I just found out that my partner has HPV. What does it mean for my health?

Partners usually share HPV. If you have been with your partner for a long time, you probably have HPV already. Most sexually active adults will have HPV at some time in their lives. Men with healthy immune systems rarely develop health problems from HPV. But you should check regularly for any abnormalities on your penis. If you have a weak immune system or HIV, ask your doctor about checking for anal and penile cancers.

If your partner is new, condoms may lower your chances of getting HPV or developing HPV-related diseases. But not having sex is the only sure way to avoid HPV.

Sources

American Cancer Society (ACS). Detailed Guide: Anal Cancer. What are the Key Statistics about Anal Cancer?

ACS. Detailed Guide: Penile Cancer. What are the Key Statistics about Penile Cancer?

ACS. Detailed Guide: Cervical Cancer. What are the Key Statistics about Cervical Cancer?

Centers for Disease Control and Prevention. Sexually Transmitted Diseases Treatment Guidelines 2006. *MMWR* 2006;55(no. RR-11).

Ho GYF, Bierman R, Beardsley L, Chang CJ, Burk RD. Natural history of cervicovaginal papilloma virus infection in young women. *N Engl J Med* 1998;338:423–28.

Koutsky LA, Kiviat NB. Genital human papillomavirus. In: K. Holmes, P. Sparling, P. Mardh et al (eds). *Sexually Transmitted Diseases*, 3rd edition. New York: McGraw-Hill, 1999, p. 347–59.

Kiviat NB, Koutsky LA, Paavonen J. Cervical neoplasia and other STD-related genital tract neoplasias. In: K. Holmes, P. Sparling, P. Mardh et al (eds). *Sexually Transmitted Diseases*, 3rd edition. New York: McGraw-Hill, 1999, p. 811–31.

Myers ER, McCrory DC, Nanda K, Bastian L, Matchar DB. Mathematical model for the natural history of human papillomavirus infection and cervical carcinogenesis. *American Journal of Epidemiology* 2000; 151(12):1158–71.

Watts DH, Brunham RC. Sexually transmitted diseases, including HIV infection in pregnancy. In: K. Holmes, P. Sparling, P. Mardh et al (eds). *Sexually Transmitted Diseases*, 3rd edition. New York: McGraw-Hill, 1999, 1089–1132.

Weinstock H, Berman S, Cates W. Sexually transmitted disease among American youth: Incidence and prevalence estimates, 2000. *Perspectives on Sexual and Reproductive Health 2004*; 36: 6–10.

Section 33.9

Pubic Lice (Crabs)

"Facts about Pubic Lice" is reprinted from "Pubic 'Crab' Lice Fact Sheet" and "Treatment" is reprinted from "Pubic 'Crab' Lice Treatment," Centers for Disease Control and Prevention, May 16, 2008.

Facts about Pubic Lice

What are pubic lice?

Also called crab lice or "crabs," pubic lice are parasitic insects found primarily in the pubic or genital area of humans. Pubic lice infestation is found worldwide and occurs in all races, ethnic groups, and levels of society.

What do pubic lice look like?

Pubic lice have forms: the egg (also called a nit), the nymph, and the adult.

Nit: Nits are lice eggs. They can be hard to see and are found firmly attached to the hair shaft. They are oval and usually yellow to white. Pubic lice nits take about six to ten days to hatch.

Nymph: The nymph is an immature louse that hatches from the nit (egg). A nymph looks like an adult pubic louse but it is smaller. Pubic lice nymphs take about two to three weeks after hatching to mature into adults capable of reproducing. To live, a nymph must feed on blood.

Adult: The adult pubic louse resembles a miniature crab when viewed through a strong magnifying glass. Pubic lice have six legs; their two front legs are very large and look like the pincher claws of a crab. This is how they got the nickname "crabs." Pubic lice are tan to grayish-white in color. Females lay nits and are usually larger than males. To live, lice must feed on blood. If the louse falls off a person, it dies within one to two days.

Where are pubic lice found?

Pubic lice usually are found in the genital area on pubic hair; but they may occasionally be found on other coarse body hair, such as hair on the legs, armpits, mustache, beard, eyebrows, or eyelashes. Pubic lice on the eyebrows or eyelashes of children may be a sign of sexual exposure or abuse. Lice found on the head are generally head lice, not pubic lice.

Animals do not get or spread pubic lice.

What are the signs and symptoms of pubic lice?

Signs and symptoms of pubic lice include the following:

- Itching in the genital area
- Visible nits (lice eggs) or crawling lice

How did I get pubic lice?

Pubic lice usually are spread through sexual contact and are most common in adults. Pubic lice found on children may be a sign of sexual exposure or abuse. Occasionally, pubic lice may be spread by close personal contact or contact with articles such as clothing, bed linens, or towels that have been used by an infested person. A common misunderstanding is that pubic lice are spread easily by sitting on a toilet seat. This would be extremely rare because lice cannot live long away from a warm human body and they do not have feet designed to hold onto or walk on smooth surfaces such as toilet seats.

Persons infested with pubic lice should be investigated for the presence of other sexually transmitted diseases.

How is a pubic lice infestation diagnosed?

A pubic lice infestation is diagnosed by finding a "crab" louse or egg (nit) on hair in the pubic region or, less commonly, elsewhere on the body (eyebrows, eyelashes, beard, mustache, armpit, perianal area, groin, trunk, scalp). Pubic lice may be difficult to find because there may be only a few. Pubic lice often attach themselves to more than one hair and generally do not crawl as quickly as head and body lice. If crawling lice are not seen, finding nits in the pubic area strongly suggests that a person is infested and should be treated. If you are unsure about infestation or if treatment is not successful, see a health care provider for a diagnosis. Persons infested with pubic lice should be investigated for the presence of other sexually transmitted diseases.

Although pubic lice and nits can be large enough to be seen with the naked eye, a magnifying lens may be necessary to find lice or eggs.

Treatment

A lice-killing lotion containing 1 percent permethrin or a mousse containing pyrethrins and piperonyl butoxide can be used to treat pubic ("crab") lice. These products are available over-the-counter without a prescription at a local drug store or pharmacy. These medications are safe and effective when used exactly according to the instructions in the package or on the label.

Lindane shampoo is a prescription medication that can kill lice and lice eggs. However, lindane is not recommended as a first-line therapy. Lindane can be toxic to the brain and other parts of the nervous system; its use should be restricted to patients who have failed treatment with or cannot tolerate other medications that pose less risk. Lindane should not be used to treat premature infants, persons with a seizure disorder, women who are pregnant or breastfeeding, persons who have very irritated skin or sores where the lindane will be applied, infants, children, the elderly, and persons who weigh less than 110 pounds.

Malathion lotion 0.5% (Ovide®) is a prescription medication that can kill lice and some lice eggs; however, malathion lotion (Ovide) currently has not been approved by the U.S. Food and Drug Administration (FDA) for treatment of pubic ("crab") lice.

Ivermectin has been used successfully to treat lice; however, ivermectin currently has not been approved by the FDA for treatment of lice.

How to Treat Pubic Lice Infestations

Warning: See special instructions for treatment of lice and nits on eyebrows or eyelashes. The lice medications described in this section should not be used near the eyes.

1. Wash the infested area; towel dry.
2. Carefully follow the instructions in the package or on the label. Thoroughly saturate the pubic hair and other infested areas with lice medication. Leave medication on hair for the time recommended in the instructions. After waiting the recommended time, remove the medication by following carefully the instructions on the label or in the box.
3. Following treatment, most nits will still be attached to hair shafts. Nits may be removed with fingernails or by using a fine-toothed comb.
4. Put on clean underwear and clothing after treatment.
5. To kill any lice or nits remaining on clothing, towels, or bedding, machine-wash and machine-dry those items that the infested person used during the two to three days before treatment. Use hot water (at least 130°F) and the hot dryer cycle.
6. Items that cannot be laundered can be dry-cleaned or stored in a sealed plastic bag for two weeks.
7. All sex partners from within the previous month should be informed that they are at risk for infestation and should be treated.
8. Persons should avoid sexual contact with their sex partner(s) until both they and their partners have been successfully treated and reevaluated to rule out persistent infestation.
9. Repeat treatment in nine to ten days if live lice are still found.
10. Persons with pubic lice should be evaluated for other sexually transmitted diseases (STDs).

Special instructions for treatment of lice and nits found on eyebrows or eyelashes:

- If only a few live lice and nits are present, it may be possible to remove these with fingernails or a nit comb.
- If additional treatment is needed for lice or nits on the eyelashes, careful application of ophthalmic-grade petrolatum ointment (only available by prescription) to the eyelid margins two to four times a day for ten days is effective. Regular Vaseline should not be used because it can irritate the eyes.

Section 33.10

Scabies

Reprinted from "Scabies," Centers for Disease Control and Prevention, February 4, 2008.

What is scabies?

Scabies is an infestation of the skin with the microscopic mite *Sarcoptes scabiei*. Infestation is common, found worldwide, and affects people of all races and social classes. Scabies spreads rapidly under crowded conditions where there is frequent skin-to-skin contact between people, such as in hospitals, institutions, child-care facilities, and nursing homes.

What are the signs and symptoms of scabies infestation?

- Pimple-like irritations, burrows, or rash of the skin, especially the webbing between the fingers; the skin folds on the wrist, elbow, or knee; the penis, the breast, or shoulder blades.
- Intense itching, especially at night and over most of the body.
- Sores on the body caused by scratching. These sores can sometimes become infected with bacteria.

How did I get scabies?

By direct, prolonged, skin-to-skin contact with a person already infested with scabies. Contact generally must be prolonged (a quick handshake or hug will usually not spread infestation). Infestation is easily spread to sexual partners and household members. Infestation may also occur by sharing clothing, towels, and bedding.

Who is at risk for severe infestation?

People with weakened immune systems and the elderly are at risk for a more severe form of scabies, called Norwegian or crusted scabies. Scabies is spread more easily by persons who have Norwegian, or crusted, scabies than by persons with other types of scabies.

How long will mites live?

Once away from the human body, mites usually do not survive more than forty-eight to seventy-two hours. When living on a person, an adult female mite can live up to a month.

Did my pet spread scabies to me?

No. Pets become infested with a different kind of scabies mite. If your pet is infested with scabies, (also called mange) and they have close contact with you, the mite can get under your skin and cause itching and skin irritation. However, the mite dies in a couple of days and does not reproduce. The mites may cause you to itch for several days, but you do not need to be treated with special medication to kill the mites. Until your pet is successfully treated, mites can continue to burrow into your skin and cause you to have symptoms.

How soon after infestation will symptoms begin?

For a person who has never been infested with scabies, symptoms may take four to six weeks to begin. For a person who has had scabies before, symptoms appear within several days.

How is scabies infestation diagnosed?

Diagnosis is most commonly made by looking at the burrows or rash. A skin scraping may be taken to look for mites, eggs, or mite fecal matter (scybala) to confirm the diagnosis. Even if a skin scraping or biopsy is taken and returns negative, it is still possible that you may be infested. Typically, there are fewer than ten mites on the entire body of an infested person; this makes it easy for an infestation to be missed. However, persons with Norwegian, or crusted, scabies can be infested with thousands of mites and should be considered highly infectious.

Can scabies be treated?

Yes. Several creams or lotions that are available by prescription are approved by the U.S. Food and Drug Administration (FDA) to treat scabies. Always follow the directions provided by your physician or the directions on the package label or insert. Apply the medication to a clean body from the neck down to the toes. After leaving the medication on the body for the recommended time, take a bath or shower to wash off the cream or lotion. Put on clean clothes. All clothes, bedding, and towels used by the infested person during the three days before treatment should be washed in hot water and dried in a hot dryer. A second treatment of the body with the same cream or lotion may be necessary. Pregnant women and children are often treated with milder scabies medications such as 5 percent permethrin cream.

Who should be treated for scabies?

Anyone who is diagnosed with scabies, as well as his or her sexual partners and persons who have close, prolonged contact with the infested person should also be treated. If your health care provider has instructed family members to be treated, everyone should receive treatment at the same time to prevent reinfestation.

How soon after treatment will I feel better?

Itching may continue for two to three weeks, and does not mean that you are still infested. Your health care provider may prescribe additional medication to relieve itching if it is severe.

Section 33.11

Syphilis

Excerpted from "Syphilis," Centers for Disease Control and Prevention, January 4, 2008.

What is syphilis?

Syphilis is a sexually transmitted disease (STD) caused by the bacterium *Treponema pallidum*. It has often been called "the great imitator" because so many of the signs and symptoms are indistinguishable from those of other diseases.

How common is syphilis?

In the United States, health officials reported over 36,000 cases of syphilis in 2006, including 9,756 cases of primary and secondary (P&S) syphilis. In 2006, half of all P&S syphilis cases were reported from twenty counties and two cities; and most P&S syphilis cases occurred in persons twenty to thirty-nine years of age. The incidence of P&S syphilis was highest in women twenty to twenty-four years of age and in men thirty-five to thirty-nine years of age. In 2006, 64 percent of the reported P&S syphilis cases were among men who have sex with men (MSM).

How do people get syphilis?

Syphilis is passed from person to person through direct contact with a syphilis sore. Sores occur mainly on the external genitals, vagina, anus, or in the rectum. Sores also can occur on the lips and in the mouth. Transmission of the organism occurs during vaginal, anal, or oral sex. Pregnant women with the disease can pass it to the babies they are carrying. Syphilis cannot be spread through contact with toilet seats, doorknobs, swimming pools, hot tubs, bathtubs, shared clothing, or eating utensils.

What are the signs and symptoms in adults?

Many people infected with syphilis do not have any symptoms for years, yet remain at risk for late complications if they are not treated.

Although transmission occurs from persons with sores who are in the primary or secondary stage, many of these sores are unrecognized. Thus, transmission may occur from persons who are unaware of their infection.

Primary stage: The primary stage of syphilis is usually marked by the appearance of a single sore (called a chancre), but there may be multiple sores. The time between infection with syphilis and the start of the first symptom can range from ten to ninety days (average twenty-one days). The chancre is usually firm, round, small, and painless. It appears at the spot where syphilis entered the body. The chancre lasts three to six weeks, and it heals without treatment. However, if adequate treatment is not administered, the infection progresses to the secondary stage.

Secondary stage: Skin rash and mucous membrane lesions characterize the secondary stage. This stage typically starts with the development of a rash on one or more areas of the body. The rash usually does not cause itching. Rashes associated with secondary syphilis can appear as the chancre is healing or several weeks after the chancre has healed. The characteristic rash of secondary syphilis may appear as rough, red, or reddish brown spots both on the palms of the hands and the bottoms of the feet. However, rashes with a different appearance may occur on other parts of the body, sometimes resembling rashes caused by other diseases. Sometimes rashes associated with secondary syphilis are so faint that they are not noticed. In addition to rashes, symptoms of secondary syphilis may include fever, swollen lymph glands, sore throat, patchy hair loss, headaches, weight loss, muscle aches, and fatigue. The signs and symptoms of secondary syphilis will resolve with or without treatment, but without treatment, the infection will progress to the latent and possibly late stages of disease.

Late and latent stages: The latent (hidden) stage of syphilis begins when primary and secondary symptoms disappear. Without treatment, the infected person will continue to have syphilis even though there are no signs or symptoms; infection remains in the body. This latent stage can last for years. The late stages of syphilis can develop in about 15 percent of people who have not been treated for syphilis, and can appear ten to twenty years after infection was first acquired. In the late stages of syphilis, the disease may subsequently damage the internal organs, including the brain, nerves, eyes, heart, blood vessels, liver, bones, and joints. Signs and symptoms of the late stage of syphilis include difficulty coordinating muscle movements, paralysis, numbness, gradual blindness, and dementia. This damage may be serious enough to cause death.

How does syphilis affect a pregnant woman and her baby?

The syphilis bacterium can infect the baby of a woman during her pregnancy. Depending on how long a pregnant woman has been infected, she may have a high risk of having a stillbirth (a baby born dead) or of giving birth to a baby who dies shortly after birth. An infected baby may be born without signs or symptoms of disease. However, if not treated immediately, the baby may develop serious problems within a few weeks. Untreated babies may become developmentally delayed, have seizures, or die.

How is syphilis diagnosed?

Some health care providers can diagnose syphilis by examining material from a chancre (infectious sore) using a special microscope called a dark-field microscope. If syphilis bacteria are present in the sore, they will show up when observed through the microscope.

A blood test is another way to determine whether someone has syphilis. Shortly after infection occurs, the body produces syphilis antibodies that can be detected by an accurate, safe, and inexpensive blood test. A low level of antibodies will likely stay in the blood for months or years even after the disease has been successfully treated. Because untreated syphilis in a pregnant woman can infect and possibly kill her developing baby, every pregnant woman should have a blood test for syphilis.

What is the link between syphilis and human immunodeficiency virus (HIV)?

Genital sores (chancres) caused by syphilis make it easier to transmit and acquire HIV infection sexually. There is an estimated two- to five-fold increased risk of acquiring HIV if exposed to that infection when syphilis is present.

Ulcerative STDs that cause sores, ulcers, or breaks in the skin or mucous membranes, such as syphilis, disrupt barriers that provide protection against infections. The genital ulcers caused by syphilis can bleed easily, and when they come into contact with oral and rectal mucosa during sex, increase the infectiousness of and susceptibility to HIV. Having other STDs is also an important predictor for becoming

HIV infected because STDs are a marker for behaviors associated with HIV transmission.

What is the treatment for syphilis?

Syphilis is easy to cure in its early stages. A single intramuscular injection of penicillin, an antibiotic, will cure a person who has had syphilis for less than a year. Additional doses are needed to treat someone who has had syphilis for longer than a year. For people who are allergic to penicillin, other antibiotics are available to treat syphilis. There are no home remedies or over-the-counter drugs that will cure syphilis. Treatment will kill the syphilis bacterium and prevent further damage, but it will not repair damage already done.

Because effective treatment is available, it is important that persons be screened for syphilis on an ongoing basis if their sexual behaviors put them at risk for STDs.

Persons who receive syphilis treatment must abstain from sexual contact with new partners until the syphilis sores are completely healed. Persons with syphilis must notify their sex partners so that they also can be tested and receive treatment if necessary.

Will syphilis recur?

Having syphilis once does not protect a person from getting it again. Following successful treatment, people can still be susceptible to re-infection. Only laboratory tests can confirm whether someone has syphilis. Because syphilis sores can be hidden in the vagina, rectum, or mouth, it may not be obvious that a sex partner has syphilis. Talking with a health care provider will help to determine the need to be re-tested for syphilis after being treated.

How can syphilis be prevented?

The surest way to avoid transmission of sexually transmitted diseases, including syphilis, is to abstain from sexual contact or to be in a long-term mutually monogamous relationship with a partner who has been tested and is known to be uninfected.

Avoiding alcohol and drug use may also help prevent transmission of syphilis because these activities may lead to risky sexual behavior. It is important that sex partners talk to each other about their HIV status and history of other STDs so that preventive action can be taken.

Genital ulcer diseases, like syphilis, can occur in both male and female genital areas that are covered or protected by a latex condom, as well as in areas that are not covered. Correct and consistent use of latex condoms can reduce the risk of syphilis, as well as genital herpes and chancroid, only when the infected area or site of potential exposure is protected.

Condoms lubricated with spermicides (especially Nonoxynol-9 or N-9) are no more effective than other lubricated condoms in protecting against the transmission of STDs. Use of condoms lubricated with N-9 is not recommended for STD/HIV prevention. Transmission of an STD, including syphilis, cannot be prevented by washing the genitals, urinating, and/or douching after sex. Any unusual discharge, sore, or rash, particularly in the groin area, should be a signal to refrain from having sex and to see a doctor immediately.

Sources

Centers for Disease Control and Prevention. Sexually transmitted diseases treatment guidelines 2006. *MMWR* 2006;55(no. RR-11).

Centers for Disease Control and Prevention. *Sexually Transmitted Disease Surveillance, 2006*. Atlanta, GA: U.S. Department of Health and Human Service, November 2007.

K. Holmes, P. Mardh, P. Sparling et al (eds). *Sexually Transmitted Diseases*, 3rd Edition. New York: McGraw-Hill, 1999, chapters 33–37.

Section 33.12

Trichomoniasis

Reprinted from "Trichomoniasis," Centers for Disease Control and Prevention, December 17, 2007.

What is trichomoniasis?

Trichomoniasis is a common sexually transmitted disease (STD) that affects both women and men, although symptoms are more common in women.

How common is trichomoniasis?

Trichomoniasis is the most common curable STD in young, sexually active women. An estimated 7.4 million new cases occur each year in women and men.

How do people get trichomoniasis?

Trichomoniasis is caused by the single-celled protozoan parasite *Trichomonas vaginalis*. The vagina is the most common site of infection in women, and the urethra (urine canal) is the most common site of infection in men.

The parasite is sexually transmitted through penis-to-vagina intercourse or vulva-to-vulva (the genital area outside the vagina) contact with an infected partner. Women can acquire the disease from infected men or women, but men usually contract it only from infected women.

What are the signs and symptoms of trichomoniasis?

Most men with trichomoniasis do not have signs or symptoms; however, some men may temporarily have an irritation inside the penis, mild discharge, or slight burning after urination or ejaculation.

Some women have signs or symptoms of infection which include a frothy, yellow-green vaginal discharge with a strong odor. The infection also may cause discomfort during intercourse and urination, as well as irritation and itching of the female genital area. In rare cases, lower abdominal pain can occur. Symptoms usually appear in women within five to twenty-eight days of exposure.

What are the complications of trichomoniasis?

The genital inflammation caused by trichomoniasis can increase a woman's susceptibility to human immunodeficiency virus (HIV) infection if she is exposed to the virus. Having trichomoniasis may increase the chance that an HIV-infected woman passes HIV to her sex partner(s).

How does trichomoniasis affect a pregnant woman and her baby?

Pregnant women with trichomoniasis may have babies who are born early or with low birth weight (low birth weight is less than 5.5 pounds).

How is trichomoniasis diagnosed?

For both men and women, a health care provider must perform a physical examination and laboratory test to diagnose trichomoniasis. The parasite is harder to detect in men than in women. In women, a pelvic examination can reveal small red ulcerations (sores) on the vaginal wall or cervix.

What is the treatment for trichomoniasis?

Trichomoniasis can usually be cured with prescription drugs, either metronidazole or tinidazole, given by mouth in a single dose. The symptoms of trichomoniasis in infected men may disappear within a few weeks without treatment. However, an infected man, even a man who has never had symptoms or whose symptoms have stopped, can continue to infect or re-infect a female partner until he has been treated. Therefore, both partners should be treated at the same time to eliminate the parasite. Persons being treated for trichomoniasis should avoid sex until they and their sex partners complete treatment and have no symptoms. Metronidazole can be used by pregnant women.

Having trichomoniasis once does not protect a person from getting it again. Following successful treatment, people can still be susceptible to re-infection.

How can trichomoniasis be prevented?

The surest way to avoid transmission of sexually transmitted diseases is to abstain from sexual contact, or to be in a long-term mutually monogamous relationship with a partner who has been tested and is known to be uninfected.

Latex male condoms, when used consistently and correctly, can reduce the risk of transmission of trichomoniasis.

Any genital symptom such as discharge or burning during urination or an unusual sore or rash should be a signal to stop having sex and to consult a health care provider immediately. A person diagnosed with trichomoniasis (or any other STD) should receive treatment and should notify all recent sex partners so that they can see a health care provider and be treated. This reduces the risk that the sex partners will develop complications from trichomoniasis and reduces the risk that the person with trichomoniasis will become re-infected. Sex should be stopped until the person with trichomoniasis and all of his or her recent partners complete treatment for trichomoniasis and have no symptoms.

Sources

Centers for Disease Control and Prevention. Sexually transmitted diseases treatment guidelines 2006. *MMWR* 2006: 55 (No. RR-11).

Krieger JN and Alderete JF. Trichomonas vaginalis and trichomoniasis. In: K. Holmes, P. Markh, P. Sparling et al (eds). *Sexually Transmitted Diseases*, 3rd Edition. New York: McGraw-Hill, 1999, 587–604.

Weinstock H, Berman S, Cates W. Sexually transmitted disease among American youth: Incidence and prevalence estimates, 2000. *Perspectives on Sexual and Reproductive Health* 2004; 36: 6–10.

Chapter 34

Sexual Dysfunction

Chapter Contents

Section 34.1

Erectile Dysfunction

Excerpted from "Erectile Dysfunction," National Institute of Diabetes and Digestive and Kidney Diseases, National Institutes of Health, NIH Publication No. 06-3923, December 2005.

Erectile dysfunction, sometimes called "impotence," is the repeated inability to get or keep an erection firm enough for sexual intercourse. The word "impotence" may also be used to describe other problems that interfere with sexual intercourse and reproduction, such as lack of sexual desire and problems with ejaculation or orgasm. Using the term erectile dysfunction makes it clear that those other problems are not involved.

Erectile dysfunction, or ED, can be a total inability to achieve erection, an inconsistent ability to do so, or a tendency to sustain only brief erections. These variations make defining ED and estimating its incidence difficult. Estimates range from fifteen million to thirty million, depending on the definition used.

In older men, ED usually has a physical cause, such as disease, injury, or side effects of drugs. Any disorder that causes injury to the nerves or impairs blood flow in the penis has the potential to cause ED. Incidence increases with age: About 5 percent of forty-year-old men and between 15 and 25 percent of sixty-five-year-old men experience ED. But it is not an inevitable part of aging.

ED is treatable at any age, and awareness of this fact has been growing. More men have been seeking help and returning to normal sexual activity because of improved, successful treatments for ED.

How does an erection occur?

The penis contains two chambers called the corpora cavernosa, which run the length of the organ. A spongy tissue fills the chambers. The corpora cavernosa are surrounded by a membrane, called the tunica albuginea. The spongy tissue contains smooth muscles, fibrous tissues, spaces, veins, and arteries. The urethra, which is the channel for urine and ejaculate, runs along the underside of the corpora cavernosa and is surrounded by the corpus spongiosum.

Erection begins with sensory or mental stimulation, or both. Impulses from the brain and local nerves cause the muscles of the corpora cavernosa to relax, allowing blood to flow in and fill the spaces. The blood creates pressure in the corpora cavernosa, making the penis expand. The tunica albuginea helps trap the blood in the corpora cavernosa, thereby sustaining erection. When muscles in the penis contract to stop the inflow of blood and open outflow channels, erection is reversed.

What causes erectile dysfunction (ED)?

Since an erection requires a precise sequence of events, ED can occur when any of the events is disrupted. The sequence includes nerve impulses in the brain, spinal column, and area around the penis, and response in muscles, fibrous tissues, veins, and arteries in and near the corpora cavernosa.

Damage to nerves, arteries, smooth muscles, and fibrous tissues, often as a result of disease, is the most common cause of ED. Diseases—such as diabetes, kidney disease, chronic alcoholism, multiple sclerosis, atherosclerosis, vascular disease, and neurologic disease—account for about 70 percent of ED cases. Between 35 and 50 percent of men with diabetes experience ED.

Lifestyle choices that contribute to heart disease and vascular problems also raise the risk of erectile dysfunction. Smoking, being overweight, and avoiding exercise are possible causes of ED.

Also, surgery (especially radical prostate and bladder surgery for cancer) can injure nerves and arteries near the penis, causing ED. Injury to the penis, spinal cord, prostate, bladder, and pelvis can lead to ED by harming nerves, smooth muscles, arteries, and fibrous tissues of the corpora cavernosa.

In addition, many common medicines—blood pressure drugs, antihistamines, antidepressants, tranquilizers, appetite suppressants, and cimetidine (an ulcer drug)—can produce ED as a side effect.

Experts believe that psychological factors such as stress, anxiety, guilt, depression, low self-esteem, and fear of sexual failure cause 10 to 20 percent of ED cases. Men with a physical cause for ED frequently experience the same sort of psychological reactions (stress, anxiety, guilt, depression). Other possible causes are smoking, which affects blood flow in veins and arteries, and hormonal abnormalities, such as not enough testosterone.

How is ED diagnosed?

Patient history: Medical and sexual histories help define the degree and nature of ED. A medical history can disclose diseases that lead to ED, while a simple recounting of sexual activity might distinguish among problems with sexual desire, erection, ejaculation, or orgasm.

Using certain prescription or illegal drugs can suggest a chemical cause, since drug effects account for 25 percent of ED cases. Cutting back on or substituting certain medications can often alleviate the problem.

Physical examination: A physical examination can give clues to systemic problems. For example, if the penis is not sensitive to touching, a problem in the nervous system may be the cause. Abnormal secondary sex characteristics, such as hair pattern or breast enlargement, can point to hormonal problems, which would mean that the endocrine system is involved. The examiner might discover a circulatory problem by observing decreased pulses in the wrist or ankles. And unusual characteristics of the penis itself could suggest the source of the problem—for example, a penis that bends or curves when erect could be the result of Peyronie disease.

Laboratory tests: Several laboratory tests can help diagnose ED. Tests for systemic diseases include blood counts, urinalysis, lipid profile, and measurements of creatinine and liver enzymes. Measuring the amount of free testosterone in the blood can yield information about problems with the endocrine system and is indicated especially in patients with decreased sexual desire.

Other tests: Monitoring erections that occur during sleep (nocturnal penile tumescence) can help rule out certain psychological causes of ED. Healthy men have involuntary erections during sleep. If nocturnal erections do not occur, then ED is likely to have a physical rather than psychological cause. Tests of nocturnal erections are not completely reliable, however. Scientists have not standardized such tests and have not determined when they should be applied for best results.

Psychosocial examination: A psychosocial examination, using an interview and a questionnaire, reveals psychological factors. A man's sexual partner may also be interviewed to determine expectations and perceptions during sexual intercourse.

How is ED treated?

Most physicians suggest that treatments proceed from least to most invasive. For some men, making a few healthy lifestyle changes may solve the problem. Quitting smoking, losing excess weight, and increasing physical activity may help some men regain sexual function.

Cutting back on any drugs with harmful side effects is considered next. For example, drugs for high blood pressure work in different ways. If you think a particular drug is causing problems with erection, tell your doctor and ask whether you can try a different class of blood pressure medicine.

Psychotherapy and behavior modifications in selected patients are considered next if indicated, followed by oral or locally injected drugs, vacuum devices, and surgically implanted devices. In rare cases, surgery involving veins or arteries may be considered.

Psychotherapy: Experts often treat psychologically based ED using techniques that decrease the anxiety associated with intercourse. The patient's partner can help with the techniques, which include gradual development of intimacy and stimulation. Such techniques also can help relieve anxiety when ED from physical causes is being treated.

Drug therapy: Drugs for treating ED can be taken orally, injected directly into the penis, or inserted into the urethra at the tip of the penis. In March 1998, the Food and Drug Administration (FDA) approved Viagra, the first pill to treat ED. Since that time, vardenafil hydrochloride (Levitra®) and tadalafil (Cialis®) have also been approved. Additional oral medicines are being tested for safety and effectiveness.

Viagra, Levitra, and Cialis all belong to a class of drugs called phosphodiesterase (PDE) inhibitors. Taken an hour before sexual activity, these drugs work by enhancing the effects of nitric oxide, a chemical that relaxes smooth muscles in the penis during sexual stimulation and allows increased blood flow.

While oral medicines improve the response to sexual stimulation, they do not trigger an automatic erection as injections do. The recommended dose for Viagra is 50 mg, and the physician may adjust this dose to 100 mg or 25 mg, depending on the patient. The recommended dose for either Levitra or Cialis is 10 mg, and the physician may adjust this dose to 20 mg if 10 mg is insufficient. A lower dose of 5 mg is available for patients who take other medicines or have conditions that may decrease the body's ability to use the drug. Levitra is also available in a 2.5 mg dose.

None of these PDE inhibitors should be used more than once a day. Men who take nitrate-based drugs such as nitroglycerin for heart problems should not use either drug because the combination can cause a sudden drop in blood pressure. Also, tell your doctor if you take any drugs called alpha-blockers, which are used to treat prostate enlargement or high blood pressure. Your doctor may need to adjust your ED prescription. Taking a PDE inhibitor and an alpha-blocker at the same time (within four hours) can cause a sudden drop in blood pressure.

Oral testosterone can reduce ED in some men with low levels of natural testosterone, but it is often ineffective and may cause liver damage. Patients also have claimed that other oral drugs—including yohimbine hydrochloride, dopamine and serotonin agonists, and trazodone—are effective, but the results of scientific studies to substantiate these claims have been inconsistent.

Many men achieve stronger erections by injecting drugs into the penis, causing it to become engorged with blood. Drugs such as papaverine hydrochloride, phentolamine, and alprostadil (marketed as Caverject®) widen blood vessels. These drugs may create unwanted side effects, however, including persistent erection (known as priapism) and scarring. Nitroglycerin, a muscle relaxant, can sometimes enhance erection when rubbed on the penis.

A system for inserting a pellet of alprostadil into the urethra is marketed as Muse®. The system uses a prefilled applicator to deliver the pellet about an inch deep into the urethra. An erection will begin within eight to ten minutes and may last thirty to sixty minutes. The most common side effects are aching in the penis, testicles, and area between the penis and rectum; warmth or burning sensation in the urethra; redness from increased blood flow to the penis; and minor urethral bleeding or spotting.

Vacuum devices: Mechanical vacuum devices cause erection by creating a partial vacuum, which draws blood into the penis, engorging and expanding it. The devices have three components: a plastic cylinder, into which the penis is placed; a pump, which draws air out of the cylinder; and an elastic band, which is placed around the base of the penis to maintain the erection after the cylinder is removed and during intercourse by preventing blood from flowing back into the body.

One variation of the vacuum device involves a semirigid rubber sheath that is placed on the penis and remains there after erection is attained and during intercourse.

Surgery: Surgery usually has one of three goals: to implant a device that can cause the penis to become erect, to reconstruct arteries to increase flow of blood to the penis, or to block off veins that allow blood to leak from the penile tissues.

Implanted devices, known as prostheses, can restore erection in many men with ED. Possible problems with implants include mechanical breakdown and infection, although mechanical problems have diminished in recent years because of technological advances.

Malleable implants usually consist of paired rods, which are inserted surgically into the corpora cavernosa. The user manually adjusts the position of the penis and, therefore, the rods. Adjustment does not affect the width or length of the penis.

Inflatable implants consist of paired cylinders, which are surgically inserted inside the penis and can be expanded using pressurized fluid. Tubes connect the cylinders to a fluid reservoir and a pump, which are also surgically implanted. The patient inflates the cylinders by pressing on the small pump, located under the skin in the scrotum. Inflatable implants can expand the length and width of the penis somewhat. They also leave the penis in a more natural state when not inflated.

Surgery to repair arteries can reduce ED caused by obstructions that block the flow of blood. The best candidates for such surgery are young men with discrete blockage of an artery because of an injury to the crotch or fracture of the pelvis. The procedure is almost never successful in older men with widespread blockage.

Surgery to veins that allow blood to leave the penis usually involves an opposite procedure—intentional blockage. Blocking off veins (ligation) can reduce the leakage of blood that diminishes the rigidity of the penis during erection. However, experts have raised questions about the long-term effectiveness of this procedure, and it is rarely done.

Section 34.2

Premature Ejaculation

"Premature Ejaculation (PE)," is reprinted with permission from www.urologyhealth.org.

Premature ejaculation (PE), is also known as rapid ejaculation, premature climax, or early ejaculation. In the United States, PE affects about one in five men ages eighteen to fifty-nine. Although the problem is often assumed to be psychological, biology also may play a role.

How does ejaculation occur?

Ejaculation, controlled by the central nervous system, happens when sexual stimulation and friction provide impulses that are delivered to the spinal cord and into the brain.

Ejaculation has two phases.

Phase I (emission): The vas deferens (the tubes that store and transport sperm from the testes) contract to squeeze the sperm toward the base of the penis through the prostate gland. The seminal vesicles release secretions that combine with the sperm to make semen. The ejaculation is unstoppable at this stage.

Phase II (ejaculation): The muscles at the base of the penis contract forcing semen out of the penis (ejaculation and orgasm) while the bladder neck contracts. Orgasm can occur without the delivery of semen (ejaculation) from the penis. Normally, erections are lost following ejaculation.

What is premature ejaculation?

Premature ejaculation (PE) is characterized by a lack of voluntary control over ejaculation. Many men occasionally ejaculate sooner than they or their partner would like during sexual activities. PE is a frustrating problem that can reduce the enjoyment of sex, harm relationships, and affect quality of life. Occasional instances of PE might not be cause for concern. However, when the problem occurs frequently and causes distress to the man or his partner, treatment may be of benefit.

What causes premature ejaculation?

Although the exact cause of premature ejaculation (PE) is not known, new studies suggest that serotonin, a natural substance produced by nerves, is important. A breakdown of the actions of serotonin in the brain may be a cause. Studies have found that high amounts of serotonin in the brain slow the time to ejaculation while low amounts of serotonin can produce a condition like PE.

Psychological factors also commonly contribute to PE. Temporary depression, stress, unrealistic expectations about performance, a history of sexual repression, or an overall lack of confidence can cause PE. Interpersonal dynamics may contribute to sexual function. PE can be caused by a lack of communication between partners, hurt feelings, or unresolved conflicts that interfere with the ability to achieve emotional intimacy.

Can premature ejaculation develop later in life?

Premature ejaculation (PE) can occur at any age. Surprisingly, aging appears not to be a cause of PE. However, the aging process typically causes changes in erectile function and ejaculation. Erections may not be as firm or as large. Erections may be maintained for a shorter period before ejaculating. The feeling that an ejaculation is about to happen may be shorter. These factors can result in an older man having an ejaculation earlier than when he was younger.

Can both premature ejaculation and erectile dysfunction affect a man at the same time?

Sometimes premature ejaculation (PE) may be a problem in men who have erectile dysfunction (ED)—the inability to achieve and/or maintain an erection sufficient for satisfactory sexual performance. Some men do not understand that the loss of erection normally occurs after ejaculation and may wrongly complain to their doctor that they have ED when the actual problem is PE. It is recommended that the ED be treated first if you experience both ED and PE, since the PE may resolve on its own once the ED has been adequately treated.

When should a doctor be seen?

When premature ejaculation (PE) happens so frequently that it interferes with your sexual pleasure, it becomes a medical problem requiring the care of a doctor. To understand the problem, the doctor will need to ask questions about your sexual history such as the following:

- How often does the PE occur?
- How long have you had this problem?
- Is the problem specific to one partner? Or does it happen with every partner?
- Does PE occur with all or just some attempts at sexual relations?
- How much stimulation results in PE?
- What type of sexual activity (i.e., foreplay, masturbation, intercourse, use of visual clues, etc.) is engaged in and how often?
- How has PE affected sexual activity?
- What is the quality of your personal relationships?
- How does PE affect your quality of life?
- Are there any factors that make PE worse or better (i.e., drugs, alcohol, etc.)?

Usually, laboratory testing is not necessary unless the history and a physical examination reveal something more complicated.

How to talk to your partner about premature ejaculation?

Premature ejaculation (PE) affects not only you but also your partner and your sexual relationship. In an episode of PE, the intimacy shared with a partner suddenly comes to a quick end. You might feel angry, ashamed, and frustrated, and turn away from your partner. At the same time, your partner may be upset with the rapid emotional change, or the outcome of the sexual encounter.

Communication is not only important to successful diagnosis and treatment, but can also help a partner understand the feelings of the individual. Sometimes couple counseling or sex therapy may be useful. Together a couple might develop techniques (for example, the squeeze technique) that may prolong an erection. Most importantly, the couple should try to relax. Anxiety (especially performance anxiety) only makes this condition worse.

What treatments are available?

There are several treatment choices for premature ejaculation: psychological therapy, behavioral therapy, and medications. Be sure to discuss these treatments with your doctor and together decide which of the following options is best for you:

- Psychological therapy addresses feelings a man may have about sexuality and sexual relationships.
- Behavioral therapy makes use of exercises to help a man develop tolerance to stimulation and, as a result, delay ejaculation.
- Medical therapy includes medications that are commonly used to treat depression. In addition, topical anesthetic creams may be used.

Psychological therapies: Psychological therapy can be used as the only treatment or can be used together with medical therapy or behavioral therapy. The focus of psychological therapy is to help you to identify and solve any difficulties in your relationships that may have added to the cause of premature ejaculation (PE). This therapy can also help couples to talk about problems with intimacy that occurred after PE began. Psychological therapy can also help a man learn to be less anxious about his sexual performance and have greater sexual confidence. Typically, a man will receive specific advice on how to enhance his and his partner's sexual satisfaction.

Behavioral therapies: Behavioral therapy can play a key part in the usual treatment of premature ejaculation. Exercises are effective; however, they may not always provide a lasting solution to the problem. Also, they rely heavily on the cooperation of the partner, which in some cases may be a problem.

With the squeeze method, an exercise developed by Masters and Johnson, the partner stimulates the man's penis until he is close to ejaculation. At the point when he is about to ejaculate, the partner squeezes the penis hard enough to make him partially lose his erection. The goal of this technique is to teach the man to become aware of the sensations leading up to orgasm, and then begin to control and delay his orgasm on his own.

With the stop-start method, the partner stimulates the man's penis until just before ejaculation. The partner should then stop all stimulation until the urge to ejaculate subsides. As the man regains control, he instructs the partner to begin stimulating his penis again. This procedure is repeated three times before allowing the man to ejaculate on the fourth time. The couple repeats this exercise three times a week, until the man has gained good control.

Medical therapies: Although not approved by the U.S. Food and Drug Administration (FDA) for this purpose, drugs used for depression and anesthetic creams have been shown to delay ejaculation in men with premature ejaculation (PE).

Medications are a relatively new form of treatment for PE. Doctors first noticed that men and women who were taking drugs for the treatment of depression (antidepressants) also had delayed orgasms. Doctors then began to use these drugs "off-label" (this implies using a medication for a different illness than what it was originally manufactured for) to treat PE. These medications include antidepressants that affect serotonin such as fluoxetine, paroxetine, sertraline and clomipramine.

If one medication fails to work, a second one is usually recommended. If the second one fails, trying a third medication will not likely be beneficial. An alternative is to combine medication with behavioral therapy and/or creams.

For use in PE, the doses of antidepressants are usually lower than those recommended for the treatment of depression. Common side effects of antidepressants can include nausea, dry mouth, drowsiness, and reduced desire for sexual activity.

These drugs can be taken either every day or only taken before sexual activity. Your doctor will decide how you should take the medication based on the frequency of intercourse. The best time for taking the antidepressant medications before sexual activity has not been established, but most doctors will recommend from two to six hours depending on the medication. Because PE can recur when the medication is not taken, you most likely will need to take it on a continuing basis.

Local anesthetic creams can be used to treat PE. These creams are applied to the head of the penis about twenty to thirty minutes before intercourse to lessen the sensitivity. Prior to sexual intercourse, a condom (if used) may be removed and the penis washed clean of any remaining cream. A loss of erection can occur if the anesthetic cream is left on the penis for a longer period of time than recommended. Also, the anesthetic cream should not be left on the exposed penis during vaginal intercourse since it may cause vaginal numbness.

See your urologist for evaluation and treatment for the biological aspects of premature ejaculation.

Section 34.3

Retrograde Ejaculation

Excerpted from "Retrograde Ejaculation," © 2009 A.D.A.M., Inc. Reprinted with permission.

Retrograde ejaculation refers to the entry of semen into the bladder instead of going out through the urethra during ejaculation.

Causes

Retrograde ejaculation may be caused by prior prostate or urethral surgery, diabetes, some medications, including some drugs used to treat hypertension (high blood pressure), and some mood-altering drugs.

The condition is relatively uncommon and may occur either partially or completely. The presence of semen in the bladder is harmless. It mixes with the urine and leaves the body with normal urination. Men with diabetes and those who have had genitourinary tract surgery are at increased risk of developing the condition.

Symptoms

- Little or no semen discharged from the urethra in conjunction with the male sexual climax (during ejaculation)
- Possible infertility
- Cloudy urine after sexual climax

Exams and Tests

A urinalysis performed on a urine specimen that is obtained shortly after ejaculation will reveal a large amount of sperm in the urine.

Treatment

If retrograde ejaculation is caused by drugs, your doctor may recommend that you stop taking such drugs. This can make the problem go away.

Retrograde ejaculation caused by diabetes or after genitourinary tract surgery may be treated with epinephrine-like drugs (such as pseudoephedrine or imipramine).

Outlook (Prognosis)

If retrograde ejaculation is caused by medications, discontinuation of the medication often restores normal ejaculation. If retrograde ejaculation is caused by surgery or diabetes, it is often not correctable.

Possible Complications

The condition may cause infertility.

When to Contact a Medical Professional

Call for an appointment with your health care provider if you are having difficulty conceiving a child or you are concerned about retrograde ejaculation.

Prevention

Maintaining good blood sugar control may help prevent this condition in men who have diabetes. Avoiding drugs that cause retrograde ejaculation will also prevent this condition.

Chapter 35

Penile Disorders

Chapter Contents

Section 35.1

Peyronie Disease

Reprinted from "Peyronie's Disease," National Institute of Diabetes and Digestive and Kidney Diseases, National Institutes of Health, NIH Publication No. 07-3902, September 2005.

Peyronie disease, a condition of uncertain cause, is characterized by a plaque, or hard lump, that forms on the penis. The plaque develops on the upper or lower side of the penis in layers containing erectile tissue. It begins as a localized inflammation and can develop into a hardened scar.

Cases of Peyronie disease range from mild to severe. Symptoms may develop slowly or appear overnight. In severe cases, the hardened plaque reduces flexibility, causing pain and forcing the penis to bend or arc during erection. In many cases, the pain decreases over time, but the bend in the penis may remain a problem, making sexual intercourse difficult. The sexual problems that result can disrupt a couple's physical and emotional relationship and lead to lowered self-esteem in the man. In a small percentage of patients with the milder form of the disease, inflammation may resolve without causing significant pain or permanent bending.

The plaque itself is benign, or noncancerous. A plaque on the top of the shaft (most common) causes the penis to bend upward; a plaque on the underside causes it to bend downward. In some cases, the plaque develops on both top and bottom, leading to indentation and shortening of the penis. At times, pain, bending, and emotional distress prohibit sexual intercourse.

One study found Peyronie disease in 1 percent of men. Although the disease occurs mostly in middle age, younger and older men can develop it. About 30 percent of men with Peyronie disease develop fibrosis (hardened cells) in other elastic tissues of the body, such as on the hand or foot. A common example is a condition known as Dupuytren contracture of the hand. In some cases, men who are related by blood tend to develop Peyronie disease, which suggests that genetic factors might make a man vulnerable to the disease.

Men with Peyronie disease usually seek medical attention because of painful erections and difficulty with intercourse. Since the cause of the disease and its development are not well understood, doctors treat the disease empirically; that is, they prescribe and continue methods that seem to help. The goal of therapy is to keep the Peyronie patient sexually active. Providing education about the disease and its course often is all that is required. No strong evidence shows that any treatment other than surgery is effective. Experts usually recommend surgery only in long-term cases in which the disease is stabilized and the deformity prevents intercourse.

A French surgeon, François de la Peyronie, first described Peyronie disease in 1743. The problem was noted in print as early as 1687. Early writers classified it as a form of impotence, now called erectile dysfunction (ED). Peyronie disease can be associated with ED; however, experts now recognize ED as only one factor associated with the disease—a factor that is not always present.

Course of the Disease

Many researchers believe the plaque of Peyronie disease develops following trauma (hitting or bending) that causes localized bleeding inside the penis. Two chambers known as the corpora cavernosa run the length of the penis. The inner-surface membrane of the chambers is a sheath of elastic fibers. A connecting tissue, called a septum, runs between the two chambers and attaches at the top and bottom.

If the penis is abnormally bumped or bent, an area where the septum attaches to the elastic fibers may stretch beyond a limit, injuring the lining of the erectile chamber and, for example, rupturing small blood vessels. As a result of aging, diminished elasticity near the point of attachment of the septum might increase the chances of injury.

The damaged area might heal slowly or abnormally for two reasons: repeated trauma and a minimal amount of blood flow in the sheath-like fibers. In cases that heal within about a year, the plaque does not advance beyond an initial inflammatory phase. In cases that persist for years, the plaque undergoes fibrosis, or formation of tough fibrous tissue, and even calcification, or formation of calcium deposits.

While trauma might explain acute cases of Peyronie disease, it does not explain why most cases develop slowly and with no apparent traumatic event. It also does not explain why some cases disappear quickly or why similar conditions such as Dupuytren contracture do not seem to result from severe trauma.

Some researchers theorize that Peyronie disease may be an autoimmune disorder.

Diagnosis and Evaluation

Doctors can usually diagnose Peyronie disease based on a physical examination. The plaque is visible and palpable whether the penis is flaccid or erect. Full evaluation, however, may require examination during erection to determine the severity of the curvature. The erection may be induced by injecting medicine into the penis or through self-stimulation. Some patients may eliminate the need to induce an erection in the doctor's office by taking a digital or Polaroid picture in the home. The examination may include an ultrasound scan of the penis to pinpoint the location and extent of the plaque and evaluate blood flow throughout the penis.

Treatment

Because the course of Peyronie disease is different in each patient and because some patients experience improvement without treatment, medical experts suggest waiting one to two years or longer before attempting to correct it surgically. During that wait, patients often are willing to undergo treatments whose effectiveness has not been proven.

Experimental treatments: Some researchers have given vitamin E orally to men with Peyronie disease in small-scale studies and have reported improvements. Yet, no controlled studies have established the effectiveness of vitamin E therapy. Similar inconclusive success has been attributed to oral application of para-aminobenzoate, a substance belonging to the family of B-complex molecules.

Researchers have injected chemical agents such as verapamil, collagenase, steroids, calcium channel blockers, and interferon alpha-2b directly into the plaques. These interventions are still considered unproven because studies included small numbers of patients and lacked adequate control groups. Steroids, such as cortisone, have produced unwanted side effects, such as the atrophy or death of healthy tissues. Another intervention involves iontophoresis, the use of a painless current of electricity to deliver verapamil or some other agent under the skin into the plaque.

Radiation therapy, in which high-energy rays are aimed at the plaque, has also been used. Like some of the chemical treatments, radiation appears to reduce pain, but it has no effect at all on the plaque itself and can cause unwelcome side effects. Although the variety of agents and methods used points to the lack of a proven treatment, new insights into the wound healing process may one day yield more effective therapies.

Surgery: Peyronie disease has been treated surgically with some success. The two most common surgical procedures are removal or expansion of the plaque followed by placement of a patch of skin or artificial material, and removal or pinching of tissue from the side of the penis opposite the plaque, which cancels out the bending effect. The first method can involve partial loss of erectile function, especially rigidity. The second method, known as the Nesbit procedure, causes a shortening of the erect penis.

Some men choose to receive an implanted device that increases rigidity of the penis. In some cases, an implant alone will straighten the penis adequately. In other cases, implantation is combined with a technique of incisions and grafting or plication (pinching or folding the skin) if the implant alone does not straighten the penis.

Most types of surgery produce positive results. But because complications can occur, and because many of the phenomena associated with Peyronie disease (for example, shortening of the penis) are not corrected by surgery, most doctors prefer to perform surgery only on the small number of men with curvature so severe that it prevents sexual intercourse.

Section 35.2

Balanitis, Phimosis, Priapism, and Other Penis Problems

Lumps, foreskin problems, and inflammation of the penis are common problems men can experience. Men who are not circumcised can experience problems with their foreskin. Most inflammations and lumps are not too serious and can easily be treated; however, some penis problems can increase the risk of penis cancer. Priapism is an erection that lasts more than three hours, and can cause damage to the penis so must be treated promptly. If you have any changes in the skin or foreskin of your penis, see your local doctor.

The Foreskin

At birth, the foreskin and the glans penis are joined. As boys start growing, an increase in hormones contributes to the foreskin and glans separating and the foreskin is then able to be pulled back. This happens in most boys at around three years of age.

The foreskin of an uncircumcised child should not forcibly be pulled back as this can cause bleeding and injury. By forcefully retracting the foreskin, scarring can happen which can then cause problems with the foreskin retracting, which is called phimosis.

All uncircumcised adult men should have a genital examination by their doctor and have their foreskin retracted to check for signs of penis cancer.

Penis Lumps

There are different types of lumps and bumps that can appear on the penis; many of them are harmless. If you are concerned about any lumps on your penis, see your doctor to rule out sexually transmitted infections and penis cancer, albeit rare. Some common lumps include the following.

Cysts: Sometimes the sebaceous glands on the penis and scrotum can become enlarged and blocked, turning into cysts. These do not usually need any treatment. Sometimes they can become painful and infected if they continue to grow.

Ulcers: These appear as craters in the skin and often have a clear liquid or pus in the crater (red wound or a sore).

A single ulcer is often quite serious and should be checked by a doctor immediately. Causes of a single ulcer include syphilis, tropical diseases, and penile cancer.

Multiple ulcers are more common and are less serious, but should still be checked by a doctor straight away. Herpes is the most common cause of multiple penile ulcers.

Papules: These are small lumps that are raised on the skin and most do not have a serious cause. One of the most common types of papules is called pearly penile papules and these appear as one or more rows of small, smooth lumps located in a circumference around the back of the glans penis (head of the penis). These look very similar to, and are often mistaken for, genital warts. These papules are not infectious and do not need to be treated.

Causes of other papules include psoriasis and sexually transmitted infections such as genital warts. Genital warts are caused by the human papillomavirus (HPV). Warts can often happen in clusters and can be very tiny. Genital warts are spread through skin-to-skin contact, so it is important to use condoms if you or your partner are infected. In women, HPV is associated with precancerous changes in the cervix. Genital warts are treated by freezing them with liquid nitrogen. Although this gets rid of the warts, it does not get rid of the virus and warts may reappear on the skin or occur in the eye of the penis. This may need an inspection of the inside of the penis to fully treat the warts.

Plaques: Plaques are raised lumps that are bigger than one centimeter in diameter. They do not usually have a serious cause, but some are infectious and can develop into more serious conditions such as penile cancer. Some causes of plaques include balanitis (see below) and eczema.

Balanitis

What is balanitis?

Balanitis is a very common inflammation of the glans penis (helmet of the penis) that can affect males at any age. This inflammation can affect circumcised males, however, it is more common in men who have not been circumcised.

What causes balanitis?

Balanitis often happens when the foreskin is not pulled back, or is unable to be pulled back due to scarring, and the inside of the foreskin is not kept clean. Inflammation caused by a bacteria or fungus is common and can be caused if the sensitive skin under the foreskin collects sweat, dead skin, and bacteria. Balanitis can also be caused by irritation from chemicals in soap, clothing, and the latex in condoms. Allergies to certain drugs, viruses such as human papillomavirus (which can cause genital warts), and obesity can also contribute to balanitis.

In adults, balanitis can be a sign of diabetes. After urinating, some urine may become trapped under the foreskin. The combination of a moist area and glucose in the urine can lead to bacteria growing and then infection. If you have balanitis and the condition keeps happening, speak to your doctor and ask to be tested for diabetes.

What are some of the signs of balanitis?

Men with balanitis may experience the following complaints:

- Inability to pull back the foreskin
- Itchiness
- Rash
- Sore or tender glans penis
- Redness or swelling
- Discharge from the penis

How is balanitis treated?

Treatment for balanitis depends on the cause of the inflammation. Most often, washing the penis and under the foreskin with soap and warm water is recommended. If the cause is from allergic reactions, try using different brands and other chemicals. If there is an infection, the doctor may prescribe antibiotics or antifungal medication. In severe cases of balanitis, circumcision may be recommended.

To avoid future bouts of balanitis, do not use strong soaps and chemicals, and pull back the foreskin and clean it daily.

What is balanitis xerotica obliterans (BXO)?

Balanitis xerotica obliterans (BXO) is not to be confused with balanitis (inflammation of the glans penis). BXO is a rare condition where scar tissue forms in the foreskin. A ring of white tissue develops at the tip of the foreskin, tightening the foreskin at the tip, and this may prevent the foreskin from retracting (phimosis). BXO may spread to the glans penis, but this is not common.

It is important to speak to your doctor if you are concerned about white scarring of your foreskin, to distinguish BXO from early penis cancer. BXO is a progressive disease and it is usually treated by circumcision.

Phimosis

What is phimosis?

Phimosis is when the foreskin is too tight, or the tip of the foreskin narrows and is unable to be pulled back to expose the head of the penis.

What causes phimosis?

Phimosis is often seen in children or young adults (primary or congenital phimosis). The condition is at its highest incidence rate before puberty.

Phimosis can also happen because of injury or damage that causes the foreskin to tear (secondary or acquired phimosis). As the tear heals, scar tissue forms which reduces the elasticity of the foreskin. This scar tissue can then stop the foreskin from stretching open far enough to pull back. The scarring from BXO can also cause phimosis.

Phimosis can often follow infection or inflammation such as balanitis. Adult men with phimosis should be checked for balanitis, diabetes, and cancer.

Are there any other symptoms with phimosis?

Severe phimosis can cause pain when urinating, urinary retention, urinary tract infections, and the skin on the penis can become infected. In older men with severe phimosis, the foreskin can look swollen.

How is phimosis treated?

Phimosis can be treated with steroid creams applied once or twice daily for a couple of weeks. Studies have shown that the creams have a success rate of more than 85 percent, and this can increase if the foreskin is gently stretched together with the cream application.

If the steroid creams do not work and phimosis is severe, circumcision is another option to consider.

Paraphimosis

What is paraphimosis?

Paraphimosis happens when the foreskin has been retracted behind the head of the penis and cannot go back to its original position. If the foreskin stays in this position, it can cause pain, swelling, and can stop blood flow to the penis. This is a serious medical problem and must be treated immediately or the penis can sustain long-term or permanent damage.

What causes paraphimosis?

Paraphimosis can happen at any age, and can be caused by injury to the head of the penis. It can also happen to infants if parents pull back their foreskin and do not pull it forward again afterward.

How is paraphimosis treated?

The glans penis and the foreskin often swell up with paraphimosis. It is important to apply ice to reduce the swelling and then try and move the foreskin forward to the usual position. Other methods used to reduce swelling include injecting medicine that lessens swelling, or inserting a needle and releasing some blood. If the foreskin does not return to its normal position, a surgeon may have to cut the foreskin to release it, or circumcision may be necessary.

Priapism

What is priapism?

Priapism is an erection that lasts for more than three hours and is usually very painful. Blood becomes trapped in the penis and does not return to circulation; it is not necessarily because of, or related to, sexual stimulation. If priapism is not treated, it can lead to permanent damage to the erectile tissue and the inability to get an erection at all. Priapism can happen to males at any age.

What causes it?

The most common cause of priapism is drug treatments for erectile dysfunction, in particular, penile injection treatments. About a quarter of other cases of priapism are associated with medical conditions such as advanced cancer, leukemia, and sickle cell anemia. Other possible causes include damage to the nervous system, injury to the penis, the use of some medicines, and illegal drugs. Sometimes the cause of priapism is unknown.

How is it treated?

It is important to see a doctor straight away because the sooner the prolonged erection is treated, the less damage will be done to the erectile tissue. If treatment is sought within four to six hours, the doctor may provide a decongestant medication to help the erection go down. Another option is for the doctor to use a needle and syringe to release the extra blood trapped in the penis. If this does not work, surgery may be needed to try and avoid permanent damage to the penis.

If priapism was caused by erectile dysfunction drugs, alternative treatments should be used instead. Also, if priapism has been caused by other medications, trying a different medication may help.

Section 35.3

Penile Trauma

"Penile Trauma" is reprinted with permission from www.urologyhealth.org, Reviewed by David A. Cooke, M.D., March 2009.

While the penis is one of the least injured organs, it is not risk-free. What can put it at risk? And how is it repaired? The following information should tell you when it is imperative to see your doctor about problems.

How does the penis normally function?

The two main functions of the penis are urinary and reproductive. Inside the penis there are three tubes. One is called the urethra. It is hollow and allows urine to flow from the bladder through the hole in the prostate through the penis and to the outside. The two other tubes are called the corpora cavernosa. The three tubes are wrapped together by a very tough fibrous sheath called the tunica albuginea. The corpora cavernosa are spongy tubes that are soft until filled with blood during an erection. At the time of sexual activity the erection of the penis allows it to be inserted into the woman's vagina. In this situation, the urethra acts as a channel for semen to be ejaculated into the vagina. The penis facilitates conception and pregnancy and also serves as a source of sexual pleasure for the man and his partner.

What are the causes and symptoms of penile injury?

The penis is much less frequently injured than other parts of the body such as the abdomen, legs, arms, and head. However, it can be wounded as a result of various injuries, including automobile accidents, gunshot wounds, burns, sexual activity, and, in the case of mental disturbance, self-mutilation.

Perhaps the most common injury to the penis occurs during sexual activity. In the flaccid state, injury to the penis is rare because of the mobility and flexibility of the organ. During an erection, arterial blood flow causes the penis to be come rigid, thus placing it at higher risk for injury. Although there is no bone in the penis, urologists frequently refer to the injury as a penile "fracture." During vigorous thrusting, the erect penis may accidentally slip out of the vagina. Due to the fast action, the penis strikes the outside of the woman instead of being reinserted into the vagina. The penis may then bend sharply despite the erection. A typical sign of this problem is a sharp pain in the penis joined by a "popping" sound. The pain and sound are produced by a rupture of the tunica albuginea, which is stretched tightly during the time of an erection. The pain may last for a short time or it may continue. The penis develops a collection of blood under the skin called a hematoma, which can distort the appearance of the penis (eggplant deformity). The injury is usually limited to one or both of the corpora cavernosa and, on rare occasions, the urethra.

The penis can also be injured by tearing the suspensory ligament, the structure that supports the organ at its base. Attached to the pelvic bone, this ligament can rip if an erect penis is pushed down suddenly, causing pain and bleeding.

Further injuries can occur if a man places a rubber tube or other instrument around the base of the penis that is too tight or on for too long. Cutting off the blood supply, it can produce a wound known as a strangulation lesion. Also, if an object is inserted into the urethra, both it and/or the penis can be injured.

How are injuries to the penis treated?

If a person sustains a penile injury, a urologist will take a thorough medical history and complete a physical examination along with blood and urine tests. The focus of any initial examination is to define the injury and assess the damage to the penis. Given that information, the doctor may call for other tests, including a retrograde urethrogram if he or she thinks the urethra is involved. This test is performed by injecting a liquid radio contrast solution through the opening at the top of the penis and then taking x-rays. If the x-ray shows any leakage outside the urethra, it may indicate damage to that part of the urinary tract.

Additional imaging techniques might include an ultrasound of the penis, magnetic resonance imaging (MRI), or a special test called a cavernosogram. In the latter test, a thin hypodermic needle is inserted into one area of the penis before a radio contrast solution is injected and x-rays taken.

If the injury is amputation of the penis, the amputated portion should be wrapped in gauze soaked in sterile saline solution and placed in a plastic bag. The plastic bag should then be put into a second bag or cooler with an ice water slush. If reattachment of the penis is possible, the lower temperature produced by the slush will increase the likelihood of successful reattachment. Penile reattachment even after sixteen hours has been reported to be successful.

Historically, treatment for a penis fractured during sexual activity was nonsurgical management (e.g., cold compresses, pressure dressings, penile splinting, and anti-inflammatory medications). Today, the treatment of choice will probably be for the individual to undergo surgery since it has the best long-term results by lowering complication rates often linked to nonsurgical approaches. The most common surgical technique is to "deglove" the penis by making a cut around the shaft near the glans penis and peeling back the skin to the base to examine the inner surface. The surgeon will then evacuate any hematoma that helps to make examination of any tears in the tunica albuginea easier. If tears exist, they are repaired before the skin is sewn back into position. A Foley catheter may be placed through the penile urethra into the bladder to drain urine and allow the penis to heal. With the entire penis bandaged, the patient will probably remain in the hospital for one or two days, and go home with or without the catheter. They may be given antibiotics and pain medication and will probably be asked to make a follow-up office visit with their doctor.

For massive injuries to the penis, major reconstruction is frequently possible by urologists experienced with this difficult surgery. How closely the reconstructed penis can return to normal urinary or sexual function varies greatly.

What can be expected after treatment for injuries to the penis?

Most cases of fractured penis caused by sexual activity and most other minor penile injuries will heal without problems. However, complications can and do occur. Possible complications include: infection, erectile dysfunction due to blockage of the nerve or blood supply to the penis, priapism in which the penis becomes erect and stays erect to the point of pain, fistula formation in which urine may leak out of the urethra and through the skin of the penis to the outside, curvature (chordee) of the penis after the injury has healed, or major loss of skin, portion of the urethra, or corpora cavernosum. Failure for the return of sufficient sexual function is dependent upon the degree of injury to the arteries, nerves, and corpora cavernosum and whether the patient was experiencing erectile dysfunction just prior to the injury.

How frequent are penile injuries?

Unfortunately, doctors have not been able to gather meaningful statistics as to how many penile injuries actually occur in the United States.

How does a Foley catheter work?

Ever since E. B. Foley, a Minneapolis urologist, first introduced the catheter bearing his name; doctors have had an effective way to efficiently and continuously drain the urinary tract. Held in place by its own configuration—primarily with a sterile, liquid-filled balloon—the Foley can be inserted simply by passing the rubber tubing through the urethra into the bladder. It remains there until the penis is healed.

How do I prevent penile injury?

Penile injuries related to sexual intercourse can be prevented in most cases if your partner is simply aware of the possibility. If your penis is erect and inadvertently slips from the vagina of your partner, stop the thrusting immediately. For other injuries, caution on the job, especially near machinery; defensive driving; and gun safety are obvious precautions for the other types of injuries.

Chapter 36

Non-Cancerous Prostate Disorders

Chapter Contents

Section 36.1

Benign Prostatic Hyperplasia

Excerpted from "Understanding Prostate Changes: A Health Guide for Men," National Cancer Institute, September 15, 2004. Revised by David A. Cooke, M.D., April 2009.

What Is Enlarged Prostate or BPH?

BPH stands for benign prostatic hyperplasia.

Benign means "not cancer," and hyperplasia means too much growth. The result is that the prostate becomes enlarged. BPH is not linked to cancer and does not raise your chances of getting prostate cancer—yet the symptoms for BPH and prostate cancer can be similar.

BPH Symptoms

BPH symptoms usually start after the age of fifty. They can include the following:

- Trouble starting a urine stream or making more than a dribble
- Passing urine often, especially at night
- Feeling that the bladder has not fully emptied
- A strong or sudden urge to pass urine
- Weak or slow urine stream
- Stopping and starting again several times while passing urine
- Pushing or straining to begin passing urine

At its worst, BPH can lead to the following:

- A weak bladder
- Backflow of urine causing bladder or kidney infections
- Complete block in the flow of urine
- Kidney failure

BPH affects most men as they get older. It can lead to urinary problems like those with prostatitis. By age sixty, many men have signs of BPH. By age seventy, almost all men have some prostate enlargement.

The prostate starts out about the size of a walnut. By the time a man is forty, it may have grown slightly larger, to the size of an apricot. By age sixty, it may be the size of a lemon.

As a normal part of aging, the prostate enlarges and can press against the bladder and the urethra. This can slow down or block urine flow. Some men might find it hard to start a urine stream, even though they feel the need to go. Once the urine stream has started, it may be hard to stop. Other men may feel like they need to pass urine all the time or are awakened during sleep with the sudden need to pass urine.

Early BPH symptoms take many years to turn into bothersome problems. These early symptoms are a cue to see your doctor.

How Can BPH Be Treated?

About half the men with BPH eventually have symptoms that are bothersome enough to need treatment. BPH cannot be cured, but drugs or surgery can often relieve its symptoms. BPH symptoms do not always grow worse.

There are three ways to manage BPH:

- Watchful waiting (regular follow-up with your doctor)
- Drug therapy
- Surgery

Talk with your doctor about the best choice for you. Your symptoms may change over time, so be sure to tell your doctor about any new changes.

Watchful Waiting

Men with mild symptoms of BPH who do not find them bothersome often choose this approach.

Watchful waiting means getting annual checkups. The checkups can include digital rectal exams (DREs) and other tests. Treatment is started only if symptoms become too much of a problem.

If you choose to live with symptoms, these simple steps can help:

- Limit drinking in the evening, especially drinks with alcohol or caffeine.

- Empty the bladder all the way when you pass urine.
- Use the restroom often. Don't wait for long periods without passing urine.

Some medications can make BPH symptoms worse, so talk with your doctor or pharmacist about any medicines you are taking, including the following:

- Over-the-counter cold and cough medicines (especially antihistamines)
- Tranquilizers
- Antidepressants
- Blood pressure medicine

Drug Therapy

Millions of American men with mild to moderate BPH symptoms have chosen prescription drugs over surgery since the early 1990s.

There are two main types of drugs used. One type relaxes muscles near the prostate while the other type shrinks the prostate gland. There is evidence that shows that taking both drugs together may work best to keep BPH symptoms from getting worse.

Alpha-blockers: These drugs help relax muscles near the prostate to relieve pressure and let urine flow more freely, but they don't shrink the size of the prostate. For many men, the drug can improve urine flow and reduce symptoms within days. Possible side effects include dizziness, headache, and fatigue.

5-alpha-reductase inhibitors: These drugs shrink the prostate. They relieve symptoms by blocking an enzyme that acts on the male hormone testosterone to boost organ growth. When the enzyme is blocked, growth slows down. This helps shrink the prostate, reduce blockage, and limit the need for surgery. Currently, two drugs of this type are available: finasteride and dutasteride.

Taking one of these drugs for at least six months to one year can increase urine flow and reduce your symptoms. They seem to work best for men with very large prostates. You must continue to take the drug to prevent symptoms from coming back.

One of the two drugs, finasteride, is also used to treat baldness in men. It can cause these side effects in a small percentage of men:

- Decreased interest in sex
- Trouble getting or keeping an erection
- Smaller amount of semen with ejaculation

It's important to note that taking these drugs can lower your prostate specific antigen (PSA) test levels. There is also evidence that finasteride lowers the risk of getting prostate cancer, but whether it lowers the risk of dying from prostate cancer is still unclear.

Table 36.1. BPH Medications

Category	Activity	Generic Name	Brand Name
Alpha-blockers	Relax muscles near prostate	doxazosin tamsulosin alfuzosin terazosin prazosin	Cardura® Flomax® Uroxatral® Hytrin® Minipress®
5-alpha-reductase inhibitors	Slows prostate growth, shrinks prostate	finasteride dutasteride	Proscar® or Propecia® Avodart®

BPH surgery: The number of prostate surgeries has gone down over the years. But operations for BPH are still one of the most common surgeries for American men. Surgery is used when symptoms are severe or drug therapy has not worked well.

Types of surgeries include the following:

- *Transurethral resection of the prostate (TURP):* This is the most common surgery for BPH. It accounts for 90 percent of all BPH surgeries. It takes about ninety minutes. The doctor passes an instrument through the urethra and trims away extra prostate tissue. A spinal block is used to numb the area. Tissue is sent to the laboratory to check for prostate cancer. TURP generally avoids the two main dangers linked to other prostate surgeries, incontinence (not being able to hold in urine) and impotence (not being able to have an erection). The recovery period for TURP is much shorter as well.
- *Transurethral incision of the prostate (TUIP):* This is similar to TURP. It is used on slightly enlarged prostate glands. The surgeon

places one or two small cuts in the prostate. This relieves pressure without trimming away tissue. It has a low risk of side effects. Like TURP, this treatment helps with urine flow by widening the urethra.

- *Transurethral needle ablation (TUNA):* This burns away excess prostate tissue using radio waves. It helps with urine flow, relieves symptoms, and may have fewer side effects than TURP. Most men need a catheter to drain urine for a period of time after the procedure.
- *Transurethral microwave thermotherapy (TUMT):* This uses microwaves sent through a catheter to destroy excess prostate tissue. This can be an option for men who should not have major surgery because they have other medical problems.
- *Transurethral electro-evaporation of the prostate (TUVP):* This uses electrical current to vaporize prostate tissue.
- *Open prostatectomy:* This means the surgeon removes the prostate through a cut in the lower abdomen. This is done only in very rare cases when obstruction is severe, the prostate is very large, or other procedures can't be done. General or spinal anesthesia is used and a catheter remains for three to seven days after the surgery. This surgery carries a higher risk of complications than medical treatment. Tissue is sent to the laboratory to check for prostate cancer.

Be sure to discuss options with your doctor and ask about the potential short- and long-term benefits and risks with each procedure.

Section 36.2

Prostatitis

Excerpted from "Prostatitis: Disorders of the Prostate," National Institute of Diabetes and Digestive and Kidney Diseases, National Institutes of Health, NIH Publication No. 08-4553, January 2008.

Prostatitis is a frequently painful condition that affects mostly young and middle-aged men. Doctors may have difficulty diagnosing prostatitis because the symptoms are not the same for every patient, and many of the symptoms—such as painful or burning urination and incomplete emptying of the bladder—could be signs of another disease.

What is the prostate?

The prostate is a walnut-sized gland that forms part of the male reproductive system. The gland is made of two lobes, or regions, enclosed by an outer layer of tissue. As Figure 36.1 and Figure 36.2 show, the prostate is located in front of the rectum and just below the bladder, where urine is stored. The prostate also surrounds the urethra, the canal through which urine and semen pass out of the body. The prostate squeezes fluid into the urethra to help make up semen as sperm move through during sexual climax.

Researchers estimate that 10 to 12 percent of men experience prostatitis-like symptoms.[1] The term "prostatitis" means inflammation of the prostate, but doctors use the term to describe four different disorders.

What are the types of prostatitis?

Acute bacterial prostatitis: This is the least common of the four types and is potentially life threatening. Fortunately, it is the easiest to diagnose and treat effectively. Men with this disease often have chills; fever; pain in the lower back and genital area; urinary frequency and urgency, often at night; burning or painful urination; body aches; and a demonstrable infection of the urinary tract as evidenced by white blood cells and bacteria in the urine. The treatment is an antimicrobial, a medicine that kills microbes—organisms that can be seen only with a microscope, including bacteria, viruses, and fungi. Antimicrobials include antibiotics and related medicines.

Chronic bacterial prostatitis: This is also relatively uncommon, and occurs when bacteria find a spot on the prostate where they can survive. Men have urinary tract infections that seem to go away but then come back with the same bacteria. Treatment usually requires the use of antimicrobials for a prolonged period of time. However, antimicrobials do not always cure this condition.

Chronic prostatitis/chronic pelvic pain syndrome: This is the most common but least understood form of prostatitis. It may be found in men of any age. Its symptoms go away and then return without warning, and it may be inflammatory or noninflammatory. In the inflammatory form, urine, semen, and prostatic fluid contain the kinds of cells the body usually produces to fight infection, but no bacteria can be found. In the noninflammatory form, not even the infection-fighting cells are present.

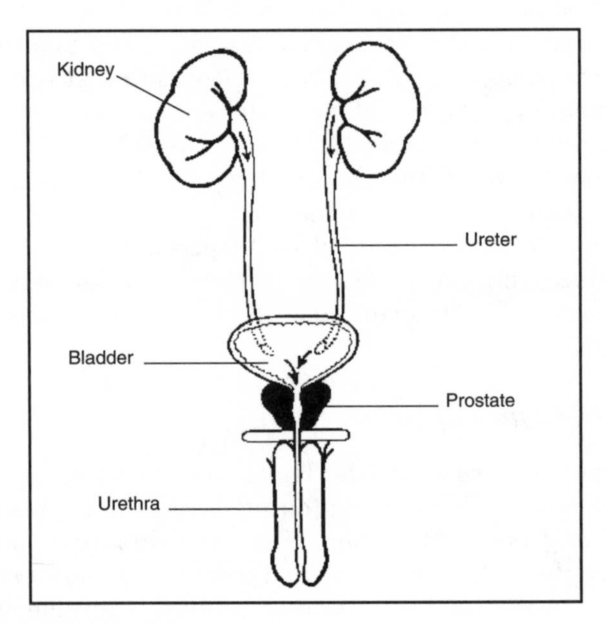

Figure 36.1. *Prostate, front view.*

Asymptomatic inflammatory prostatitis: This is the diagnosis given when the patient does not complain of pain or discomfort but has infection-fighting cells in his prostate fluid and semen. Doctors usually find this form of prostatitis when looking for causes of infertility or testing for prostate cancer.

How is prostatitis diagnosed?

A doctor performs a digital rectal exam (DRE) by inserting a gloved and lubricated finger into the patient's rectum, just behind the prostate. The doctor can feel the prostate to see if it is swollen or tender in spots.

The doctor can diagnose the bacterial forms of prostatitis by examining a urine sample with a microscope. The sample may also be sent to a laboratory to perform a culture. In a urine culture, the bacteria are allowed to grow so they can be identified and tested for their resistance to different types of antimicrobials.

To confirm the prostate infection, the doctor may obtain two urine samples—before and after prostate massage. To perform a prostate massage, the doctor will insert a gloved and lubricated finger into the

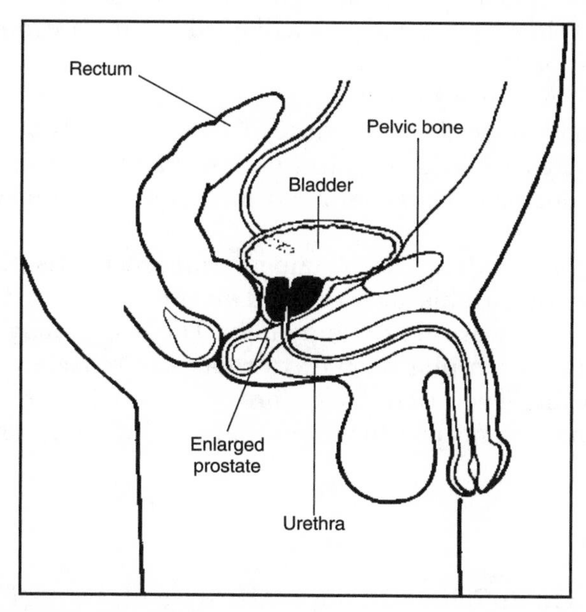

Figure 36.2. *Prostate, side view.*

rectum, as in a DRE, and stroke the prostate to release fluids from the gland. The post-massage urine sample will contain prostate fluid. If that second urine sample contains bacteria or infection-fighting cells that were not present in the pre-massage urine sample, this suggests the prostate contains infection.

To diagnose chronic prostatitis/chronic pelvic pain syndrome, the doctor must rule out all other possible causes of urinary symptoms, such as kidney stones, bladder disorders, and infections. Since many different conditions must be considered, the doctor may order a full range of tests, including ultrasound or magnetic resonance imaging (MRI), biopsy, blood tests, and tests of bladder function.

If all other possible causes of a patient's symptoms are ruled out, the doctor may then diagnose chronic prostatitis/chronic pelvic pain syndrome. To aid in understanding the symptoms and measuring the effects of treatment, the doctor may ask a series of questions from a standard questionnaire, the NIH-Chronic Prostatitis Symptom Index.

How is prostatitis treated?

The bacterial forms of prostatitis are treated with antimicrobials. Acute prostatitis may require a short hospital stay so that fluids and antimicrobials can be given through an intravenous, or IV, tube. After the initial therapy, the patient will need to take antimicrobials for two to four weeks.

Chronic bacterial prostatitis requires a longer course of therapy. The doctor may prescribe a low dose of antimicrobials for six months to prevent recurrent infection. If a patient has trouble emptying his bladder, the doctor may recommend medicine or surgery to correct blockage.

Antimicrobials will not help nonbacterial prostatitis. Each patient will have to work with his doctor to find an effective treatment. Changing diet or taking warm baths may help. The doctor may prescribe a medicine called an alpha blocker to relax the muscle tissue in the prostate. No single solution works for everyone with this condition.

No treatment is needed for asymptomatic inflammatory prostatitis.

Reference

1. McNaughton-Collins M, Joyce GF, Wise M, Pontari MA. Prostatitis. In: Litwin MS, Saigal CS, editors. *Urologic Diseases in*

America. U.S. Department of Health and Human Services, Public Health Service, National Institutes of Health, National Institute of Diabetes and Digestive and Kidney Diseases. Washington, DC: U.S. Government Publishing Office, 2007; NIH Publication No. 07–5512 pp. 9–42.

Chapter 37

Disorders of the Scrotum and Testicles

Chapter Contents

Section 37.1

Epididymitis and Orchitis

"Epididymitis and Orchitis" is reprinted with permission from www.urologyhealth.org.

If you are a male and experiencing pain the scrotum or testicle, then it might be attributed to epididymitis, orchitis or a combination of the two. The information below will give you a head start in learning more about these conditions and aid in you in your discussions with a urologist.

What are epididymitis, orchitis, and epididymo-orchitis?

Epididymitis is inflammation of the epididymis—the coiled tube that collects sperm from the testicle and passes it on to the vas deferens. There are two forms of this disease, acute and chronic. Acute epididymitis comes on suddenly with severe symptoms and subsides with treatment. Chronic epididymitis is a long-standing condition, usually of gradual onset, for which the symptoms can be improved with treatment but may not completely be eradicated. Most cases of epididymitis occur in adults.

Orchitis is inflammation of the testicle. It almost always comes on suddenly and subsides with treatment. Chronic orchitis is not well defined, and instead is considered to be one of the many conditions related to chronic testicular pain (orchalgia).

Epididymo-orchitis is the sudden inflammation of both the epididymis and the testicle.

What are the causes of such conditions?

Acute epididymitis is usually caused by a bacterial infection. In children who haven't reached puberty, the infection usually starts in the bladder or kidney and then spreads to the testicle. This is often associated with a birth-related abnormality that predisposes to urinary tract infection. In sexually active men, the most common infection causing epididymitis is a sexually transmitted disease such as gonorrhea or chlamydia infection. These infections start in the urethra, causing urethritis, which can then move into the testicle. In men over forty years of age, the most common cause is bacteria from the urinary tract. Other causes can include: bladder outlet obstruction due to enlargement of the prostate; partial blockage of the urethra; or recent catheterization of the urethra. In any of these cases, the original infection may not cause symptoms, and the first sign of a problem may be epididymitis. Bacterial epididymitis rarely occurs when a bacterial infection spreads from the bloodstream into the epididymis, although this is the typical way that tuberculosis infection can involve the epididymis. Epididymitis is occasionally due to causes other than infection. Chemical epididymitis occurs when sterile urine flows backward from the urethra to the epididymis, which most commonly occurs with heavy lifting or straining. The urine causes inflammation without infection. The drug amiodarone also can cause a noninfectious epididymitis, and there are other cases of noninfectious epididymitis without known cause.

Chronic epididymitis may develop after several episodes of acute epididymitis that do not subside, but also can occur without any symptomatic episodes of acute epididymitis or prior infection—in which case the cause is unknown.

In most cases of acute orchitis, the testicle is inflamed due to the spread of a bacterial infection from the epididymis, and therefore "epididymo-orchitis" is the correct term. Although orchitis without epididymitis can occur from a bacterial infection, orchitis without epididymitis usually results from an infection related to the mumps virus. "Mumps orchitis" occurs in approximately one-third of males who contract mumps after puberty.

Acute epididymo-orchitis is usually a primary bacterial or tuberculous infection of the epididymis that has spread to the testicle to involve both structures. Rarely, it can start in the testicle and spread to the epididymis. Mumps orchitis does not spread to the epididymis.

What are the symptoms and how are they diagnosed?

Acute epididymitis and acute epididymo-orchitis: Symptoms occur not only from the local infection, but also from the original source of the infection. Common symptoms from the original source of the infection include: urethral discharge and urethral pain or itching (from urethritis); pelvic pain and urinary frequency, urgency or painful/burning urination (from infection of the bladder, called cystitis); fever, perineal pain, urinary frequency, urinary urgency, or painful/burning urination (from infection of the prostate, called prostatitis); fever and flank pain (from infection of the kidney, called pyelonephritis). In some cases, pain in the scrotum from the local infection is the only noticeable symptom. The pain starts at the back of one testicle but can soon spread to the entire testicle, the scrotum, and occasionally the groin. Swelling, tenderness, redness, firmness, and warmth of the skin may also accompany the pain. The entire scrotum can swell up with fluid (hydrocele). To make the diagnosis, the doctor will ask you about your medical history and examine you. The doctor may test a urine sample and look at it under the microscope to assess for bacterial infection, culture a urine sample as a more definitive way to see if there is bacterial infection, or examine a swab obtained from the urethra (if urethritis is suggested by your symptoms). If your pain came on very suddenly and severely, then an ultrasound, which is a noninvasive test that uses sound waves to look at the epididymis and measure blood flow, might be used to distinguish epididymitis from another condition called testicular torsion. This is managed very differently than epididymitis, so making the distinction is very important. Tuberculous epididymitis presents in the same way, although chemical and amiodarone epididymitis are less severe.

Chronic epididymitis: The pain occurs only in the scrotal contents, and is less severe and more localized than acute epididymitis. Swelling, tenderness, redness, and warmth of the skin do not occur. Additional tests may be used as for acute epididymitis, but are less frequently required. In acute epididymitis the urine is usually infected, whereas in chronic epididymitis it is usually not.

Acute orchitis: During the acute phase of mumps orchitis, symptoms include pain of varying severity, tenderness, and swelling. The parotiditis (swelling of facial glands) of mumps usually precedes orchitis by three to seven days. Isolated orchitis from bacterial infection has the same symptoms of acute epididymitis or epididymo-orchitis.

What are the treatment options?

Acute epididymitis and acute epididymo-orchitis: Treatment in cases suspected to be from bacteria (most) includes at least two weeks of antibiotics. Most cases can be treated with oral antibiotics as an outpatient. Your doctor can choose one of several, including: doxycycline, azithromycin, ofloxacin, ciprofloxacin, levofloxacin, or trimethoprim-sulfamethoxazole. Tuberculous epididymitis is treated with anti-tuberculous medications, although in many cases surgical removal of the testicle (orchiectomy, which includes removal of the epididymis) is required because the damage is so severe. Cases of severe infection, with intractable pain, vomiting, very high fever, or overall severe illness, may require admission to the hospital. Aside from treatment of amiodarone epididymitis by reducing the dose or stopping the drug, there is no specific therapy for noninfectious epididymitis. General therapy for epididymitis includes bed rest for one to two days combined with elevation of the scrotum. The aim is to get the inflamed epididymis above the level of the heart. This improves blood flow out of the testicle, which promotes more rapid healing and reduces swelling and discomfort. Intermittent application of ice might also be of assistance and, in cases due to infection, intake of plenty of fluids. Nonsteroidal anti-inflammatory drugs such as ibuprofen or naproxen are useful since they not only relieve pain but also reduce the inflammation that is the cause of the pain.

Chronic epididymitis: Primary therapy is with medications and other treatments directed towards reducing the discomfort. Nonsteroidal anti-inflammatory medications and local application of heat are the mainstays of treatment. If symptoms persist, your physician may recommend other medications to alter the perception of pain in the area, or might refer you to a specialist in pain management. If all else fails the epididymis can be surgically removed (epididymectomy) while leaving the testicle in place.

Acute orchitis: There is no specific treatment for acute mumps orchitis. In cases of bacterial infection, treatment is as for acute epididymitis and acute epididymo-orchitis.

What can be expected after treatment?

Acute epididymitis and acute epididymo-orchitis: In the typical infectious case, it will take two to three days for you to notice improvement. If the redness does not subside and you do not start to feel better by that time, contact your physician. Complete resolution of symptoms will take longer. Discomfort can persist until the entire course of antibiotics is completed, and the firmness and swelling can takes months to resolve. Following the instructions to stay at bed rest with scrotal elevation for the first one to two days will help speed recovery. You should follow up with your physician after treatment. In cases of tuberculous epididymitis that do not require orchiectomy, it takes months to resolve on medications, and there will likely be some shrinking of the testicle. Amiodarone epididymitis improves after reducing the dose or stopping the drug, without any residual problems. Chemical epididymitis also resolves completely.

Chronic epididymitis: Treatment is ongoing, and not curative. You may need to take medications for years, or until the symptoms resolve spontaneously. If epididymectomy is performed, relief of symptoms occurs in three out of four patients after a few weeks for surgical recovery. If surgery has not resolved your symptoms, then your doctor will try medical therapy again.

Acute orchitis: Following the acute phase of mumps orchitis, the pain resolves but there is often atrophy of the testicle.

What if the swelling and pain do not get better after the first three days of antibiotics?

Most cases of acute epididymitis or epididymo-orchitis are treated well by antibiotics, but in some cases a different antibiotic needs to be used. Tuberculous epididymitis should also be considered when symptoms do not resolve appropriately. On occasion, surgery needs to be performed. If an abscess (pocket of pus) has formed, antibiotics alone are rarely sufficient and surgery to drain the abscess or remove part or all of the epididymis and testicle might be required. Other complications that might require surgery include testicular infarction (death of the testicle due to destruction of the blood vessels) and cutaneous fistula (infection that continues to drain out through the skin).

Can I pass the infection to my sexual partner?

If the acute epididymitis or epididymo-orchitis is from a sexually transmitted disease (usually in sexually active men under forty years of age), then your sexual partner needs to be treated as well since the infection can be passed back and forth through sexual contact. The urinary tract bacteria that cause other cases of epididymitis or epididymo-orchitis are not sexually transmitted. Treatment of your partner is not required, and there is no risk of infecting your partner.

Will the ability to father children be reduced?

The atrophy associated with mumps orchitis and tuberculous epididymitis is associated with reduced production of sperm in the affected testicle in some cases. After an episode of acute epididymitis or epididymo-orchitis there can rarely be blockage of the epididymis, which would reduce delivery of sperm from that testicle. In any of these cases, if the other testicle is unaffected then most men are able to father a child normally.

Will hormone production by the testicle be affected?

The ability of the affected testicle to produce testosterone is lost in some men with atrophy associated with mumps orchitis and tuberculous epididymitis. The rare epididymal blockage that occurs after acute epididymitis or epididymo-orchitis does not affect hormone production.

Do epididymal or testicular infections lead to cancer?

There is no association of these infections with cancer.

Section 37.2

Hydrocele and Inguinal Hernia

Hydrocele

Alternative Names

Processus vaginalis; patent processus vaginalis

Definition

A hydrocele is a fluid-filled sack along the spermatic cord within the scrotum.

Causes

Hydroceles are common in newborn infants.

During normal development, the testicles descend down a tube from the abdomen into the scrotum. Hydroceles result when this tube fails to close. Fluid drains from the abdomen through the open tube. The fluid builds up in the scrotum, where it becomes trapped. This causes the scrotum to become swollen.

Hydroceles normally go away a few months after birth, but their appearance may worry new parents. Occasionally, a hydrocele may be associated with an inguinal hernia.

Hydroceles may also be caused by inflammation or injury of the testicle or epididymis, or by fluid or blood blockage within the spermatic cord. This type of hydrocele is more common in older men.

Symptoms

The main symptom is a painless, swollen testicle, which feels like a water balloon. A hydrocele may occur on one or both sides.

Exams and Tests

During a physical exam, the doctor usually finds a swollen scrotum that is not tender. Often, the testicle cannot be felt because of the surrounding fluid. The size of the fluid-filled sack can sometimes be increased and decreased by pressure to the abdomen or the scrotum.

If the size of the fluid collection varies, it is more likely to be associated with an inguinal hernia.

Hydroceles can be easily demonstrated by shining a flashlight (transillumination) through the enlarged portion of the scrotum. If the scrotum is full of clear fluid, as in a hydrocele, the scrotum will light up.

An ultrasound may be done to confirm the diagnosis.

Treatment

Hydroceles are usually not dangerous, and they are usually only treated when they cause discomfort or embarrassment, or if they are large enough to threaten the testicle's blood supply.

One option is to remove the fluid in the scrotum with a needle, a process called aspiration. However, surgery is generally preferred. Aspiration may be the best alternative for people who have certain surgical risks.

Sclerosing (thickening or hardening) medications may be injected after aspiration to close off the opening. This helps prevent the future buildup of fluid.

Hydroceles associated with an inguinal hernia should be repaired surgically as quickly as possible. Hydroceles that do not go away on their own over a period of months should be evaluated for possible surgery. A surgical procedure, called a hydrocelectomy, is often performed to correct a hydrocele.

Outlook (Prognosis)

Generally, a simple hydrocele goes away without surgery. If surgery is necessary, it is a simple procedure for a skilled surgeon, and usually has an excellent outcome.

Possible Complications

Complications may occur from hydrocele treatment.

Risks related to hydrocele surgery may include:

- blood clots;
- infection;
- injury to the scrotal tissue or structures.

Risks related to aspiration and sclerosing may include:

- infection;
- fibrosis;
- mild to moderate pain in the scrotal area;
- return of the hydrocele.

When to Contact a Medical Professional

Call for an appointment with your health care provider if you have symptoms of hydrocele (to rule out other causes of a testicle lump).

Acute pain in the scrotum or testicles is a surgical emergency. If enlargement of the scrotum is associated with acute pain, seek medical attention immediately.

References

Behrman RE. *Nelson Textbook of Pediatrics*. 17th ed. Philadelphia, Pa: WB Saunders; 2004.

Wein AJ. Campbell. *Walsh Urology*. 9th ed. St. Louis, Mo: WB Saunders; 2007.

Inguinal Hernia

What is an inguinal hernia?

An inguinal hernia is an abnormal bulge, or protrusion, that can be seen and felt in the groin area (the area between the abdomen and the thigh). An inguinal hernia develops when a portion of an internal organ such as the intestine, along with fluid, bulges through a weakened area in the muscle wall of the abdomen.

Who is at risk for an inguinal hernia?

Some people, especially men, are born with a weakness in their groin muscles. Ninety percent of the newborns who have inguinal hernias are boys. With or without this weakness, an inguinal hernia can be caused by increasing pressure in the abdomen. Risk factors include:

- Being moderately to severely overweight
- Pregnancy
- Lifting heavy objects
- Persistent coughing, such as smoker's cough
- Sneezing a lot, which may be common in a person with allergies
- Straining during bowel movement, which may be caused by constipation or diarrhea
- For men, trying to urinate when there is a blockage caused by an enlarged prostate

What are the symptoms of inguinal hernia?

Inguinal hernias are characterized by pain in the groin area when coughing, sneezing, or lifting. Some people may notice a slight bulge or protrusion in the groin area that can be pushed back in. Other symptoms include constipation and blood in the stool.

How is an inguinal hernia diagnosed?

A physician's physical examination is often enough to diagnose a hernia. Sometimes hernia swelling is visible when you stand upright.

Usually, the hernia can be felt if you place your hand directly over it and then bear down. Ultrasound may be used to see certain types of hernias, and abdominal x-rays and computed axial tomography (CAT) scans may be ordered to identify a bowel obstruction.

How is an inguinal hernia treated?

If the hernia bulge can be pushed back in and the symptoms are tolerable, you may not need surgery. Your physician may suggest that you wear a special belt or binder to support the area, and avoid heavy lifting.

If the inguinal hernia symptoms are painful, the treatment is elective surgery. The surgery to correct the condition is performed under general anesthesia, either on an outpatient basis or in the hospital. (In some cases, the surgery may be performed under a local anesthesia.) The surgery, called herniorrhaphy, repairs the opening in the muscle wall. Inguinal herniorrhaphy is performed using a laparoscope, a thin, telescope-like instrument that requires a small incision and involves a short recovery time.

During laparoscopic surgery, three to six small (5 to 10 millimeter) incisions are made in the abdomen. The laparoscope and surgical instruments are inserted through these incisions. The surgeon is guided by the laparoscope, which transmits a picture of the internal organs on a monitor. The advantages of laparoscopic surgery include smaller incisions, less risk of infection, less pain and scarring, and a more rapid recovery.

Sometimes the weak area is reinforced with mesh or wire. This operation is called hernioplasty.

Incarcerated and strangulated hernias: If the weakness in the abdominal wall is small to moderate in size, a portion of intestine may get trapped, or incarcerated. This is called an incarcerated hernia and can cause problems such as severe pain, nausea, vomiting, or absence of bowel movements.

If the intestine becomes incarcerated or trapped in the abdominal wall defect, blood flow to the intestines may become blocked. This is called a strangulated hernia. This type of hernia is often painful and requires prompt surgery.

Surgery may be needed to remove part of the intestine if the hernia is incarcerated or strangulated. This surgery is called bowel resection. (Bowel is another word for intestine.) Bowel resection can also be performed laparoscopically.

Recovering from surgery: Many patients are able to walk around the day after hernia surgery. Generally, there are no dietary restrictions and the patient can resume his or her regular activities within a week (with the exception of lifting). Complete recovery will take three to four weeks, and hard labor and heavy lifting should be avoided for at least three months after surgery. Surgery is no guarantee that your hernia will not return, so preventive measures are especially important to avoid a recurrence.

How can I prevent an inguinal hernia?

- If you are overweight, follow your physician's advice for losing weight.
- Avoid lifting, pulling, and pushing heavy objects. Use proper lifting, pulling, and pushing techniques when needed. Bend at your knees and lift using your legs rather than your back.
- Stop smoking and try to avoid coughing.
- Use deep breathing techniques to help control your coughing. Obtain a medical prescription to treat the condition causing your cough.
- Take medication to reduce allergies and sneezing.
- Avoid constipation by eating foods that are high in fiber, using stool softeners, or drinking a natural stimulant beverage such as prune juice. Use laxatives or enemas only if recommended by your physician.
- For males, wear a jock strap or similar groin support.
- Adjust your occupational duties, if necessary.

When should I call the doctor?

If you have been diagnosed with a hernia, and you have the following symptoms—nausea, vomiting, unable to have a bowel movement, or pass gas—you may have a strangulated hernia or an obstruction. These are medical emergencies. Call your doctor immediately.

Section 37.3

Spermatocele

The male reproductive tract is responsible for the production, maturation of sperm, and delivery of sperm. This tract is a complex and highly integrated entity. Sperm are produced in the testicles and then are transported through the genital ductal system to the penis and out of the urethra during ejaculation. Each component of the reproductive tract is highly specialized.

Abnormalities within the male reproductive tract may appear as scrotal masses. Masses may be of little significance or may represent life-threatening illnesses. It is necessary to follow a set course of action to determine the nature of the masses and the most appropriate treatment option. For example, testicular cancer is a source of great concern and uniformly requires prompt intervention. Other masses, such as varicoceles, can cause pain or impair reproductive function. Spermatoceles are benign and generally painless masses that grow at the top of the testicle. Thus, it is important for a patient to seek prompt medical attention when he identifies a scrotal mass or abnormality while performing testicular self-examination. The following information will assist you when talking to a urologist about spermatoceles.

What is a spermatocele?

Spermatoceles, also known as spermatic cysts, are typically painless, noncancerous (benign) cysts that grow from the epididymis near the top of the testicle. Spermatoceles are typically smooth and they are usually filled with a milky or clear colored fluid containing sperm. Over time, spermatoceles may remain stable in size or they may grow. If in fact the size becomes bothersome, or results in pain, then there are several treatment options to rectify the problem. Spermatoceles are generally no more than a nuisance rather than a serious medical condition.

What can cause spermatoceles?

The precise cause of spermatoceles is not known. While spermatoceles may form as a result of trauma or inflammation, these conditions are certainly not required for spermatocele formation. Others suggest that blockage of the efferent ducts and epididymis result in spermatocele formation. Additionally, in utero exposure to diethylstilbestrol (DES), a synthetic form of estrogen, has also been suggested as a possible cause.

How common are spermatoceles?

The precise incidence of spermatoceles is unknown, but an estimated 30 percent of all men have this condition. Incidence increases with age, with peak rates for the diagnosis of spermatoceles occurring in men in their forties and fifties. No racial or ethnic predispositions to spermatocele formation are known.

What are the symptoms of spermatoceles?

Men with spermatoceles usually have no symptoms. However, when associated symptoms are present, they may include scrotal heaviness and/or pain.

How are spermatoceles diagnosed?

Spermatoceles are typically discovered through a man's self-examination of his testicles or at the time of an evaluation by a physician. Light can be shined through a spermatocele (transillumination), indicating that the mass is not a solid tumor but more likely a benign cyst. Ultrasound examination remains a very reliable means of evaluation and is a relatively quick, noninvasive, and inexpensive test. Other diagnostic imaging tests are not generally used although magnetic resonance imaging (MRI) can also be used as an adjunct in cases where scrotal ultrasound is inconclusive.

How are spermatoceles treated?

Since spermatoceles generally do not cause discomfort and often go unnoticed by patients, they rarely require treatment. Nevertheless, some affected individuals do experience significant associated symptoms, such as bothersome size or pain. When intervention is indicated, the available treatment options include:

- **Medical therapy:** Oral analgesics or anti-inflammatory agents may be used to relieve pain associated with symptomatic spermatoceles. No other type of medical therapy is specifically indicated for the treatment of spermatoceles.
- **Surgical therapy:** Spermatocelectomy involves surgical removal of the spermatocele from the adjoining epididymal tissue. The overall goal of surgical therapy is removal of the spermatocele with preservation of the continuity of the male reproductive tract.
- **Other therapies:** Aspiration and sclerotherapy are two less commonly utilized approaches to treat spermatoceles. Aspiration involves puncture of the spermatocele with a needle and withdrawal of its contents into a syringe. Sclerotherapy is performed with subsequent injection of an irritating agent directly into the spermatocele sac to cause it to heal or scar closed, removing the spermatocele space and decreasing the odds of fluid reaccumulation. Although several reports describe the effectiveness and tolerability of these treatment options, they are generally not recommended. Spermatocele recurrence is a common complication with both approaches, and chemical epididymitis and pain are common complications with sclerotherapy. Furthermore, aspiration and sclerotherapy have limited applicability in men of reproductive age, due to the significant risk of epididymal damage potentially leading to obstruction and resultant subfertility.

What can be expected after surgical treatment?

Spermatocelectomy is typically performed as an outpatient procedure, under a variety of possible anesthetic agents. Patients are generally discharged home with a pressure dressing consisting of an athletic supporter filled with fluffy gauze. Ice packs are applied for two to three days to minimize swelling. Oral pain medications are generally used for one to two days postoperatively. Patients may shower twenty-four to forty-eight hours after surgery, and a follow-up visit is scheduled for one to two weeks after the procedure.

Potential complications of spermatocelectomy include fever, infection, bleeding (scrotal hematoma), and persistent pain. Furthermore, inadvertent epididymal obstruction may result, which can lead to subfertility or infertility. Therefore, intervention should be avoided in men who still desire children. These complications may potentially be minimized by use of meticulous surgical technique (including use of an operating microscope or optical magnification).

Do spermatoceles lead to testicular cancer?

Spermatoceles are benign epididymal lesions. They are separate and distinct from the testicle. Patients with spermatoceles do not have an identified increased risk of testicular cancer.

Are any medications available to cure my spermatocele or prevent the formation of additional ones?

Medications are available to treat associated discomfort or pain, but no medication will lead to resolution or prevention of spermatoceles.

How often should I perform scrotal self-exams?

These exams should be performed at least once per month. Your physician can instruct you in the specific technique. If you detect any suspicious changes, such as increasing size or unusual firmness of scrotal structures, contact your physician.

Section 37.4

Testicular Failure

Reprinted from "Testicular Failure,"

Alternative Names

Primary hypogonadism—male

Definition

Testicular failure is the inability of the testicles to produce sperm or male hormones.

Causes

Testicular failure is uncommon. Causes include:

- certain drugs, including glucocorticoids, ketoconazole, and opioids;
- chromosome problems;
- diseases that affect the testicle, including mumps, orchitis, and testicular cancer;
- injury to the testicles;
- testicular torsion.

The following things increase the risk for testicular failure:

- Activities that may cause constant, low-level injury to the scrotum, such as riding a motorcycle
- Frequent and heavy use of marijuana
- Undescended testicles at birth

Symptoms

- Decrease in height

- Enlarged breasts (gynecomastia)
- Infertility
- Lack of muscle mass
- Lack of sex drive (libido)
- Loss of armpit and pubic hair
- Slow development or absence of secondary male sex characteristics (growth and distribution of hair, scrotal enlargement, penis enlargement, voice changes)

Men may also notice they do not need to shave as frequently.

Exams and Tests

A physical examination may reveal:

- genitals that do not clearly look either male or female (usually noted in infancy);
- abnormally small testicle;
- tumor or mass (group of cells) on or near the testicle.

Further testing may show decreased bone mineral density and fractures. Blood tests may reveal low levels of testosterone and high levels of follicle-stimulating hormone (FSH) and luteinizing hormone (LH).

Testicular failure and low testosterone levels may be difficult to diagnose in older men because testosterone levels normally fall with age. The level of testosterone at which replacement therapy would be likely to improve symptoms and other outcomes is unpredictable and variable.

Treatment

Male hormone supplements may successfully treat some forms of testicular failure. Men who take testosterone replacement therapy need to be carefully monitored by a doctor. Testosterone may cause overgrowth of the prostate gland and an abnormal increase in red blood cells.

Avoiding a specific drug or activity known to cause the problem may result in return of normal testicular function.

Outlook (Prognosis)

Many forms of testicular failure cannot be reversed. Hormone replacement therapy can help reverse symptoms, although it may not restore fertility.

Possible Complications

Testicular failure before the onset of puberty will stop normal body growth, specifically the development of adult male characteristics.

When to Contact a Medical Professional

Call for an appointment with your health care provider if you have symptoms of testicular failure.

Prevention

Avoid higher-risk activities if possible.

References

Bhasin S, Cunningham GR, Hayes FJ, et al. Testosterone therapy in adult men with androgen deficiency syndromes: an Endocrine Society clinical practice guideline. *J Clin Endocrinol Metab*. 2006 Jun;91(6):1995–2010.

Section 37.5

Testicular Torsion

Reprinted from "Testicular Torsion,"

Alternative Names

Torsion of the testis; testicular ischemia; testicular twisting

Definition

Testicular torsion is the twisting of the spermatic cord, which cuts off the blood supply to the testicle and surrounding structures within the scrotum.

Causes

Some men may be predisposed to testicular torsion as a result of inadequate connective tissue within the scrotum. However, the condition can result from trauma to the scrotum, particularly if significant swelling occurs. It may also occur after strenuous exercise or may not have an obvious cause.

The condition is more common during infancy (first year of life) and at the beginning of adolescence (puberty).

Symptoms

- Sudden onset of severe pain in one testicle, with or without a previous predisposing event
- Swelling within one side of the scrotum (scrotal swelling)
- Nausea or vomiting
- Light-headedness

Additional symptoms that may be associated with this disease:

- Testicle lump
- Blood in the semen
- Extremely tender and enlarged testicular region—more common on the right
- The testicle on the affected side is higher

Treatment

Surgery is usually required and should be performed as soon as possible after symptoms begin. If surgery is performed within six hours, most testicles can be saved.

During surgery, the testicle on the other (non-affected) side is usually also anchored as a preventive measure. This is because the non-affected testicle is at risk of testicular torsion in the future.

Outlook (Prognosis)

If the condition is diagnosed quickly and immediately corrected, the testicle may continue to function properly. After six hours of torsion (impaired blood flow), the likelihood that the testicle will need to be removed increases. However, even with less than six hours of torsion, the testicle may lose its ability to function.

Possible Complications

If the blood supply is cut off to the testicle for a prolonged period of time, it may atrophy (shrink) and need to be surgically removed. Atrophy of the testicle may occur days to months after the torsion has been corrected. Severe infection of the testicle and scrotum is also possible if the blood flow is restricted for a prolonged period.

When to Contact a Medical Professional

Go to the emergency room or call the local emergency number (such as 911) if testicular torsion symptoms occur.

Prevention

Use precautions to avoid trauma to the scrotum. Many cases are not preventable.

References

Expert Panel on Urologic Imaging. Acute onset of scrotal pain (without trauma, without antecedent mass). Reston, Va: American College of Radiology; 2005. 4 p.

Ringdahl E. Testicular Torsion. *Am Fam Physician*. Nov 2006; 74(10): 1739–43.

Wein AJ. *Campbell- Walsh Urology*. 9th ed. St. Louis, Mo: WB Saunders; 2007.

Section 37.6

Undescended Testicle

"Undescended Testicle (Cryptorchidism)," by Christopher Cooper, M.D. Reprinted with permission of the University of Iowa Department of Urology, © 2006.

What is an undescended testicle?

When the testicle is formed it is located in the abdomen. In most boys it comes down into the scrotum by birth. Even after birth some testicles will still come down to the normal position in the scrotum (most of these come down by four months of age). If a testicle is not in the scrotum by six months of age, it is unlikely that it will come down. This testicle is called an undescended testicle. If the testicle can't be felt at all, it is called a "cryptorchid testicle." An undescended testicle requires surgery, called "orchidopexy," to place it in the scrotum.

Why is surgery necessary?

There are several reasons for placing an undescended testicle in the scrotum.

Fertility: The temperature in the scrotum is less than up in the abdomen. We know that the sperm-producing cells in the testicle do better if they are in the cooler scrotal environment. Bringing the testicle down into the scrotum at an early age may improve the semen quality and chances of fertility later in life.

Cancer: Undescended testicles have an increased chance of developing cancer later in life. It is unclear if early placement of the testicle in the scrotum decreases this chance of cancer. Placement of the testicle in the scrotum does permit self-examination of the testicle and earlier detection of testicular cancer should it occur.

Hernia: A hernia sac is almost always associated with an undescended testicle. During the operation to bring the testicle down, this hernia is routinely identified and fixed.

Protection: A testicle left in the abdomen may be at increased risk for injury or torsion (twisting and cutting of its blood supply).

Cosmoses: Placement of the testicle in the scrotum makes the scrotum look normal.

When should surgery be performed?

Since some testicles that are not descended at birth will come down, it is best to wait until around six months of age. By this age if a testicle cannot be felt or is very high, it is unlikely that it will come down.

What is the surgery like?

In most cases the child will go home on the same day the surgery is performed. A small incision is made in the groin and on the scrotum. No stitches will need to be removed. In some boys when the testicle can't be felt (known as "cryptorchidism"), laparoscopy may be used. Laparoscopy involves making an incision in the abdomen and placing a lighted telescope through this incision to look for the missing testicle. If it is found (some testicles are absent), laparoscopy is used for bringing it down into the scrotum.

What are some of the specific complications with orchidopexy?

Wound infection or bleeding may occur with any operation. Injury to the testicular blood vessels or vas deferens (the tube that carries sperm) may occur when performing an orchidopexy. These structures are delicate and avoidance of injury requires delicacy and precision while performing the surgery. Rarely, there are some testicles that don't reach the scrotum after the first surgery and require a second surgery (about a year later) to bring them into their normal scrotal position.

Section 37.7

Varicocele

Excerpted from "Varicocele," April 2007, reprinted with permission from www.kidshealth.org. Copyright © 2007 The Nemours Foundation. This information was provided by KidsHealth, one of the largest resources online for medically reviewed health information written for parents, kids, and teens. For more articles like this one, visit www.KidsHealth.org, or www.TeensHealth.org.

What is a varicocele?

In all guys, there's a structure that contains arteries, veins, nerves, and tubes—called the spermatic cord—that provides a connection and circulates blood to and from the testicles. Veins carry the blood flowing from the body back toward the heart, and a bunch of valves in the veins keep the blood flowing one way and stop it from flowing backward. In other words, the valves regulate your blood flow and make sure everything is flowing in the right direction.

But sometimes these valves can fail. When this happens, some of the blood can flow in reverse. This backed-up blood can collect in pools in the veins, which then causes the veins to stretch and get bigger, or become swollen. This is called a varicocele (pronounced: var-uh-ko-seel).

Who gets them?

Although they don't happen to every guy, varicoceles are fairly common. They appear in about 15 percent of guys between fifteen and twenty-five years old, and they mostly occur during puberty. That's because during puberty, the testicles grow rapidly and need more blood delivered to them. If the valves in the veins in the scrotum aren't functioning quite as well as they should, the veins can't handle transporting this extra blood from the testicles. So, although most of the blood continues to flow correctly, blood begins to back up, creating a varicocele.

An interesting fact is that varicoceles occur mostly on the left side of the scrotum. This is because a guy's body is organized so that blood flow on that side of the scrotum is greater, so varicoceles happen more often in the left testicle than the right. Although it's less common, they can sometimes occur on both sides.

What are the signs and symptoms?

In most cases, guys have no symptoms at all. A guy might not even be aware that he has a varicocele. However, if there are symptoms, they tend to occur during hot weather, after heavy exercise, or when a guy has been standing or sitting for a long time. Signs include:

- a dull ache in the testicle(s);
- a feeling of heaviness or dragging in the scrotum;
- dilated veins in the scrotum that can be felt (described as feeling like worms or spaghetti);
- discomfort in the testicle or on that particular side of the scrotum;
- the testicle is smaller on the side where the dilated veins are (due to difference in blood flow).

What do doctors do?

It's a good idea to get a testicular exam regularly, which is normally part of a guy's regular checkup. In addition to visually checking for any unusual lumps or bumps, the doctor generally feels the testicles and the area around them to make sure a guy's equipment is in good shape and there are no problems.

A testicular exam may be done while a guy is standing up so that the scrotum is relaxed. (Some abnormalities like a varicocele can be more easily felt in a standing position.) The doctor checks things like the size, weight, and position of the testicles, and gently rolls each testicle back and forth to feel for lumps or swelling. The doctor also feels for any signs of tenderness along the epididymis, the tube that transports sperm from the testicles.

The spermatic cord is also examined for any indication of swelling. If the doctor suspects a varicocele, he or she might confirm suspicions by using a stethoscope to hear the blood flowing backward through the faulty veins or might even use an ultrasound, which can identify malfunction of the veins and also measure blood flow.

Do varicoceles cause permanent damage?

Although there is no way to prevent a varicocele, it usually needs no special treatment. A varicocele is usually harmless and more than likely won't affect a guy's ability to father a child. Some experts believe, though, that in some cases a varicocele might damage the testicle or decrease sperm production. In those cases, a doctor will probably recommend surgery.

What if the doctor finds a varicocele?

Varicoceles are generally harmless, but if there is any pain and swelling the doctor may prescribe an anti-inflammatory medication to relieve it. If the varicocele is causing discomfort or aching, wearing snug underwear (like briefs) or a jock strap for support may bring relief. If pain is persistent and support doesn't help, the doctor may recommend a varicocelectomy (a surgical procedure to remove the varicocele).

A varicocelectomy is done by a urologist (pronounced: yoo-rah-luh-jist), a doctor who specializes in urinary and genital problems. The procedure is usually done on an outpatient basis (meaning there's no need for an overnight stay in hospital). The patient usually undergoes general or local anesthesia. To fix the problem, the doctor simply ties off the affected vein to redirect the flow of blood into other normal veins.

After surgery, the doctor probably will recommend that a guy wears a scrotal support and places an ice pack on the area to bring down any swelling. There may be discomfort in the testicle for a few weeks, but after that, any aches and pains will go away and everything should be back in full working order.

Part Four

Other Common Health Concerns in Men

Chapter 38

Violence and Abuse

Chapter Contents

Section 38.1

Violence Is a Concern for Men

Reprinted from "Violence Prevention,"
National Women's Health Information Center, July 17, 2008.

Consider the following:

- 86 percent of homicide deaths for victims eighteen to twenty-four years of age are males.
- Homicide is the fifth leading cause of death for black males.
- Males are almost four times more likely than females to be murdered.
- Suicide is the eighth leading cause of death for all U.S. men.

The statistics on violent deaths tell only part of the story, however. Many more survive violence and are left with permanent physical and emotional scars. Men also are more likely than women to commit acts of violence. One nationwide survey found male students more likely to have been involved in a physical fight than female students in the twelve months preceding the survey.

Many people don't talk about the fact that men are sometimes victims of intimate partner violence or sexual violence. Only 20 to 50 percent of all the different forms of intimate partner violence are reported to the police, and even fewer against men are reported. Although women are more likely to be victims of sexual violence than men, this finding may be influenced by the reluctance of men to report sexual violence. Rape is a serious issue among incarcerated men. Many times, men who are victims of these crimes remain silent and suffer alone.

Get Help for Violence in Your Life

Intimate Partner Violence—Including Domestic Violence and Sexual Violence

Violence against anyone, in any form, is a crime, regardless of who committed the violent act. It is always wrong, whether the abuser is a family member; someone you date; a current or past spouse, boyfriend, or girlfriend; an acquaintance; or a stranger. You are not at fault. You did not cause the abuse to occur, and you are not responsible for the violent behavior of someone else. If you or someone you know has been sexually, physically, or emotionally abused, seek help from other family members and friends or community organizations. Reach out for support or counseling. Talk with a doctor, especially if you have been physically hurt. Learn how to minimize your risk of becoming a victim of sexual assault or sexual abuse before you find yourself in an uncomfortable or threatening situation. Keep in mind, if you're a victim of violence at the hands of someone you know or love or you are recovering from an assault by a stranger, you are not alone.

Are You Violent?

Maybe you abuse somebody you love. Perhaps you lash out physically at others when angry. If you want to stop the cycle of violence in your life, talk to your doctor. Your doctor can help you find a mental health professional who can help you deal with your abuse.

Help Prevent Violence among Youth

Acts of violence have terrible and costly results for everyone involved, including families, communities, and society. Preventing violence is a top public health priority in the United States. You can do your part by being a good role model to the young men in your life. Teach them early and often that there is no place for violence in a relationship, and that violence of any kind is always wrong. Whether you are a father, coach, teacher, uncle, older brother, or mentor, you can make a real difference in a boy's life. Many young men need advice and direction on how to behave toward women and their peers, and they want to talk to you about it. You can share your experiences and let them know what you've learned.

Section 38.2

Men Can Be Victims of Sexual Assault

"Male Survivors: Men Who Have Been Sexually Assaulted," © 2001 Men Can Stop Rape (www.mencanstoprape.org). Reprinted with permission. Reviewed for currency in 2009.

Rape is a men's issue for many reasons. For one, we don't often talk about the fact that men are sexually assaulted. We need to start recognizing the presence of male survivors and acknowledging their unique experience.

The following questions and answers can help us all learn about male survivors so that we stop treating them as invisible and start helping them heal.

How often are men sexually assaulted?

While the numbers vary from study to study, most research suggests that 10 to 20 percent of males will be sexually violated at some point in their lifetimes. That translates into tens of thousands of boys and men assaulted each year alongside hundreds of thousands of girls and women.

If there are so many male survivors, why don't I know any?

Like female survivors, most male survivors never report being assaulted. Perhaps worst of all, men fear being blamed for the assault because they were not "man enough" to protect themselves in the face of an attack.

Can a woman sexually assault a man?

Yes, but it's not nearly as common as male-on-male assault. A recent study shows that more than 86 percent of male survivors are sexually abused by another male. That is not to say, however, that we should overlook boys or men who are victimized by females. It may be tempting to dismiss such experiences as wanted sexual initiation (especially in the case of an older female assaulting a younger male), but the reality is that the impact of female-on-male assault can be just as damaging.

Don't only men in prison get raped?

While prison rape is a serious problem and a serious crime, many male survivors are assaulted in everyday environments often by people they know—friends, teammates, relatives, teachers, clergy, bosses, or partners. As with female survivors, men are also sometimes raped by strangers. These situations tend to be more violent and more often involve a group of attackers rather than a single attacker.

How does rape affect men differently from women?

Rape affects men in many ways similar to women. Anxiety, anger, sadness, confusion, fear, numbness, self-blame, helplessness, hopelessness, suicidal feelings, and shame are common reactions of both male and female survivors.

In some ways, though, men react uniquely to being sexually assaulted. Immediately after an assault, men may show more hostility and aggression rather than tearfulness and fear. Over time, they may also question their sexual identity, act out in a sexually aggressive manner, and even downplay the impact of the assault.

Don't men who get raped become rapists?

No! This is a destructive myth that often adds to the anxiety a male survivor feels afterwards. Because of this myth, it is common for a male survivor to fear that he is now destined to do to others what was done to him.

While many convicted sex offenders have a history of being sexually abused, most male survivors do not become offenders. The truth is that the great majority of male survivors have never and will never sexually assault anyone.

If a man is raped by another man, does it mean he's gay?

No! A man getting raped by another man says nothing about his sexual orientation before the assault, nor does it change his sexual orientation afterwards.

Rape is prompted by anger or a desire to intimidate or dominate, not by sexual attraction or a rapist's assumption about his intended victim's sexual preference.

Because of society's confusion about the role that attraction plays in sexual assault and whether victims are responsible for provoking an assault, even heterosexual male survivors may worry that they somehow gave off "gay vibes" that the rapist picked up and acted upon. This is hardly the case.

How should I respond if a man tells me he has been assaulted?

The basics of supporting female survivors are the same for males. Believe him. Don't push and don't blame. Be cautious about physical contact until he's ready. Ask him if he wants to report it to the authorities and if he wants to talk to a counselor. If you need to, get counseling for yourself as well.

Where can male survivors go for help?

Most community resources—local or campus-based rape crisis centers—have on-site counselors trained in working with male survivors. Or they can refer survivors to professionals who can help. Know the resources in your area to help male survivors heal.

Section 38.3

Are You Being Abused?

"Male Victims of Domestic Abuse," © 2008 Domestic Abuse Helpline for Men and Women. Reprinted with permission. The Domestic Abuse Helpline for Men and Women offers a national 24-hour helpline for information and support, referrals to other programs and resources, and other supportive services. For additional information, call the Helpline at 888-7HELPLINE (888-743-5754) or visit www.dahmw.info.

Have You Been Abused?

- Does your partner block an exit to keep you from leaving during an argument? Open personal mail? Keep you from seeing friends or family? Use name-calling?

- Does your partner denigrate you in the presence of others? Say no one else would want you? Threaten suicide if you were to leave?
- Do you feel like you're "walking on eggshells" around your partner? Does she act like two different people (e.g., Dr. Jekyll/Mr. Hyde)?
- Does she threaten that if you leave you will never see the children again? Destroy or threaten to destroy your property?
- Have you been shoved, slapped, punched, bitten, or kicked? Even once?
- Does your partner anger easily, especially when drinking or on drugs?

If any number of these factors are true in your relationship, there is a problem. Victims of intimate partner violence come from all walks of life–all cultures, incomes, professions, ages, and religions. Intimate partner violence is not always defined by who's the stronger and/or bigger person in the relationship. However, it is about one person having and maintaining power and control over another person through physical, psychological, and/or verbally abusive means.

Why Men Don't Tell

Men typically face disbelief and ridicule when reporting abuse. As a result, male victims of domestic abuse tend to make excuses for injuries—"It was an accident"—when questioned by friends or medical personnel, which only allows perpetrators to continue the abuse.

Abusers are experts at making their victims feel like no one is on their side. Feeling like no one cares can create a spiral of isolation—the more you withdraw from friends and family, the less those who care about you will be able to help.

Though you may have been injured far worse on an athletic field, it is not the same thing as being physically attacked by your intimate partner, which hurts emotionally as well as physically. Allowing this pattern to continue can result in depression, substance abuse, loss of confidence, and even suicide.

For over thirty years, domestic violence has been defined as "the chronic abuse of power that men use to control women." Public awareness campaigns have focused solely on men as the perpetrators, never as victims. And yet, a Department of Justice study indicates that over 834,000 men report being domestically assaulted annually. The general public has been desensitized by sit-coms and commercials depicting men being hit over the head with frying pans, kicked in the groin, and slapped in the face by their intimate female partners. What message does this give society? A woman hitting a man is humorous and acceptable behavior. But it's not. No one deserves to be abused, whether man, woman, or child.

What You Can Do

- Keep a record of incidents of abuse.
- Take photographs.
- Always seek medical attention for your injuries, and be truthful about what caused them.
- Tell family and friends what is happening.
- Avoid being provoked into physical retaliation. When it is safe for you to do so, leave.
- Document! Document! Document!

Reasons Why Men Stay in Abusive Relationships

- **Shame:** What will people think? OR I don't want to be laughed at OR No one will believe me.
- **Self-worth:** I probably deserved it.
- **Denial:** I can handle it, it's not that bad OR All I have to do is leave the house until she cools down OR It's premenstrual syndrome; the kids are giving her a hard time.
- **Reluctance to give up the good:** She is a really creative, or loving, or wonderful person most of the time OR She didn't mean it.
- **Inertia:** It's too hard to do anything about it OR I'm not ready to change my life OR I'll deal with it later.

Chapter 39

Mental Health Concerns

Chapter Contents

Section 39.1

Depression in Men

Reprinted with permission from "Men and Depression," a publication of the Royal College of Psychiatrists, http://www.rcpsych.ac.uk.

Introduction

This section is for any man who is depressed, their friends and their family. Men seem to suffer from depression just as often as women, but they are less likely to ask for help. This section gives some basic facts about depression, how it affects men in particular, and how to get help.

Why Is It Important?

Depression causes a huge amount of suffering. It is a major reason for people taking time off work. Many people who kill themselves have been depressed—so it is potentially fatal. However, it is easy to treat, and this is best done as early as possible.

What's the Difference Between Just Feeling Miserable and Being Depressed?

Everyone has times in their lives when they feel down or depressed. It is usually for a good reason, does not dominate your life, and does not last for a long time. However, if the depression goes on for a long time, or becomes very severe, you may find yourself stuck and unable to lift yourself out of the depression. This is what doctors call a "depressive illness." Some people suffer from manic depression (also called bipolar affective disorder). They have periods of bad depression, but also times of great "elation" and overactivity. These can be just as harmful as the periods of depression.

What Are the Signs and Symptoms?

If you are depressed, you will probably notice some of the following:

- Mind:
  - You feel unhappy, miserable, down, depressed. It just won't go away and can be worse at a particular time of day, often first thing in the morning.
  - You can't enjoy anything.
  - You can't concentrate properly.
  - You feel guilty about things that have nothing to do with you.
  - You become pessimistic.
  - You start to feel hopeless, and perhaps even suicidal.
- Body:
  - You can't get to sleep, and wake early in the morning and/or throughout the night.
  - You lose interest in sex.
  - You can't eat.
  - You lose weight.

Other people may notice that you:

- perform less well at work;
- seem unusually quiet and unable to talk about things;
- worry about things more than usual;
- are more irritable than usual;
- complain more about vague physical problems;
- are not looking after yourself properly—you may not bother to shave, wash your hair, look after your clothes.

How Is Depression Different for Men?

There is no evidence for a completely separate type of "male depression." However, there is evidence that some symptoms of depression are more common in men than in women. These include the following:

- Irritability
- Sudden anger
- Increased loss of control

- Greater risk-taking
- Aggression

Men are also more likely to commit suicide.

Getting Help

Men seem to suffer from depression just as often as women, but are less likely to ask for help. It may also be that men try to deal with their depression by using drugs and alcohol. This might account for the fact that, although men are diagnosed as having depression less than women, they abuse drugs and alcohol rather more.

Men's Attitudes and Behavior

Compared with women, men tend to be more competitive and concerned with power and success. Most men don't like to admit that they feel fragile or that they need help. They feel that they should rely on themselves, and that it is somehow weak to have to depend on someone else, even for a short time. So they are less likely to talk about their feelings with their friends, their loved ones, or their doctors. This may be why they don't get the help they need.

This traditional view of how men should be—always tough and self-reliant—is also held by some women. Some men worry that, if they talk about their feelings of depression, their partner may reject them. Even professionals may share this view, and do not spot depression in men as often as they should.

How Do Men Cope?

Instead of talking about how they feel, men may use alcohol or drugs to feel better. This usually makes things worse, certainly in the long run. Your work will suffer and alcohol often leads to irresponsible, unpleasant, or dangerous behavior. Men may also focus more on their work than their relationships or home life. This can cause conflicts with your wife or partner. All of these things make depression more likely.

Relationships

For married men, research has shown that trouble in a marriage or long-term relationship is the single most common problem associated with depression. Men can't cope with disagreements as well as women. Arguments actually make men feel very physically uncomfortable. They try to avoid arguments or difficult discussions. The partner will want to talk about a problem, but he will do his best to avoid it. The partner then feels ignored and tries to talk about it more, which makes the man feel he is being nagged. So, he withdraws further, which makes his partner feel even more ignored and so on. This vicious circle can destroy a relationship.

Separation and Divorce

Men have traditionally seen themselves as being in control of their families' lives. However, the process of separation and divorce is most often started by women. Of all men, those who are divorced are most likely to kill themselves, probably because depression is more common and more severe in this group. This may be because, as well as losing their main relationship:

- they often lose touch with their children;
- they may have to move to live in a different place;
- they often find themselves short of money.

These are stressful events in themselves, quite apart from the stress of the breakup, and may bring on depression.

Sex

When men are depressed, they feel less good about their bodies and less sexy. Many go off sex completely. Several recent studies suggest that, in spite of this, men who are depressed have intercourse just as often, but they don't feel as satisfied as usual. A few depressed men actually report an increase in sexual drive and intercourse, possibly as a way of trying to make themselves feel better. Another problem may be that some antidepressant drugs reduce sex drive in a small number of men. However, the good news is that, as the depression improves, so will sexual desire, performance, and satisfaction.

It's worth remembering that it can happen the other way around. Impotence (difficulty in getting or keeping an erection) can bring about depression. Again, this is a problem for which it is usually possible to find effective help.

Pregnancy and Children

We have known for many years that some mothers feel severely depressed after having a baby. It is only recently that we have realized that more than one in ten fathers also suffer psychological problems during this time. This shouldn't really be surprising. We know that major events in people's lives, even good ones like moving house, can make you depressed. And this particular event changes your life more than any other. Suddenly, you have to spend much more of your time looking after your partner, and possibly other children, and you may be very tired.

On an intimate level, new mothers tend to be less interested in sex for a number of months. Simple tiredness is the main problem, although you may take it personally and feel that you are being rejected. You may have to adjust, perhaps for the first time, to taking second place in your partner's affections. You may also find that you can't spend so much time at work.

New fathers are more likely to become depressed if their partner is depressed, if they aren't getting along with their partner, or if they are unemployed. This isn't important just from the father's point of view. It will affect the mother and may have an impact on how the baby grows and develops in the first few months.

Unemployment and Retirement

Leaving work, for any reason, can be stressful. Recent research has shown that up to one in seven men who become unemployed will develop a depressive illness in the next six months.

After relationship difficulties, unemployment is the thing most likely to push a man into a serious depression—work is often the main source of a man's sense of worth and self-esteem. You may lose the signs of your success, such as the company car. You may have to adjust to being at home, looking after children, while your wife or partner becomes the breadwinner.

From a position of being in control, you may face a future over which you have little, especially if it takes a long time to find another job.

You are more likely to become depressed if you are shy, if you don't have a close relationship, or if you don't manage to find another job. Depression itself can make it harder to get another job.

Even retiring from work at the usual age can be difficult for many men, especially if your partner continues to work. It can be hard to adjust to losing the structure of your day and your contact with colleagues.

Gay Men and Depression

On the whole, gay men do not suffer from depression any more than straight men. However, it seems that gay teenagers and young adults are more likely to become depressed, possibly due to the stress of "coming out."

Suicide

Men are around three times more likely to kill themselves than women. Suicide is commonest among men who are separated, widowed, or divorced and is more likely if someone is a heavy drinker.

Over the last few years, men have become more likely to kill themselves, particularly those aged between sixteen and twenty-four years and those between thirty-nine and fifty-four years. We don't yet know the reason for this.

We do know that around half the people who kill themselves will have seen their doctor in the previous four weeks—although not necessarily to discuss their emotional state. However, fewer men than women will have seen their doctor in the year before their suicide. We also know that about two out of three people who kill themselves will have talked about it to friends or family.

Asking someone if he is feeling suicidal will not put the idea into his head or make it more likely that he will kill himself. Even if someone is not very good at talking about how he is feeling, it is important to ask if you have any suspicion—and to take such ideas seriously.

For a man who feels suicidal, there is nothing more demoralizing than to feel that others do not take him seriously. He will often have taken some time to pluck up the courage to tell anyone about it.

If you find yourself feeling so bad that you have thought about suicide, it can be a great relief to talk about it.

Violence

Some studies have shown that men who commit violent crimes are more likely to get depressed than men who don't. However, we don't know if the depression makes their violence more likely, or if it's just the way they lead their lives.

Helping Men

Many men find it difficult to ask for help when they are depressed—it can feel unmanly and weak. It may be easier for men to ask for help if those who give that help take into account men's special needs.

Men who are depressed are more likely to talk about the physical symptoms of their depression than the emotional and psychological ones. This may be one reason why doctors sometimes don't diagnose it. If you are feeling wretched, don't hold back—tell your doctor.

It can help to see depression as a result of chemical changes in the brain and/or as the inevitable cost of living in a demanding and difficult world. It is nothing to do with being weak or unmanly and it can be helped. Both talking and medication can be important ways to help you get better.

If a depressed man is married, or in a steady relationship—straight or gay—his partner should be involved so that she/he can understand what is happening. This will make it less likely for the depression to interfere with their relationship.

Some men don't feel comfortable talking about themselves, and so may be reluctant to consider psychotherapy. However, it is a powerful way of relieving depression and works well for many men.

Helping Yourself

Don't bottle things up—if you've had a major upset in your life, try to tell someone how you feel about it.

Keep active—get out of doors and get some exercise, even if it's only a walk. This will help to keep you physically fit and you will sleep better. It can also help you not to dwell on painful thoughts and feelings.

Eat properly—you may not feel very hungry, but you should eat a balanced diet, with lots of fruit and vegetables. It's easy to lose weight and run low on vitamins when you are depressed.

Avoid alcohol and drugs—alcohol may make you feel better for a couple of hours, but it will make you more depressed in the long run. The same goes for street drugs, particularly amphetamines, cocaine, and ecstasy.

Don't get upset if you can't sleep—do something restful that you enjoy, like listening to the radio or watching television. Use relaxation techniques—if you feel tense all the time, try exercise, yoga, massage, aromatherapy etc.

Do something you enjoy—set some time aside regularly each week to do something you really enjoy: exercise, reading, a hobby.

Check out your lifestyle—a lot of people who have depression are perfectionists and tend to drive themselves too hard. You may need to set yourself more realistic targets and reduce your workload.

Take a break—this may be easier said than done, but it can be really helpful to get away and out of your normal routine for a few days. Even a few hours can be helpful.

Read about depression—there are now many books and websites about depression. Not only can they help you to cope, but they may also help friends and relatives to understand what you are going through.

Remember, in the long run, depression can be helpful—some people come out of it stronger and coping better than before. You may see situations and relationships more clearly, and may now have the strength and wisdom to make important decisions and changes that you were avoiding before.

Finding More Help

The best place to start is your doctor, who can go over your options and discuss any worries you have about confidentiality.

Depression may be due to physical illness, so you need to get a proper physical check-up. If you are already being treated for a physical illness, your doctor will need to know.

Any worries about confidentiality should be discussed with your doctor.

Depression can be as much of an illness as pneumonia or breaking your leg. You shouldn't feel embarrassed or ashamed about it. The most important thing to remember is to ask for the help you need, when you need it.

Remember—depression is common, it is treatable, and you are entitled to the help you need.

References

Thase, F.E. Natural history and preventative treatment of recurrent mood disorders. *Annual Review of Medicine* (1999). http://med.annualreviews.org/cgi/content/full/50/1/453

NICE Clinical guideline 23: Depression—Management of depression in primary and secondary care. December 2004 National Institute for Clinical Excellence, London. http://www.nice.org.uk/page.aspx?o=235213

Anderson, I.M., et al. Effectiveness of antidepressants: evidence based guidelines for treating depressive disorders with antidepressants. *Journal of Psychopharmacology* (2000) 14 (1):3–20. http://www.sagepub.co.uk/journals/details/j0102.html

Haddad, P., Lejoyeux, M., and Young, A., Problems stopping: antidepressant discontinuation reactions. *British Medical Journal* (1998) 316:1105–06. http://bmj.com/cgi/content/full/316/7138/1105

Luoma, J., Martin, C.E., and Pearson, J.L. Contact with mental health and primary care providers before suicide: a review of the evidence. *American Journal of Psychiatry* (2002) 159:6 909–16.

Moller-Leimkuhler, A.M., Barriers to help-seeking by men: a review of sociocultural and clinical literature with particular reference to depression. *Journal of Affective Disorders* (September 2002) Vol. 71, Issues 1–3:1–9.

Winkler, D. et al. Gender differences in the psychopathology of depressed inpatients. *European Archives of Psychiatry and Clinical Neurosciences* (2003) 254, 209–14.

Ramchandani P., Stein A., Evans J., O'Connor T.G., Paternal depression in the postnatal period and child development: a prospective population study. *The Lancet* (25 June 2005) Vol. 365, Issue 9478:2201–05.

Section 39.2

Obsessive-Compulsive Disorder

Excerpted from "Anxiety Disorders," National Institute of Mental Health, National Institutes of Health, NIH Publication No. 06-3879, 2007.

People with obsessive-compulsive disorder (OCD) have persistent, upsetting thoughts (obsessions) and use rituals (compulsions) to control the anxiety these thoughts produce. Most of the time, the rituals end up controlling them.

For example, if people are obsessed with germs or dirt, they may develop a compulsion to wash their hands over and over again. If they develop an obsession with intruders, they may lock and relock their doors many times before going to bed. Being afraid of social embarrassment may prompt people with OCD to comb their hair compulsively in front of a mirror—sometimes they get "caught" in the mirror and can't move away from it. Performing such rituals is not pleasurable. At best, it produces temporary relief from the anxiety created by obsessive thoughts.

Other common rituals are a need to repeatedly check things, touch things (especially in a particular sequence),or count things. Some common obsessions include having frequent thoughts of violence and harming loved ones, persistently thinking about performing sexual acts the person dislikes, or having thoughts that are prohibited by religious beliefs. People with OCD may also be preoccupied with order and symmetry, have difficulty throwing things out (so they accumulate), or hoard unneeded items.

Healthy people also have rituals, such as checking to see if the stove is off several times before leaving the house. The difference is that people with OCD perform their rituals even though doing so interferes with daily life and they find the repetition distressing. Although most adults with OCD recognize that what they are doing is senseless, some adults and most children may not realize that their behavior is out of the ordinary.

OCD affects about 2.2 million American adults,[1] and the problem can be accompanied by eating disorders,[6] other anxiety disorders, or depression.[2,4] It strikes men and women in roughly equal numbers and usually appears in childhood, adolescence, or early adulthood.[2] One-third of adults with OCD develop symptoms as children, and research indicates that OCD might run in families.[3]

The course of the disease is quite varied. Symptoms may come and go, ease over time, or get worse. If OCD becomes severe, it can keep a person from working or carrying out normal responsibilities at home. People with OCD may try to help themselves by avoiding situations that trigger their obsessions, or they may use alcohol or drugs to calm themselves.[4,5]

OCD usually responds well to treatment with certain medications and/or exposure-based psychotherapy, in which people face situations that cause fear or anxiety and become less sensitive (desensitized) to them. The National Institute of Mental Health (NIMH) is supporting research into new treatment approaches for people whose OCD does not respond well to the usual therapies. These approaches include combination and augmentation (add-on) treatments, as well as modern techniques such as deep brain stimulation.

References

1. Kessler RC, Chiu WT, Demler O, Walters EE. Prevalence, severity, and comorbidity of twelvemonth DSM-IV disorders in the National Comorbidity Survey Replication (NCS-R). *Archives of General Psychiatry*. 2005; 62(6):617–27.

2. Robins LN, Regier DA, eds. *Psychiatric Disorders in America: the Epidemiologic Catchment Area Study*. New York: The Free Press, 1991.

3. The NIMH Genetics Workgroup. Genetics and mental disorders, NIH Publication No. 98-4268. Rockville, MD: National Institute of Mental Health, 1998.

4. Regier DA, Rae DS, Narrow WE, et al. Prevalence of anxiety disorders and their comorbidity with mood and addictive disorders. *British Journal of Psychiatry Supplement*. 1998;34:24–28.

5. Kushner MG, Sher KJ, Beitman BD. The relation between alcohol problems and the anxiety disorders. *American Journal of Psychiatry*. 1990;147(6):685–95.

6. Wonderlich SA, Mitchell JE. Eating disorders and comorbidity: Empirical, conceptual, and clinical implications. *Psychopharmacology Bulletin*. 1997;33(3):381–90.

Section 39.3

Phobias

Excerpted from "Anxiety Disorders," National Institute of Mental Health, National Institutes of Health, NIH Publication No. 06-3879, 2007.

Social Phobia (Social Anxiety Disorder)

Social phobia, also called social anxiety disorder, is diagnosed when people become overwhelmingly anxious and excessively self-conscious in everyday social situations. People with social phobia have an intense, persistent, and chronic fear of being watched and judged by others and of doing things that will embarrass them. They can worry for days or weeks before a dreaded situation. This fear may become so severe that it interferes with work, school, and other ordinary activities, and can make it hard to make and keep friends.

While many people with social phobia realize that their fears about being with people are excessive or unreasonable, they are unable to overcome them. Even if they manage to confront their fears and be around others, they are usually very anxious beforehand, are intensely uncomfortable throughout the encounter, and worry about how they were judged for hours afterward.

Social phobia can be limited to one situation (such as talking to people, eating or drinking, or writing on a blackboard in front of others) or may be so broad (such as in generalized social phobia) that the person experiences anxiety around almost anyone other than the family.

Physical symptoms that often accompany social phobia include blushing, profuse sweating, trembling, nausea, and difficulty talking. When these symptoms occur, people with social phobia feel as though all eyes are focused on them.

Social phobia affects about fifteen million American adults.[1] Women and men are equally likely to develop the disorder,[2] which usually begins in childhood or early adolescence.[3] There is some evidence that genetic factors are involved.[4] Social phobia is often accompanied by other anxiety disorders or depression,[3,5] and substance abuse may develop if people try to self-medicate their anxiety.[5,6]

Social phobia can be successfully treated with certain kinds of psychotherapy or medications.

Specific Phobias

A specific phobia is an intense, irrational fear of something that actually poses little or no threat. Some of the more common specific phobias are heights, escalators, tunnels, highway driving, closed-in places, water, flying, dogs, spiders, and injuries involving blood. People with specific phobias may be able to ski the world's tallest mountains with ease but be unable to go above the fifth floor of an office building. While adults with phobias realize that these fears are irrational, they often find that facing, or even thinking about facing, the feared object or situation brings on a panic attack or severe anxiety.

Specific phobias affect around 19.2 million American adults[1] and are twice as common in women as men.[2] They usually appear in childhood or adolescence and tend to persist into adulthood.[1,3] The causes of specific phobias are not well understood, but there is some evidence that the tendency to develop them may run in families.[4]

If the feared situation or feared object is easy to avoid, people with specific phobias may not seek help; but if avoidance interferes with their careers or their personal lives, it can become disabling and treatment is usually pursued.

Specific phobias respond very well to carefully targeted psychotherapy.

References

1. Kessler RC, Chiu WT, Demler O, Walters EE. Prevalence, severity, and comorbidity of twelvemonth DSM-IV disorders in the National Comorbidity Survey Replication (NCS-R). *Archives of General Psychiatry*. 2005; 62(6):617–27.

2. Bourdon KH, Boyd JH, Rae DS, et al. Gender differences in phobias: Results of the ECA community survey. *Journal of Anxiety Disorders*. 1998;2:227–41.

3. Robins LN, Regier DA, eds. *Psychiatric Disorders in America: the Epidemiologic Catchment Area Study*. New York: The Free Press, 1991.

4. Kendler KS, Walters EE, Truett KR, et al. A twin family study of self-report symptoms of panic-phobia and somatization. *Behavior Genetics*. 1995;25(6):499–515.

5. Regier DA, Rae DS, Narrow WE, et al. Prevalence of anxiety disorders and their comorbidity with mood and addictive disorders. *British Journal of Psychiatry Supplement*. 1998;34:24–28.

6. Kushner MG, Sher KJ, Beitman BD. The relation between alcohol problems and the anxiety disorders. *American Journal of Psychiatry*. 1990;147(6):685–95.

Section 39.4

Posttraumatic Stress Disorder

Excerpted from "Anxiety Disorders," National Institute of Mental Health, National Institutes of Health, NIH Publication No. 06-3879, 2007.

Post-traumatic stress disorder (PTSD) develops after a terrifying ordeal that involved physical harm or the threat of physical harm. The person who develops PTSD may have been the one who was harmed, the harm may have happened to a loved one, or the person may have witnessed a harmful event that happened to loved ones or strangers.

PTSD was first brought to public attention in relation to war veterans, but it can result from a variety of traumatic incidents, such as mugging, rape, torture, being kidnapped or held captive, child abuse, car accidents, train wrecks, plane crashes, bombings, or natural disasters such as floods or earthquakes.

People with PTSD may startle easily, become emotionally numb (especially in relation to people with whom they used to be close), lose interest in things they used to enjoy, have trouble feeling affectionate, be irritable, become more aggressive, or even become violent. They avoid situations that remind them of the original incident, and anniversaries of the incident are often very difficult. PTSD symptoms seem to be worse if the event that triggered them was deliberately initiated by another person, as in a mugging or a kidnapping.

Most people with PTSD repeatedly relive the trauma in their thoughts during the day and in nightmares when they sleep. These are called flashbacks. Flashbacks may consist of images, sounds, smells, or feelings, and are often triggered by ordinary occurrences, such as a door slamming or a car backfiring on the street. A person having a flashback may lose touch with reality and believe that the traumatic incident is happening all over again.

Not every traumatized person develops full-blown or even minor PTSD. Symptoms usually begin within three months of the incident but occasionally emerge years afterward. They must last more than a month to be considered PTSD. The course of the illness varies. Some people recover within six months, while others have symptoms that last much longer. In some people, the condition becomes chronic.

PTSD affects about 7.7 million American adults,[1] but it can occur at any age, including childhood.[2] Women are more likely to develop PTSD than men,[3] and there is some evidence that susceptibility to the disorder may run in families.[4] PTSD is often accompanied by depression, substance abuse, or one or more of the other anxiety disorders.

Certain kinds of medication and certain kinds of psychotherapy usually treat the symptoms of PTSD very effectively.

References

1. Kessler RC, Chiu WT, Demler O, Walters EE. Prevalence, severity, and comorbidity of twelve-month DSM-IV disorders in the National Comorbidity Survey Replication (NCS-R). *Archives of General Psychiatry*. 2005; 62(6):617–27.

2. Margolin G, Gordis EB. The effects of family and community violence on children. *Annual Review of Psychology*. 2000;51:445–79.

3. Davidson JR. Trauma: The impact of post-traumatic stress disorder. *Journal of Psychopharmacology*. 2000;14(2 Suppl 1):S5–S12.

4. Yehuda R. Biological factors associated with susceptibility to posttraumatic stress disorder. *Canadian Journal of Psychiatry*. 1999;44(1):34–39.

Section 39.5

Schizophrenia

Excerpted from "Schizophrenia," National Institute of Mental Health, National Institutes of Health, April 3, 2008.

What Is Schizophrenia?

Schizophrenia is a chronic, severe, and disabling brain disorder that has been recognized throughout recorded history. It affects about 1 percent of Americans.[1]

People with schizophrenia may hear voices other people don't hear or they may believe that others are reading their minds, controlling their thoughts, or plotting to harm them. These experiences are terrifying and can cause fearfulness, withdrawal, or extreme agitation. People with schizophrenia may not make sense when they talk, may sit for hours without moving or talking much, or may seem perfectly fine until they talk about what they are really thinking. Because many people with schizophrenia have difficulty holding a job or caring for themselves, the burden on their families and society is significant as well.

Available treatments can relieve many of the disorder's symptoms, but most people who have schizophrenia must cope with some residual symptoms as long as they live. Nevertheless, this is a time of hope for people with schizophrenia and their families. Many people with the disorder now lead rewarding and meaningful lives in their communities. Researchers are developing more effective medications and using new research tools to understand the causes of schizophrenia and to find ways to prevent and treat it.

What Are the Symptoms of Schizophrenia?

The symptoms of schizophrenia fall into three broad categories:

- Positive symptoms are unusual thoughts or perceptions, including hallucinations, delusions, thought disorder, and disorders of movement.

- Negative symptoms represent a loss or a decrease in the ability to initiate plans, speak, express emotion, or find pleasure in everyday life. These symptoms are harder to recognize as part of the disorder and can be mistaken for laziness or depression.
- Cognitive symptoms(or cognitive deficits) are problems with attention, certain types of memory, and the executive functions that allow us to plan and organize. Cognitive deficits can also be difficult to recognize as part of the disorder but are the most disabling in terms of leading a normal life.

When Does It Start and Who Gets It?

Psychotic symptoms (such as hallucinations and delusions) usually emerge in men in their late teens and early twenties and in women in their mid-twenties to early thirties. They seldom occur after age forty-five and only rarely before puberty, although cases of schizophrenia in children as young as five have been reported. In adolescents, the first signs can include a change of friends, a drop in grades, sleep problems, and irritability. Because many normal adolescents exhibit these behaviors as well, a diagnosis can be difficult to make at this stage. In young people who go on to develop the disease, this is called the "prodromal" period.

Research has shown that schizophrenia affects men and women equally and occurs at similar rates in all ethnic groups around the world.[2]

Are People with Schizophrenia Violent?

People with schizophrenia are not especially prone to violence and often prefer to be left alone. Studies show that if people have no record of criminal violence before they develop schizophrenia and are not substance abusers, they are unlikely to commit crimes after they become ill. Most violent crimes are not committed by people with schizophrenia, and most people with schizophrenia do not commit violent crimes. Substance abuse always increases violent behavior, regardless of the presence of schizophrenia. If someone with paranoid schizophrenia becomes violent, the violence is most often directed at family members and takes place at home.

What Causes Schizophrenia?

Like many other illnesses, schizophrenia is believed to result from a combination of environmental and genetic factors. All the tools of modern science are being used to search for the causes of this disorder.

Can Schizophrenia Be Inherited?

Scientists have long known that schizophrenia runs in families. It occurs in 1 percent of the general population but is seen in 10 percent of people with a first-degree relative (a parent, brother, or sister) with the disorder. People who have second-degree relatives (aunts, uncles, grandparents, or cousins) with the disease also develop schizophrenia more often than the general population. The identical twin of a person with schizophrenia is most at risk, with a 40 to 65 percent chance of developing the disorder.[3]

Although there is a genetic risk for schizophrenia, it is not likely that genes alone are sufficient to cause the disorder. Interactions between genes and the environment are thought to be necessary for schizophrenia to develop. Many environmental factors have been suggested as risk factors, such as exposure to viruses or malnutrition in the womb, problems during birth, and psychosocial factors, like stressful environmental conditions.

Do People with Schizophrenia Have Faulty Brain Chemistry?

It is likely that an imbalance in the complex, interrelated chemical reactions of the brain involving the neurotransmitters dopamine and glutamate (and possibly others) plays a role in schizophrenia. Neurotransmitters are substances that allow brain cells to communicate with one another. Basic knowledge about brain chemistry and its link to schizophrenia is expanding rapidly and is a promising area of research.

How Is Schizophrenia Treated?

Because the causes of schizophrenia are still unknown, current treatments focus on eliminating the symptoms of the disease.

Antipsychotic Medications

Antipsychotic medications have been available since the mid-1950s. They effectively alleviate the positive symptoms of schizophrenia. While these drugs have greatly improved the lives of many patients, they do not cure schizophrenia.

Everyone responds differently to antipsychotic medication. Sometimes several different drugs must be tried before the right one is found. People with schizophrenia should work in partnership with their doctors to find the medications that control their symptoms best with the fewest side effects.

The older antipsychotic medications include chlorpromazine (Thorazine®), haloperidol (Haldol®), perphenazine (Etrafon®, Trilafon®), and fluphenazine (Prolixin®). The older medications can cause extrapyramidal side effects, such as rigidity, persistent muscle spasms, tremors, and restlessness.

In the 1990s, new drugs, called atypical antipsychotics, were developed that rarely produced these side effects. The first of these new drugs was clozapine (Clozaril®). It treats psychotic symptoms effectively even in people who do not respond to other medications, but it can produce a serious problem called agranulocytosis, a loss of the white blood cells that fight infection. Therefore, patients who take clozapine must have their white blood cell counts monitored every week or two. The inconvenience and cost of both the blood tests and the medication itself has made treatment with clozapine difficult for many people, but it is the drug of choice for those whose symptoms do not respond to the other antipsychotic medications, old or new.

Some of the drugs that were developed after clozapine was introduced—such as risperidone (Risperdal®), olanzapine (Zyprexa®), quetiapine (Seroquel®), sertindole (Serdolect®), and ziprasidone (Geodon®)—are effective and rarely produce extrapyramidal symptoms and do not cause agranulocytosis; but they can cause weight gain and metabolic changes associated with an increased risk of diabetes and high cholesterol.[4]

People respond individually to antipsychotic medications, although agitation and hallucinations usually improve within days and delusions usually improve within a few weeks. Many people see substantial improvement in both types of symptoms by the sixth week of treatment. No one can tell beforehand exactly how a medication will affect a particular individual, and sometimes several medications must be tried before the right one is found.

When people first start to take atypical antipsychotics, they may become drowsy; experience dizziness when they change positions; have blurred vision; or develop a rapid heartbeat, menstrual problems, a sensitivity to the sun, or skin rashes. Many of these symptoms will go away after the first days of treatment, but people who are taking atypical antipsychotics should not drive until they adjust to their new medication.

Length of treatment: Like diabetes or high blood pressure, schizophrenia is a chronic disorder that needs constant management. At the moment, it cannot be cured, but the rate of recurrence of psychotic episodes can be decreased significantly by staying on medication. Although responses vary from person to person, most people with schizophrenia need to take some type of medication for the rest of their lives as well as use other approaches, such as supportive therapy or rehabilitation.

Relapses occur most often when people with schizophrenia stop taking their antipsychotic medication because they feel better, or only take it occasionally because they forget or don't think taking it regularly is important. It is very important for people with schizophrenia to take their medication on a regular basis and for as long as their doctors recommend. If they do so, they will experience fewer psychotic symptoms.

No antipsychotic medication should be discontinued without talking to the doctor who prescribed it, and it should always be tapered off under a doctor's supervision rather than being stopped all at once.

There are a variety of reasons why people with schizophrenia do not adhere to treatment. If they don't believe they are ill, they may not think they need medication at all. If their thinking is too disorganized, they may not remember to take their medication every day. If they don't like the side effects of one medication, they may stop taking it without trying a different medication. Substance abuse can also interfere with treatment effectiveness. Doctors should ask patients how often they take their medication and be sensitive to a patient's request to change dosages or to try new medications to eliminate unwelcome side effects.

Psychosocial Treatment

Numerous studies have found that psychosocial treatments can help patients who are already stabilized on antipsychotic medications deal with certain aspects of schizophrenia, such as difficulty with communication, motivation, self-care, work, and establishing and maintaining relationships with others. Learning and using coping mechanisms to address these problems allows people with schizophrenia to attend school, work, and socialize. Patients who receive regular psychosocial treatment also adhere better to their medication schedule and have fewer relapses and hospitalizations. A positive relationship with a therapist or a case manager gives the patient a reliable source of information, sympathy, encouragement, and hope, all of which are essential for managing the disease. The therapist can help patients better understand and adjust to living with schizophrenia by educating them about the causes of the disorder, common symptoms or problems they may experience, and the importance of staying on medications.

Illness management skills: People with schizophrenia can take an active role in managing their own illness. Once they learn basic facts about schizophrenia and the principles of schizophrenia treatment, they can make informed decisions about their care. If they are taught how to monitor the early warning signs of relapse and make a plan to respond to these signs, they can learn to prevent relapses. Patients can also be taught more effective coping skills to deal with persistent symptoms.

Rehabilitation: Rehabilitation emphasizes social and vocational training to help people with schizophrenia function more effectively in their communities. Because people with schizophrenia frequently become ill during the critical career-forming years of life (ages eighteen to thirty-five) and because the disease often interferes with normal cognitive functioning, most patients do not receive the training required for skilled work. Rehabilitation programs can include vocational counseling, job training, money management counseling, assistance in learning to use public transportation, and opportunities to practice social and workplace communication skills.

Family education: Patients with schizophrenia are often discharged from the hospital into the care of their families, so it is important that family members know as much as possible about the disease to prevent relapses. Family members should be able to use different kinds of treatment adherence programs and have an arsenal of coping strategies and problem-solving skills to manage their ill relative effectively. Knowing where to find outpatient and family services that support people with schizophrenia and their caregivers is also valuable.

Cognitive behavioral therapy: Cognitive behavioral therapy is useful for patients with symptoms that persist even when they take medication. The cognitive therapist teaches people with schizophrenia how to test the reality of their thoughts and perceptions, how to "not listen" to their voices, and how to shake off the apathy that often immobilizes them. This treatment appears to be effective in reducing the severity of symptoms and decreasing the risk of relapse.

Addendum to Schizophrenia January 2007

Aripiprazole (Abilify®) is another atypical antipsychotic medication used to treat the symptoms of schizophrenia and manic or mixed (manic and depressive) episodes of bipolar I disorder. Aripiprazole is in tablet and liquid form. An injectable form is used in the treatment of symptoms of agitation in schizophrenia and manic or mixed episodes of bipolar I disorder.

References

1. Regier DA, Narrow WE, Rae DS, Manderscheid RW, Locke BZ, Goodwin FK. The de facto US mental and addictive disorders service system. Epidemiologic catchment area prospective 1-year prevalence rates of disorders and services. *Arch Gen Psychiatry*. 1993 Feb; 50(2):85–94.
2. Mueser KT, McGurk SR. Schizophrenia. *Lancet*. 2004 Jun 19;363(9426):2063–72.
3. Cardno AG, Gottesman II. Twin studies of schizophrenia: from bow-and-arrow concordances to star wars Mx and functional genomics. *Am J Med Genet*. 2000 Spring; 97(1):12–17.
4. Lieberman JA, Stroup TS, McEvoy JP, Swartz MS, Rosenheck RA, Perkins DO, Keefe RS, Davis SM, Davis CE, Lebowitz BD, Severe J, Hsiao JK; Clinical Antipsychotic Trials of Intervention Effectiveness (CATIE). Effectiveness of antipsychotic drugs in patients with chronic schizophrenia. *N Engl J Med*. 2005 Sep 22;353(12):1209–23.

Chapter 40

Male Menopause

Women may not be the only ones who suffer the effects of changing hormones. Some doctors are noticing that their male patients are reporting some of the same symptoms that women experience in menopause.

The medical community is currently debating whether or not men really do go through a well-defined menopause. Doctors have reported that male patients receiving hormone replacement therapy (testosterone) have reported relief of some of the symptoms associated with so-called male menopause.

What is male menopause?

Since men do not go through a well-defined period referred to as menopause, some physicians refer to this problem as androgen (testosterone) decline in the aging male. Men do experience a decline in the production of the male hormone testosterone with aging, but this also occurs with some disease states, such as diabetes. Along with the decline in testosterone, some men experience symptoms such as fatigue, weakness, depression, and sexual problems. The relationship

---

of these symptoms to the decreased testosterone levels is still controversial.

Unlike menopause in women, which represents a well-defined period in which hormone production stops completely, male hormone (testosterone) decline is a slower process. The testes, unlike the ovaries, do not stop making testosterone. In addition to testosterone, the testes of a healthy male may be able to make sperm well into his eighties or longer.

However, as a result of disease, subtle changes in the function of the testes may occur as early as forty-five to fifty years of age, and more dramatically after the age of seventy in some men.

How is male menopause diagnosed?

To make the diagnosis, the doctor will perform a physical exam and ask about symptoms. He or she may order other diagnostic tests to rule out any medical problems that may be contributing to the condition. The doctor will then order a series of blood tests, which may include several hormone levels, including a blood testosterone level.

Can male menopause be treated?

If testosterone levels are low, testosterone replacement therapy may help relieve such symptoms as loss of interest in sex (decreased libido), depression, and fatigue. But, as with hormone replacement therapy in women, testosterone replacement therapy does have some potential risks and side effects. Replacing testosterone may worsen prostate cancer, for example.

If you or a loved one is considering androgen replacement therapy, talk to a doctor to learn more. Your doctor may also recommend certain lifestyle changes, such as a new diet or exercise program, or other medications, such as an antidepressant, to help with some of the symptoms of male menopause.

Chapter 41

Male Pattern Baldness

What is baldness or hair loss?

Hair loss can happen on any part of the body for a variety of reasons, and can range from being mild to severe. Male (and female) pattern baldness is hair loss specifically from the head. Extreme forms of hair loss happen when there is hair loss all over the head and body.

What is male pattern hair loss?

Male pattern hair loss (also known as androgenetic alopecia) is a progressive hair thinning condition and is the most common type of hair loss in men.

Male pattern hair loss typically begins at the forehead, with the hairline gradually receding along the sides to form an "M" shape. The remaining hair may become finer and shorter, with hair at the crown (back) of the head also beginning to thin. The amount of hair loss can vary among men and is usually influenced by an individual's genetic makeup. In severe cases, the receding forehead hairline may eventually extend to the thinned crown, leaving a horseshoe pattern of hair around the sides of the head.

There are slight variations in how male pattern hair loss can happen:

- **Frontal baldness:** Hair loss happens from the hairline at the forehead but not at the crown.
- **Vertex baldness:** Hair loss happens at the crown but not the hairline at the forehead.

Usually, most men will have a combination of both types of hair loss patterns.

What causes hair loss?

There are many different causes of hair loss, including certain illnesses (including disorders of the immune system), stress as a result of major surgery, chemotherapy, radiotherapy, hormonal problems, fungal infections, and as a side-effect of some medications. Scarring from burns can also cause permanent hair loss.

Hair loss in patches, sudden hair loss, breaking of hair shafts, or hair loss associated with redness, scaling, or pain are likely to be caused by specific health conditions.

What causes male pattern hair loss?

While it is not completely understood why the hair follicles on men's heads stop producing new hair, the male hormone dihydrotestosterone (DHT) is thought to play a part.

Testosterone, the most important male sex hormone (androgen) in men, is responsible for the growth of bone and muscles, sexual function, and for producing physical characteristics in men including facial and body hair. In the body, testosterone is converted to DHT by an enzyme (5-alpha reductase). DHT acts on different organs in the body, including the hair follicles and cells in the prostate. For reasons we don't understand, hair follicles sometimes become more sensitive to DHT, slowing down hair production and producing weaker, shorter hair. Sometimes hair growth stops completely. It is not clear why different hair follicles are affected at different times, making the balding process gradual, or why only scalp hairs are affected.

Is thinning hair and hair loss reversible?

Thinning hair or loss of hair is not reversible, but there are medications to treat male pattern hair loss that can stop or slow baldness. Some men may even experience new hair growth with treatments.

Should I be concerned about hair loss?

Many men accept male pattern hair loss as a normal part of aging. For some men, for a variety of reasons, their concern for their hair loss prompts them to seek treatment for cosmetic reasons to try and stop or slow further hair loss.

If you start to lose your hair suddenly, if your hair loss happens in clumps or is significant enough that you notice large amounts falling out, it is not male pattern hair loss. It is recommended that you discuss these types of hair loss with your doctor. Further investigation may be needed to determine the cause.

What is the emotional impact on men experiencing hair loss?

While hair loss is a normal part of the ageing process for most men, it can be distressing for some, particularly if it is excessive or happens at an early age. Men experiencing hair loss can feel less confident, less attractive, and may think it makes them look older. While many men accept that they are losing their hair, a small number may suffer from depression as a result. It is recommended that men speak to a counselor if they are feeling upset or they are obsessing about their hair loss.

How is hair loss treated?

There are a number of treatments available for hair loss, and treatments often work well in most cases. Men usually seek treatment for cosmetic rather than medical reasons.

Wigs and hairpieces: Hair weaving, hairpieces, or a change of hairstyle may disguise hair loss and is generally the least expensive and safest treatment for male pattern hair loss.

Surgery: Hair transplantation involves removing tiny plugs of hair from areas where it continues to grow and inserting them in bald areas. This can cause minor scarring and carries some risk of skin infection. Multiple transplantation sessions are usually needed and can be expensive. Results, however, are often excellent and permanent. Choosing a surgeon with experience in this operation is recommended.

Medications: There are medications that can be used to treat male pattern hair loss that tend to have results in stopping or slowing hair loss, with new hair growth happening in some men. The two main medications used to treat male pattern hair loss are finasteride and minoxidil.

Finasteride—also known as Propecia®—is an oral medication that works by blocking the conversion of testosterone to DHT. The hair follicles are then not affected by DHT and can enlarge back to normal. About two in three men who take finasteride every day experience some hair re-growth. About one in three men experience no hair re-growth, but most don't experience any further hair loss. Finasteride has no effect in about one in one hundred men. The chances are therefore quite high that finasteride will help hair re-grow or at least stop more hair from falling out.

Most men do not notice any effects from taking finasteride for up to four months. It can take up to one to two years for full hair re-growth to happen. Any improvement in hair growth is usually greatest over the crown than over the frontal areas of the scalp. If treatment is stopped, the balding process will begin again, meaning if successful, treatment needs to be ongoing to continue hair re-growth. Side effects are uncommon, but about two in one hundred men taking finasteride experience a loss of sex drive (libido).

Finasteride taken at a higher dose (marketed as Proscar®) is also commonly taken by men to treat benign prostate enlargement, and has been found to reduce the risk of developing prostate cancer. However, research has found that men who do develop prostate cancer while taking the drug have an increased risk of the cancer being more aggressive.[1] However, whether this arises because finasteride induces more aggressive disease, or simply because finasteride makes it easier to detect more aggressive disease earlier is not certain.[2] Nevertheless, men taking finasteride for hair loss should not be worried as the dose of finasteride given for hair loss is much lower than what is used to treat prostate enlargement, but should speak to their doctor if they have any concerns. The low dose used for treating hair loss does not seem to have an effect on the development of prostate cancer.

Minoxidil—also known as Rogaine®, Hair a-gain®, Hair Retreva®—is a lotion that is rubbed onto the head. There is debate as to how well it works, but it is believed about half of the men who use minoxidil experience a delay in further balding. About fifteen in one hundred men have good hair re-growth, while hair loss continues in about one in three users.

Minoxidil needs to be rubbed onto the scalp every day, and taken continually for four months before results are noticeable. As with finasteride, treatment needs to be ongoing for hair growth to continue. Any new hair that does re-grow tends to fall out two months after treatment is stopped. Side effects are uncommon, but minoxidil can cause skin irritation or a rash in some men.

Is there a link between male pattern hair loss and prostate cancer?

Because testosterone through the action of DHT is involved in the growth of the prostate and hair growth, some preliminary studies have been done to see if men who are balding are at an increased risk of prostate cancer. An Australian study found a link between men with vertex hair loss (hair loss from the crown only) and prostate cancer.[3] There were no associations found between prostate cancer and men with frontal hair loss, or frontal hair loss together with vertex hair loss. The reason for this link between vertex hair loss and prostate cancer is not clear and further studies are needed.

What are the myths about male pattern hair loss?

Standing on your head lessens hair loss: The "blood-flow" theory, which led men to stand on their heads in the 1980s, can be found in the advertising for many of the ineffective hair loss treatments on the market, but again is an unfounded myth in the treatment of male pattern baldness. While minoxidil is suspected for working, in part, by increasing blood flow to hair follicles, there is no evidence that standing on one's head can stop hair loss or cause hair to re-grow.

Hair loss comes from your mother's side of the family: There is a myth that hair loss is a genetic trait passed down from the mother's side of the family. Genetics is the cause of male pattern hair loss, but a number of genes are responsible, and genes are most likely contributed by both parents. The condition does run in families, so if there is a close relative with male pattern hair loss, then there is a higher risk another relative will develop the condition.

Hair loss happens in men with high testosterone levels: Some men think they are losing their hair because they have higher levels of the male sex hormone testosterone. High levels of testosterone are not linked with hair loss. However, some studies have shown that men with high levels of "free" testosterone (only 2 percent of the total amount of testosterone produced by the body) are more likely to have vertex hair loss (from the crown only).

References

1. Thompson IM et al. The influence of Finasteride on the development of prostate cancer. *NEJM* 2003; 349: 213–22.

2. Lucia MS et al. Finasteride and high-grade prostate cancer in the Prostate Cancer Prevention Trial. *J Natl Cancer Inst* 2007;99:1375–83.

3. Giles GG, Severi G, Sinclair R, English DR, McCredie MRE, Johnson W, Boyle P, Hopper JL. Androgenetic alopecia and prostate cancer: findings from an Australian case-control study. *Cancer Epidemiology, Biomarkers & Prevention* 2002; 11: 549–53.

Chapter 42

Sex-Linked Genetic Disorders

Chapter Contents

Section 42.1

Color Vision Deficiency

"Color Vision Deficiency," © 2006 American Optometric Association (www.aoa.org). Reprinted with permission.

Color vision deficiency is the inability to distinguish certain shades of color or in more severe cases, see colors at all. The term "color blindness" is also used to describe this visual condition, but very few people are completely color blind.

Most people with color vision deficiency can see colors, but they have difficulty differentiating between:

- particular shades of reds and greens (most common); or
- blues and yellows (less common).

People who are totally color blind, a condition called achromatopsia, can only see things as black and white or in shades of gray.

The severity of color vision deficiency can range from mild to severe depending on the cause. It will affect both eyes if it is inherited and usually just one if the cause for the deficiency is injury or illness.

Color vision is possible due to photoreceptors in the retina of the eye known as cones. These cones have light-sensitive pigments that enable us to recognize color. Found in the macula, the central portion of the retina, each cone is sensitive to either red, green, or blue light, which the cones recognize based upon light wavelengths.

Normally, the pigments inside the cones register differing colors and send that information through the optic nerve to the brain, enabling you to distinguish countless shades of color. But if the cones lack one or more light-sensitive pigments, you will be unable to see one or more of the three primary colors, thereby causing a deficiency in your color perception.

The most common form of color deficiency is red-green. This does not mean that people with this deficiency cannot see these colors at all; they simply have a harder time differentiating between them. The difficulty they have in correctly identifying them depends on how dark or light the colors are.

Another form of color deficiency is blue-yellow. This is a rarer and more severe form of color vision loss than red-green since persons with blue-yellow deficiency frequently have red-green blindness too. In both cases, it is common for people with color vision deficiency to see neutral or gray areas where a particular color should appear.

What causes color vision deficiency?

Usually, color deficiency is an inherited condition caused by a common X-linked recessive gene, which is passed from a mother to her son. But disease or injury damaging the optic nerve or retina can also result in loss of color recognition. Some specific diseases that can cause color deficits are:

- diabetes;
- glaucoma;
- macular degeneration;
- Alzheimer disease;
- Parkinson disease;
- multiple sclerosis;
- chronic alcoholism;
- leukemia;
- sickle cell anemia.

Other causes for color vision deficiency include:

- **Medications:** Certain medications such as drugs used to treat heart problems, high blood pressure, infections, nervous disorders, and psychological problems can affect color vision.
- **Aging:** The ability to see colors can gradually lessen with age.
- **Chemical exposure:** Contact with certain chemicals such as fertilizers and styrene have been known to cause loss of color vision.

In the majority of cases, genetics is the predominate cause for color deficiency. About 8 percent of Caucasian males are born with some degree of color deficiency. Women are typically just carriers of the color deficient gene, though approximately 0.5 percent of women have color vision deficiency. When the deficiency is hereditary, the severity generally remains constant throughout life. Inherited color vision deficiency does not lead to additional vision loss or blindness.

How is color vision deficiency diagnosed?

Color deficiency can be diagnosed through a comprehensive eye examination. Testing will include the use of a series of specially designed pictures composed of colored dots, called pseudoisochromatic plates, which include hidden numbers or embedded figures that can only be correctly seen by persons with normal color vision.

Pseudoisochromatic testing plates: The patient is asked to look for numbers among the various colored dots, which help distinguish between red, green, and blue color deficiencies. Individuals with normal color vision will see a number, while those with a deficiency do not see it. On some plates, a person with normal color vision may see one number, while a person with a deficiency sees a different number.

Pseudoisochromatic plate testing can be used to determine if a color vision deficiency exists and the type of deficiency. However, additional testing may be needed to determine the exact nature and degree of color deficiency.

It is possible for a person to have poor color vision and not know it. Quite often, people with red-green deficiency aren't even aware of their problem since they've learned to see the "right" color. For example, tree leaves are green, so they call the color they see green.

Also, parents may not suspect the condition in their children until a situation causes confusion or misunderstanding. Early detection of color deficiency is vital since many learning materials rely heavily on color perception or color coding. That is one reason that the American Optometric Association recommends a comprehensive optometric examination before a child begins school.

How is color vision deficiency treated?

There is no cure for inherited color deficiency. But if the cause is an illness or eye injury, treating these conditions may improve color vision.

Using special tinted eyeglasses or wearing a red-tinted contact lens on one eye can increase some people's ability to differentiate between colors, though nothing can make you truly see the deficient color.

Most color-deficient persons compensate for their inability to distinguish certain colors with color cues and details that are not consciously evident to people with normal color vision. There are ways to work around the inability to see certain colors by:

- Organizing and labeling clothing, furniture, or other colored objects (with the help of friends or family) for ease of recognition.
- Remembering the order of things rather than their color can also increase the chances of correctly identifying colors. For example, a traffic light has red on top, yellow in the middle, and green on the bottom.

Though color vision deficiency can be a frustration and may limit participation in some occupations, in most cases it is not a serious threat to vision and can be adapted to your lifestyle with time, patience, and practice.

Section 42.2

Fragile X Syndrome

Reprinted from "Learning About Fragile X Syndrome," National Human Genome Research Institute, April 10, 2008.

What is fragile X syndrome?

Fragile X syndrome is the most common form of inherited mental retardation in males and is also a significant cause of mental retardation in females. It affects about one in four thousand males and one in eight thousand females and occurs in all racial and ethnic groups.

Nearly all cases of fragile X syndrome are caused by an alteration (mutation) in the FMR1 gene where a DNA segment, known as the CGG triplet repeat, is expanded. Normally, this DNA segment is repeated from five to about forty times. In people with fragile X syndrome, however, the CGG segment is repeated more than two hundred times. The abnormally expanded CGG segment inactivates (silences) the FMR1 gene, which prevents the gene from producing a protein called fragile X mental retardation protein. Loss of this protein leads to the signs and symptoms of fragile X syndrome. Both boys and girls can be affected, but because boys have only one X chromosome, a single fragile X is likely to affect them more severely.

What are the symptoms of fragile X syndrome?

A boy who has the full FMR1 mutation has fragile X syndrome and will have moderate mental retardation. They have a particular facial appearance, characterized by a large head size, a long face, prominent forehead and chin, and protruding ears. In addition, males who have fragile X syndrome have loose joints (joint laxity) and large testes (after puberty).

Affected boys may have behavioral problems such as hyperactivity, hand flapping, hand biting, temper tantrums, and autism. Other behaviors in boys after they have reached puberty include poor eye contact, perseverative speech, problems in impulse control, and distractibility. Physical problems that have been seen include eye, orthopedic, heart, and skin problems.

Girls who have the full FMR1 mutation have mild mental retardation.

Family members who have fewer repeats in the FMR1 gene may not have mental retardation, but may have other problems. Women with less severe changes may have premature menopause or difficulty becoming pregnant.

Both men and women may have problems with tremors and poor coordination.

What does it mean to have a fragile X premutation?

People with about fifty-five to two hundred repeats of the CGG segment are said to have an FMR1 premutation (an intermediate variation of the gene). In women, the premutation is liable to expand to more than two hundred repeats in cells that develop into eggs. This means that women with the FMR1 premutation have an increased risk of having a child with fragile X syndrome. By contrast, the premutation CGG repeat in men remains at the same size or shortens as it is passed to the next generation.

Males and females who have a fragile X premutation have normal intellect and appearance. A few individuals with a premutation have subtle intellectual or behavioral symptoms, such as learning difficulties or social anxiety. The difficulties are usually not socially debilitating, and these individuals may still marry and have children.

Males who have a premutation with fifty-nine to two hundred CGG trinucleotide repeats are usually unaffected and are at risk for fragile X–associated tremor/ataxia syndrome (FXTAS). The fragile X–associated tremor/ataxia syndrome (FXTAS) is characterized by late onset, progressive cerebellar ataxia, and intention tremor in males who have a premutation. Other neurologic findings include short-term memory loss, executive function deficits, cognitive decline, parkinsonism, peripheral neuropathy, lower-limb proximal muscle weakness, and autonomic dysfunction.

The degree to which clinical symptoms of fragile X are present (penetrance) is age related; symptoms are seen in 17 percent of males aged fifty to fifty-nine years, in 38 percent of males aged sixty to sixty-nine years, in 47 percent of males aged seventy to seventy-nine years, and in 75 percent or males aged eighty years or older. Some female premutation carriers may also develop tremor and ataxia.

Females who have a premutation usually are unaffected, but may be at risk for premature ovarian failure and FXTAS. Premature ovarian failure (POF) is defined as cessation of menses before age forty years, has been observed in carriers of premutation alleles. A review by Sherman (2005) concluded that the risk for POF was 21 percent in premutation carriers compared to a 1 percent for the general population.

How is fragile X syndrome diagnosed?

There are very few outward signs of fragile X syndrome in babies, but one is a tendency to have a large head circumference. An experienced geneticist may note subtle differences in facial characteristics. Mental retardation is the hallmark of this condition and, in females, this may be the only sign of the problem.

A specific genetic test (polymerase chain reaction [PCR]) can now be performed to diagnose fragile X syndrome. This test looks for an expanded mutation (called a triplet repeat) in the FMR1 gene.

How is fragile X syndrome treated?

There is no specific treatment available for fragile X syndrome. Supportive therapy for children who have fragile X syndrome includes the following:

- Special education and anticipatory management including avoidance of excessive stimulation to decrease behavioral problems.

- Medication to manage behavioral issues, although no specific medication has been shown to be beneficial.
- Early intervention, special education, and vocational training.
- Vision, hearing, connective tissue problems, and heart problems when present are treated in the usual manner.

Is fragile X syndrome inherited?

This condition is inherited in an X-linked dominant pattern. A condition is considered X-linked if the mutated gene that causes the disorder is located on the X chromosome, one of the two sex chromosomes. The inheritance is dominant if one copy of the altered gene in each cell is sufficient to cause the condition. In most cases, males experience more severe symptoms of the disorder than females. A striking characteristic of X-linked inheritance is that fathers cannot pass X-linked traits to their sons.

Section 42.3

Hemophilia

Reprinted from "Learning about Hemophilia," National Human Genome Research Institute, August 1, 2008.

What is hemophilia?

Hemophilia is a bleeding disorder that slows down the blood clotting process. People who have hemophilia often have longer bleeding after an injury or surgery. People who have severe hemophilia have spontaneous bleeding into the joints and muscles. Hemophilia occurs more commonly in males than in females.

The two most common types of hemophilia are hemophilia A (also known as classic hemophilia) and hemophilia B (also known as Christmas disease). People who have hemophilia A have low levels of a blood clotting factor called factor eight (FVIII). People who have hemophilia B have low levels of factor nine (FIX).

The two types of hemophilia are caused by permanent gene changes (mutations) in different genes. Mutations in the FVIII gene cause hemophilia A. Mutations in the FIX gene cause hemophilia B. Proteins made by these genes have an important role in the blood clotting process. Mutations in either gene keep clots from forming when there is an injury, causing too much bleeding that can be difficult to stop.

Hemophilia A is the most common type of this condition. One in 5,000 to 10,000 males worldwide have hemophilia A. Hemophilia B is less common, and it affects 1 in 20,000 to 34,500 males worldwide.

What are the symptoms of hemophilia?

Symptoms of hemophilia include prolonged oozing after injuries, tooth extractions. or surgery; renewed bleeding after initial bleeding has stopped; easy or spontaneous bruising; and prolonged bleeding.

In both severe hemophilia A and severe hemophilia B, the most frequent symptom is spontaneous joint bleeding. Other serious sites of bleeding include the bowel, the brain, and soft tissues. These types of bleeding can lead to throwing up blood or passing blood in the stool, stroke, and sudden severe pain in the joints or limbs. Painful bleeding into the soft tissues of the arms and legs can lead to nerve damage.

Individuals who have severe hemophilia are usually diagnosed within the first year of life. People who have moderate hemophilia do not usually have spontaneous bleeding, but they do have longer bleeding and oozing after small injuries. They are usually diagnosed before they reach five or six years.

Individuals who have mild hemophilia do not have spontaneous bleeding. If they are not treated they may have longer bleeding when they have surgery, teeth removed, or major injuries. Individuals with mild hemophilia may not be diagnosed until later in life.

How is hemophilia diagnosed?

Hemophilia A and B are diagnosed by measuring factor clotting activity. Individuals who have hemophilia A have low factor VIII clotting activity. Individuals who have hemophilia B have low factor IX clotting activity.

Genetic testing is also available for the factor VIII gene and the factor IX gene. Genetic testing of the FVIII gene finds a disease-causing mutation in up to 98 percent of individuals who have hemophilia A.

Genetic testing of the FIX gene finds disease-causing mutations in more than 99 percent of individuals who have hemophilia B.

Genetic testing is usually used to identify women who are carriers of a FVIII or FIX gene mutation, and to diagnose hemophilia in a fetus during a pregnancy (prenatal diagnosis). It is sometimes used to diagnose individuals who have mild symptoms of hemophilia A or B.

What is the treatment for hemophilia?

There is currently no cure for hemophilia. Treatment depends on the severity of hemophilia.

Treatment may involve slow injection of a medicine called desmopressin (DDAVP) by the doctor into one of the veins. DDAVP helps to release more clotting factor to stop the bleeding. Sometimes, DDAVP is given as a medication that can be breathed in through the nose (nasal spray).

People who have moderate to severe hemophilia A or B may need to have an infusion of clotting factor taken from donated human blood or from genetically engineered products called recombinant clotting factors to stop the bleeding. If the potential for bleeding is serious, a doctor may give infusions of clotting factor to avoid bleeding (preventive infusions) before the bleeding begins. Repeated infusions may be necessary if the internal bleeding is serious.

When bleeding has damaged joints, physical therapy is used to help them function better. Physical therapy helps to keep the joints moving and prevents the joints from becoming frozen or badly deformed. Sometimes the bleeding into joints damages them or destroys them. In this situation, the individual may be given an artificial joint.

When a person who has hemophilia has a small cut or scrape, using pressure and a bandage will take care of the wound. An ice pack can be used when there are small areas of bleeding under the skin.

Researchers have been working to develop a gene replacement treatment (gene therapy) for hemophilia A. Research of gene therapy for hemophilia A is now taking place. The results are encouraging. Researchers continue to evaluate the long-term safety of gene therapies. The hope is that there will be a genetic cure for hemophilia in the future.

Individuals who have hemophilia A and B are living much longer and with less disability than they did thirty years ago. This is because of the use of the intravenous infusion of factor VIII concentrate, home infusion programs, prophylactic treatment, and improved patient education.

Is hemophilia inherited?

Hemophilia is inherited in an X-linked recessive pattern. A condition is considered X-linked when the gene mutation that causes it is located on the X chromosome, one of the two sex chromosomes. In males (who have only one X chromosome), one altered copy of the gene in each cell is enough to cause the condition. Since females have two X chromosomes, a mutation must be present in both copies of the gene to cause the hemophilia. Males are affected by X-linked recessive disorders much more frequently than females. A major characteristic of X-linked inheritance is that fathers cannot pass X-linked traits to their sons.

A female who is a carrier has a one in two (50 percent) chance to pass on her X chromosome with the gene mutation for hemophilia A or B to a boy who will be affected. She has a one in two (50 percent) chance to pass on her X chromosome with the normally functioning gene to a boy who will not have hemophilia.

Section 42.4

Klinefelter Syndrome

Reprinted from "Learning about Klinefelter Syndrome," National Human Genome Research Institute, May 27, 2008.

What is Klinefelter syndrome?

Klinefelter syndrome is a condition that occurs in men as a result of an extra X chromosome. The most common symptom is infertility.

Humans have forty-six chromosomes, which contain all of a person's genes and DNA. Two of these chromosomes, the sex chromosomes, determine a person's gender. Both of the sex chromosomes in females are called X chromosomes. (This is written as XX.) Males have an X and a Y chromosome (written as XY). The two sex chromosomes help a person develop fertility and the sexual characteristics of their gender.

Most often, Klinefelter syndrome is the result of one extra X (written as XXY). Occasionally, variations of the XXY chromosome count may occur, the most common being the XY/XXY mosaic. In this variation, some of the cells in the male's body have an additional X chromosome, and the rest have the normal XY chromosome count. The percentage of cells containing the extra chromosome varies from case to case. In some instances, XY/XXY mosaics may have enough normally functioning cells in the testes to allow them to father children.

Klinefelter syndrome is found in about one out of every five hundred to one thousand newborn males. The additional sex chromosome results from a random error during the formation of the egg or sperm. About half of the time the error occurs in the formation of sperm, while the remainder are due to errors in egg development. Women who have pregnancies after age thirty-five have a slightly increased chance of having a boy with this syndrome.

What are the symptoms of Klinefelter syndrome?

Males who have Klinefelter syndrome may have the following symptoms: small, firm testes; a small penis; sparse pubic, armpit, and facial hair; enlarged breasts (called gynecomastia); tall stature; and abnormal body proportions (long legs, short trunk).

School-age children may be diagnosed if they are referred to a doctor to evaluate learning disabilities. The diagnosis may also be considered in the adolescent male when puberty is not progressing as expected. Adult males may come to the doctor because of infertility.

Klinefelter syndrome is associated with an increased risk for breast cancer, a rare tumor called extragonadal germ cell tumor, lung disease, varicose veins, and osteoporosis. Men who have Klinefelter syndrome also have an increased risk for autoimmune disorders such as lupus, rheumatoid arthritis, and Sjögren syndrome.

How is Klinefelter syndrome diagnosed?

A chromosomal analysis (karyotype) is used to confirm the diagnosis. In this procedure, a small blood sample is drawn. White blood cells are then separated from the sample, mixed with tissue culture medium, incubated, and checked for chromosomal abnormalities, such as an extra X chromosome.

The chromosome analysis looks at a number of cells, usually at least twenty, which allows for the diagnosis of genetic conditions in both the full and mosaic state. In some cases, low-level mosaicism may be missed. However, if mosaicism is suspected (based on hormone levels, sperm counts, or physical characteristics), additional cells can be analyzed from within the same blood draw.

How is Klinefelter syndrome treated?

Testosterone therapy is used to increase strength, promote muscular development, grow body hair, improve mood and self esteem, increase energy, and improve concentration.

Most men who have Klinefelter syndrome are not able to father children. However, some men with an extra X chromosome have fathered healthy offspring, sometimes with the help of infertility specialists.

Most men who have Klinefelter syndrome can expect to have a normal and productive life. Early diagnosis, in conjunction with educational interventions, medical management, and strong social support, will optimize each individual's potential in adulthood.

Section 42.5

Muscular Dystrophy

Excerpted from "Muscular Dystrophy: Hope Through Research," National Institute of Neurological Disorders and Stroke, August 19, 2008.

What is muscular dystrophy?

Muscular dystrophy (MD) refers to a group of more than thirty genetic diseases that cause progressive weakness and degeneration of skeletal muscles used during voluntary movement. The word dystrophy is derived from the Greek *dys*, which means "difficult" or "faulty," and *troph*, or "nourish." These disorders vary in age of onset, severity, and pattern of affected muscles. All forms of MD grow worse as muscles progressively degenerate and weaken. The majority of patients eventually lose the ability to walk.

Some types of MD also affect the heart, gastrointestinal system, endocrine glands, spine, eyes, brain, and other organs. Respiratory and cardiac diseases are common, and some patients may develop a swallowing disorder. MD is not contagious and cannot be brought on by injury or activity.

What causes MD?

All of the muscular dystrophies are inherited and involve a mutation in one of the thousands of genes that program proteins critical to muscle integrity. The body's cells don't work properly when a protein is altered or produced in insufficient quantity (or sometimes missing completely). Many cases of MD occur from spontaneous mutations that are not found in the genes of either parent, and this defect can be passed to the next generation.

Genes are like blueprints: they contain coded messages that determine a person's characteristics or traits. They are arranged along twenty-three rod-like pairs of chromosomes, with one half of each pair being inherited from each parent. Each half of a chromosome pair is similar to the other, except for one pair, which determines the sex of the individual. Muscular dystrophies can be inherited in three ways:

- Autosomal dominant inheritance occurs when a child receives a normal gene from one parent and a defective gene from the other parent. Autosomal means the genetic mutation can occur on any of the twenty-two non-sex chromosomes in each of the body's cells. Dominant means only one parent needs to pass along the abnormal gene in order to produce the disorder. In families where one parent carries a defective gene, each child has a 50 percent chance of inheriting the gene and therefore the disorder. Males and females are equally at risk and the severity of the disorder can differ from person to person.
- Autosomal recessive inheritance means that both parents must carry and pass on the faulty gene. The parents each have one defective gene but are not affected by the disorder. Children in these families have a 25 percent chance of inheriting both copies of the defective gene and a 50 percent chance of inheriting one gene and therefore becoming a carrier, able to pass along the defect to their children. Children of either sex can be affected by this pattern of inheritance.
- X-linked (or sex-linked) recessive inheritance occurs when a mother carries the affected gene on one of her two X chromosomes

and passes it to her son (males always inherit an X chromosome from their mother and a Y chromosome from their father, while daughters inherit an X chromosome from each parent). Sons of carrier mothers have a 50 percent chance of inheriting the disorder. Daughters also have a 50 percent chance of inheriting the defective gene but usually are not affected, since the healthy X chromosome they receive from their father can offset the faulty one received from their mother. Affected fathers cannot pass an X-linked disorder to their sons but their daughters will be carriers of that disorder. Carrier females occasionally can exhibit milder symptoms of MD.

How many people have MD?

MD occurs worldwide, affecting all races. Its incidence varies, as some forms are more common than others. Its most common forms in children, Duchenne and Becker muscular dystrophy, alone affect approximately 1 in every 3,500 to 5,000 boys, or between 400 and 600 live male births each year in the United States.[1] Some types of MD are more prevalent in certain countries and regions of the world. Most muscular dystrophies are familial, meaning there is some family history of the disease.

How does MD affect muscles?

Muscles are made up of thousands of muscle fibers. Each fiber is actually a number of individual cells that have joined together during development and are encased by an outer membrane. Muscle fibers that make up individual muscles are bound together by connective tissue.

Although MD can affect several body tissues and organs, it most prominently affects the integrity of muscle fibers. The disease causes muscle degeneration, progressive weakness, fiber death, fiber branching and splitting, phagocytosis (in which muscle fiber material is broken down and destroyed by scavenger cells), and, in some cases, chronic or permanent shortening of tendons and muscles. Also, overall muscle strength and tendon reflexes are usually lessened or lost due to replacement of muscle by connective tissue and fat.

How do the muscular dystrophies differ?

There are nine major groups of the muscular dystrophies. The disorders are classified by the extent and distribution of muscle weakness, age of onset, rate of progression, severity of symptoms, and family history (including any pattern of inheritance). Although some forms of MD become apparent in infancy or childhood, others may not appear until middle age or later. Overall, incidence rates and severity vary, but each of the dystrophies causes progressive skeletal muscle deterioration, and some types affect cardiac muscle.

There are four forms of MD that begin in childhood.

Duchenne MD: Duchenne MD is the most common childhood form of MD, as well as the most common of the muscular dystrophies overall, accounting for approximately 50 percent of all cases. It affects approximately one in 3,500 male births. Because inheritance is X-linked recessive (caused by a mutation on the X, or sex, chromosome), Duchenne MD primarily affects boys, although girls and women who carry the defective gene may show some symptoms. About one-third of the cases reflect new mutations and the rest run in families. Sisters of boys with Duchenne MD have a 50 percent chance of carrying the defective gene.

Duchenne MD usually becomes apparent when an affected child begins to walk. Progressive weakness and muscle wasting (a decrease in muscle strength and size) caused by degenerating muscle fibers begins in the upper legs and pelvis before spreading into the upper arms. Other symptoms include loss of some reflexes, a waddling gait, frequent falls and clumsiness (especially when running), difficulty when rising from a sitting or lying position or when climbing stairs, changes to overall posture, impaired breathing, lung weakness, and cardiomyopathy (heart muscle weakness that interferes with pumping ability). Many children are unable to run or jump. The wasting muscles, in particular the calf muscle (and, less commonly, muscles in the buttocks, shoulders, and arms), may be enlarged by an accumulation of fat and connective tissue, causing them to look larger and healthier than they actually are (called pseudohypertrophy). As the disease progresses, the muscles in the diaphragm that assist in breathing and coughing may weaken. Patients may experience breathing difficulties, respiratory infections, and swallowing problems. Bone thinning and scoliosis (curving of the spine) are common. Some children are mildly mentally impaired. Between ages three and six, children may show brief periods of physical improvement followed by progressive muscle degeneration. Children with Duchenne MD are typically wheelchair-bound by age twelve and usually die in their late teens or early twenties from progressive weakness of the heart muscle, respiratory complications, or infection.

Duchenne MD results from an absence of the muscle protein dystrophin. Blood tests of children with Duchenne MD show an abnormally high level of creatine kinase, which is apparent from birth.

Becker MD: Becker MD is less severe than but closely related to Duchenne MD. Persons with Becker MD have partial but insufficient function of the protein dystrophin. The disorder usually appears around age eleven but may occur as late as age twenty-five, and patients generally live into middle age or later. The rate of progressive, symmetric (on both sides of the body) muscle atrophy and weakness varies greatly among affected individuals. Many patients are able to walk until they are in their mid-thirties or later, while others are unable to walk past their teens. Some affected individuals never need to use a wheelchair. As in Duchenne MD, muscle weakness in Becker MD is typically noticed first in the upper arms and shoulders, upper legs, and pelvis.

Early symptoms of Becker MD include walking on one's toes, frequent falls, and difficulty rising from the floor. Calf muscles may appear large and healthy as deteriorating muscle fibers are replaced by fat, and muscle activity may cause cramps in some people. Cardiac and mental impairments are not as severe as in Duchenne MD.

Congenital MD: Congenital MD refers to a group of autosomal recessive muscular dystrophies that are either present at birth or become evident before age two. They affect both boys and girls. The degree and progression of muscle weakness and degeneration vary with the type of disorder. Weakness may be first noted when children fail to meet landmarks in motor function and muscle control. Muscle degeneration may be mild or severe and is restricted primarily to skeletal muscle. The majority of patients are unable to sit or stand without support, and some affected children may never learn to walk.

Patients with congenital MD may develop contractures (chronic shortening of muscles or tendons around joints, which prevents the joints from moving freely), scoliosis, respiratory and swallowing difficulties, and foot deformities. Some patients have normal intellectual development while others become severely impaired. Weakness in diaphragm muscles may lead to respiratory failure. Congenital MD may also affect the central nervous system, causing vision and speech problems, seizures, and structural changes in the brain. Some children with the disorders die in infancy while others may live into adulthood with only minimal disability.

Emery-Dreifuss MD: Emery-Dreifuss MD primarily affects boys. The disorder has two forms: one is X-linked recessive and the other is autosomal dominant.

Onset of Emery-Dreifuss MD is usually apparent by age ten, but symptoms can appear as late as the mid-twenties. This disease causes slow but progressive wasting of the upper arm and lower leg muscles and symmetric weakness. Contractures in the spine, ankles, knees, elbows, and back of the neck usually precede significant muscle weakness, which is less severe than in Duchenne MD. Contractures may cause elbows to become locked in a flexed position. The entire spine may become rigid as the disease progresses. Other symptoms include shoulder deterioration, toe-walking, and mild facial weakness. Serum creatine kinase levels may be moderately elevated. Nearly all Emery-Dreifuss MD patients have some form of heart problem by age thirty, often requiring a pacemaker or other assistive device. Female carriers of the disorder often have cardiac complications without muscle weakness. Patients often die in mid-adulthood from progressive pulmonary or cardiac failure.

Youth/adolescent-onset muscular dystrophies are classified two ways.

Facioscapulohumeral MD (FSHD): FSHD initially affects muscles of the face (facio), shoulders (scapulo), and upper arms (humera) with progressive weakness. Also known as Landouzy-Dejerine disease, this third most common form of MD is an autosomal dominant disorder. Life expectancy is normal, but some individuals become severely disabled. Disease progression is typically very slow, with intermittent spurts of rapid muscle deterioration. Onset is usually in the teenage years but may occur as late as age forty. Muscles around the eyes and mouth are often affected first, followed by weakness around the lower shoulders and chest. A particular pattern of muscle wasting causes the shoulders to appear to be slanted and the shoulder blades to appear winged. Muscles in the lower extremities may also become weakened. Reflexes are impaired only at the biceps and triceps. Changes in facial appearance may include the development of a crooked smile, a pouting look, flattened facial features, or a mask-like appearance. Some patients cannot pucker their lips or whistle and may have difficulty swallowing, chewing, or speaking. Other symptoms may include hearing loss (particularly at high frequencies) and lordosis, an abnormal swayback curve in the spine. Contractures are rare. Some FSHD patients feel severe pain in the affected limb. Cardiac muscles are not affected, and the pelvic girdle is rarely significantly involved.

An infant-onset form of FSHD can also cause retinal disease and some hearing loss.

Limb-girdle MD: Limb-girdle MD refers to more than a dozen inherited conditions marked by progressive loss of muscle bulk and symmetrical weakening of voluntary muscles, primarily those in the shoulders and around the hips. At least three forms of autosomal dominant limb-girdle MD (known as type 1) and eight forms of autosomal recessive limb-girdle MD (known as type 2) have been identified. Some autosomal recessive forms of the disorder are now known to be due to a deficiency of any of four dystrophin-glycoprotein complex proteins called the sarcoglycans.

The recessive limb-girdle muscular dystrophies occur more frequently than the dominant forms, usually begin in childhood or the teenage years, and show dramatically increased levels of serum creatine kinase. The dominant limb-girdle muscular dystrophies usually begin in adulthood. In general, the earlier the clinical signs appear, the more rapid the rate of disease progression. Limb-girdle MD affects both males and females. Some forms of the disease progress rapidly, resulting in serious muscle damage and loss of the ability to walk, while others advance very slowly over many years and cause minimal disability, allowing a normal life expectancy. In some cases, the disorder appears to halt temporarily, but symptoms then resume.

Weakness is typically noticed first around the hips before spreading to the shoulders, legs, and neck. Patients develop a waddling gait and have difficulty when rising from chairs, climbing stairs, or carrying heavy objects. Patients fall frequently and are unable to run. Contractures at the elbows and knees are rare but patients may develop contractures in the back muscles, which gives them the appearance of a rigid spine. Proximal reflexes (closest to the center of the body) are often impaired. Some patients also experience cardiomyopathy and respiratory complications. Intelligence remains normal. Most persons with limb-girdle MD become severely disabled within twenty years of disease onset.

There are three forms of MD that usually begin in adulthood.

Distal MD: Distal MD, also called distal myopathy, describes a group of at least six specific muscle diseases that primarily affect distal muscles (those farthest away from the shoulders and hips) in the forearms, hands, lower legs, and feet. Distal dystrophies are typically less severe, progress more slowly, and involve fewer muscles than other forms of MD, although they can spread to other muscles. Distal MD can affect the heart and respiratory muscles, and patients may eventually require the use of a ventilator. Patients may not be able to perform fine hand movement and have difficulty extending the fingers. As leg muscles become affected, walking and climbing stairs become difficult and some patients may be unable to hop or stand on their heels. Onset of distal MD, which affects both men and women, is typically between the ages of forty and sixty years. In one form of distal MD, a muscle membrane protein complex called dysferlin is known to be lacking.

Although distal MD is primarily an autosomal dominant disorder, autosomal recessive forms have been reported in young adults. Symptoms are similar to those of Duchenne MD but with a different pattern of muscle damage. An infantile-onset form of autosomal recessive distal MD has also been reported. Slow but progressive weakness is often first noticed around age one, when the child begins to walk, and continues to progress very slowly throughout adult life.

Myotonic MD: Myotonic MD, also known as Steinert disease and dystrophia myotonica, may be the most common adult form of MD. Myotonia, or an inability to relax muscles following a sudden contraction, is found only in this form of MD. People with myotonic MD can live a long life, with variable but slowly progressive disability. Typical disease onset is between ages twenty and thirty, but it may develop earlier. Myotonic MD affects the central nervous system and other body systems, including the heart, adrenal glands and thyroid, eyes, and gastrointestinal tract. Muscles in the face and the front of the neck are usually first to show weakness and may produce a haggard, "hatchet" face and a thin, swan-like neck. Wasting and weakness noticeably affect forearm muscles. Other symptoms include cardiac complications, difficulty swallowing, droopy eyelids (called ptosis), cataracts, poor vision, early frontal baldness, weight loss, impotence, testicular atrophy, mild mental impairment, and increased sweating. Patients may also feel drowsy and have an excess need to sleep.

This autosomal dominant disease affects both men and women. Females may have irregular menstrual periods and may be infertile. The disease occurs earlier and is more severe in successive generations. A childhood form of myotonic MD may become apparent between ages five and ten. Symptoms include general muscle weakness (particularly in the face and distal muscles), lack of muscle tone, and mental impairment.

Oculopharyngeal MD (OPMD): OPMD generally begins in a person's forties or fifties and affects both men and women. In the United States, the disease is most common in families of French-Canadian descent and among Hispanic residents of northern New Mexico. Patients first report drooping eyelids, followed by weakness in the facial muscles and pharyngeal muscles in the throat, causing difficulty swallowing. The tongue may atrophy and changes to the voice may occur. Eyelids may droop so dramatically that some patients compensate by tilting back their heads. Patients may have double vision and problems with upper gaze, and others may have retinitis pigmentosa (progressive degeneration of the retina that affects night vision and peripheral vision) and cardiac irregularities. Muscle weakness and wasting in the neck and shoulder region is common. Limb muscles may also be affected. Persons with OPMD may find it difficult to walk, climb stairs, kneel, or bend. Those persons most severely affected will eventually lose the ability to walk.

How are the muscular dystrophies diagnosed?

Both the patient's medical history and a complete family history should be thoroughly reviewed to determine if the muscle disease is secondary to a disease affecting other tissues or organs or is an inherited condition. It is also important to rule out any muscle weakness resulting from prior surgery, exposure to toxins, or current medications that may affect the patient's functional status. Thorough clinical and neurological exams can rule out disorders of the central and/or peripheral nervous systems, identify any patterns of muscle weakness and atrophy, test reflex responses and coordination, and look for contractions.

Various laboratory tests may be used to confirm the diagnosis of MD.

Blood and urine tests can detect defective genes and help identify specific neuromuscular disorders. For example:

- The level of serum aldolase, an enzyme involved in the breakdown of glucose, is measured to confirm a diagnosis of skeletal muscle disease. High levels of the enzyme, which is present in most body tissues, are noted in patients with MD and some forms of myopathy.
- Creatine kinase is an enzyme that leaks out of damaged muscle. Elevated creatine kinase levels may indicate muscle damage, including some forms of MD, before physical symptoms become

apparent. Levels are significantly increased in patients in the early stages of Duchenne and Becker MD. Testing can also determine if a young woman is a carrier of the disorder.

- Myoglobin is measured when injury or disease in skeletal muscle is suspected. Myoglobin is an oxygen-binding protein found in cardiac and skeletal muscle cells. High blood levels of myoglobin are found in patients with MD.
- Polymerase chain reaction (PCR) can detect mutations in the dystrophin gene. Also known as molecular diagnosis or genetic testing, PCR is a method for generating and analyzing multiple copies of a fragment of DNA.
- Serum electrophoresis is a test to determine quantities of various proteins in a person's DNA. A blood sample is placed on specially treated paper and exposed to an electric current. The charge forces the different proteins to form bands that indicate the relative proportion of each protein fragment.

Electron microscopy can identify changes in subcellular components of muscle fibers. Electron microscopy can also identify changes that characterize cell death, mutations in muscle cell mitochondria, and an increase in connective tissue seen in muscle diseases such as MD. Changes in muscle fibers that are evident in a rare form of distal MD can be seen using an electron microscope.

Exercise tests can detect elevated rates of certain chemicals following exercise and are used to determine the nature of the MD or other muscle disorder.

Genetic testing looks for genes known to either cause or be associated with inherited muscle disease. DNA analysis and enzyme assays can confirm the diagnosis of certain neuromuscular diseases, including MD. Genetic linkage studies can identify whether a specific genetic marker on a chromosome and a disease are inherited together. They are particularly useful in studying families with members in different generations who are affected. An exact molecular diagnosis is necessary for some of the treatment strategies that are currently being developed.

Genetic counseling can help parents who have a family history of MD determine if they are carrying one of the mutated genes that cause the disorder.

Magnetic resonance imaging (MRI) is used to examine muscle quality, any atrophy or abnormalities in size, and fatty replacement of muscle tissue, as well as to monitor disease progression.

Muscle biopsies are used to monitor the course of disease and treatment effectiveness.

Immunofluorescence testing can detect specific proteins such as dystrophin within muscle fibers. Following biopsy, fluorescent markers are used to stain the sample that has the protein of interest.

Neurophysiology studies can identify physical and/or chemical changes in the nervous system.

How are the muscular dystrophies treated?

There is no specific treatment that can stop or reverse the progression of any form of MD. All forms of MD are genetic and cannot be prevented. Treatment is aimed at keeping the patient independent for as long as possible and preventing complications that result from weakness, reduced mobility, and cardiac and respiratory difficulties. Treatment may involve a combination of approaches, including physical therapy, drug therapy, and surgery.

Assisted ventilation is often needed to treat respiratory muscle weakness that accompanies many forms of MD, especially in the later stages. Patients on a ventilator may also require the use of a gastric feeding tube.

Drug therapy may be prescribed to delay muscle degeneration. Corticosteroids such as prednisone can slow the rate of muscle deterioration in Duchenne MD and help children retain strength and prolong independent walking by as much as several years. However, these medicines have side effects such as weight gain and bone fragility that can be especially troubling in children. Immunosuppressive drugs such as cyclosporin and azathioprine can delay some damage to dying muscle cells. Drugs that may provide short-term relief from myotonia (muscle spasms and weakness) include mexiletine; phenytoin; baclofen, which blocks signals sent from the spinal cord to contract the muscles; dantrolene, which interferes with the process of muscle contraction; and quinine. (Drugs for myotonia are not effective in myotonic MD but work well for myotonia congenita, a genetic neuromuscular disorder characterized by the slow relaxation of the muscles.) Anticonvulsants, also known as antiepileptics, are used to control seizures and some muscle activity. Commonly prescribed oral anticonvulsants include carbamazepine, phenytoin, clonazepam, gabapentin, topiramate, and felbamate. Respiratory infections may be treated with antibiotics.

Physical therapy can help prevent deformities, improve movement, and keep muscles as flexible and strong as possible. Options include passive stretching, postural correction, and exercise. A program is developed to meet the individual patient's needs. Therapy should begin as soon as possible following diagnosis, before there is joint or muscle tightness.

Dietary changes have not been shown to slow the progression of MD. Proper nutrition is essential, however, for overall health. Limited mobility or inactivity resulting from muscle weakness can contribute to obesity, dehydration, and constipation. A high-fiber, high-protein, low-calorie diet combined with recommended fluid intake may help. MD patients with swallowing or breathing disorders and those persons who have lost the ability to walk independently should be monitored for signs of malnutrition.

Occupational therapy may help some patients deal with progressive weakness and loss of mobility. Some individuals may need to learn new job skills or new ways to perform tasks while other persons may need to change jobs. Assistive technology may include modifications to home and workplace settings and the use of motorized wheelchairs, wheelchair accessories, and adaptive utensils.

Corrective surgery is often performed to ease complications from MD.

- Tendon or muscle-release surgery is recommended when a contracture becomes severe enough to lock a joint or greatly impair movement.
- Patients with either Emery-Dreifuss or myotonic MD may eventually require a pacemaker to treat cardiac problems.
- Surgery to reduce the pain and postural imbalance caused by scoliosis may help some patients.
- Persons with myotonic MD often develop cataracts, a clouding of the lens of the eye that blocks light. Cataract surgery involves removing the cloudy lens to improve the person's ability to see.

What is the prognosis?

The prognosis varies according to the type of MD and the speed of progression. Some types are mild and progress very slowly, allowing normal life expectancy, while others are more severe and result in functional disability and loss of ambulation. Life expectancy may depend on the degree of muscle weakness and any respiratory and/or cardiac complications.

What research is being done?

Drug-based therapy to delay muscle wasting: Progressive loss of muscle mass is primarily responsible for reduced quality and length of life in MD. In the absence of a genetic cure, drug treatment strategies designed to slow this muscle degeneration can have substantial impact on quality of life.

Corticosteroids are known to extend the ability of Duchenne MD patients to walk by up to two years, but steroids have substantial side effects and their mechanism of action is unknown. NIH-funded scientists have established clinical standards for steroid treatment of Duchenne MD. A recent study identified one mechanism of steroid action, raising the prospect that a modified steroid may be designed to minimize or eliminate side effects.

Researchers at the National Institute of Neurological Disorders and Stroke (NINDS) and several universities are exploring the potential of using agents that inhibit enzymes that degrade muscle as a treatment for various types of MD.

Scientists are also exploring several other drugs that may help delay the loss of muscle mass.

Enhancing natural muscle repair mechanisms: Skeletal muscle has the ability to repair itself, but its regeneration and repair mechanisms are progressively depleted during the course of several types of MD. Understanding the repair mechanisms may provide new therapies to slow, and possibly stabilize, muscle degeneration.

NIH-supported studies have provided a broad understanding of the mechanisms of muscle regeneration. Additional NIH-funded studies are identifying points in the regeneration-repair pathways that can be targeted by either drug or gene therapy for muscle rescue.

Cell-based therapy: The muscle cells of MD patients often lack a critical protein, such as dystrophin in Duchenne MD or sarcoglycan in the limb-girdle MDs. Scientists are exploring the possibility that the missing protein can be replaced by introducing muscle stem cells capable of making the missing protein in new muscle cells. Such new cells would be protected from the progressive degeneration characteristic of MD and potentially restore muscle function in affected persons.

The natural regenerative capacity of muscle provides possibilities for treatment of MD. Attempts to take muscle precursor cells from fathers of Duchenne patients and implant them into patients' muscles originally failed. However, more recent studies have focused on using stem cells to try to restore missing proteins in MD patients. Researchers have shown that stem cells can be used to deliver a functional dystrophin gene to skeletal muscles of dystrophic mice.

Gene replacement therapy: A true cure for Duchenne, congenital, and limb-girdle MD might be obtained if the defective dystrophin gene could be replaced by a functional gene. The large size of the dystrophin gene and the early inability of gene-delivery systems (viral vectors) to target muscle have been substantive barriers to development of gene therapy for Duchenne MD.

Over the last several years, a mini-dystrophin gene (one that is small enough for a viral carrier to deliver it) has proven successful in animal models of Duchenne MD. Viral delivery systems are much better today than they once were (viral vector delivery can set off a serious immune response). As a result, NIH-funded researchers have made important progress in delivering a dystrophin mini-gene to muscles of a mouse model of Duchenne MD.

Scientists also are using high-throughput screening (HTS) to find drugs that increase the muscle production of the protein utrophin, which is similar to dystrophin and can help compensate for its loss. HTS lets scientists test hundreds of chemical compounds quickly to find leads for further drug development.

Genetic modification therapy to bypass inherited mutations: Approximately 80 percent of Duchenne MD patients have mutations in the dystrophin gene that causes it to function improperly and stop producing the dystrophin protein. By manipulating the protein synthesis process, production of a gene that "reads through" the genetic mutation that stops production can result in functional dystrophin.

Two strategies are currently under study to bypass dystrophin mutations. First, the antibiotic gentamicin has been shown to be effective in causing the synthesis machinery to ignore the premature stop signal and produce functional dystrophin. This strategy may be useful in about 15 percent of Duchenne MD patients. An NINDS-funded clinical trial using gentamicin in Duchenne MD patients is under way. Second, a more recent approach uses splicing technology to skip past the mutations in the dystrophin gene to a point where the genetic information is complete and can produce a functional protein. This strategy has shown promise in a mouse model of Duchenne

MD. As many as 80 percent of patients could benefit from this new technology.

References

1. Centers for Disease Control and Prevention, National Center on Birth Defects and Developmental Disabilities, July 27, 2005.

Chapter 43

Sleep Apnea

What Is Sleep Apnea?

Sleep apnea is a common disorder in which you have one or more pauses in breathing or shallow breaths while you sleep.

Breathing pauses can last from a few seconds to minutes. They often occur five to thirty times or more an hour. Typically, normal breathing then starts again, sometimes with a loud snort or choking sound.

Sleep apnea usually is a chronic (ongoing) condition that disrupts your sleep three or more nights each week. You often move out of deep sleep and into light sleep when your breathing pauses or becomes shallow.

This results in poor sleep quality that makes you tired during the day. Sleep apnea is one of the leading causes of excessive daytime sleepiness.

Overview

Sleep apnea often goes undiagnosed. Doctors usually can't detect the condition during routine office visits. Also, there are no blood tests for the condition.

Most people who have sleep apnea don't know they have it because it only occurs during sleep. A family member and/or bed partner may first notice the signs of sleep apnea.

Reprinted from "Sleep Apnea," National Heart Lung and Blood Institute, National Institutes of Health, February 2008.

The most common type of sleep apnea is obstructive sleep apnea. This most often means that the airway has collapsed or is blocked during sleep. The blockage may cause shallow breathing or breathing pauses.

When you try to breathe, any air that squeezes past the blockage can cause loud snoring. Obstructive sleep apnea happens more often in people who are overweight, but it can affect anyone.

Central sleep apnea is a less common type of sleep apnea. It happens when the area of your brain that controls your breathing doesn't send the correct signals to your breathing muscles. You make no effort to breathe for brief periods.

Central sleep apnea often occurs with obstructive sleep apnea, but it can occur alone. Snoring doesn't typically happen with central sleep apnea.

This chapter mainly focuses on obstructive sleep apnea.

Outlook

Untreated sleep apnea can do the following:

- Increase the risk for high blood pressure, heart attack, stroke, obesity, and diabetes
- Increase the risk for or worsen heart failure
- Make irregular heartbeats more likely
- Increase the chance of having work-related or driving accidents

Lifestyle changes, mouthpieces, surgery, and/or breathing devices can successfully treat sleep apnea in many people.

Other Names for Sleep Apnea

- Sleep-disordered breathing
- Cheyne-Stokes breathing

What Causes Sleep Apnea?

When you're awake, throat muscles help keep your airway stiff and open so air can flow into your lungs. When you sleep, these muscles are more relaxed. Normally, the relaxed throat muscles don't stop your airway from staying open to allow air into your lungs.

But if you have obstructive sleep apnea, your airways can be blocked or narrowed during sleep because:

- Your throat muscles and tongue relax more than normal.
- Your tongue and tonsils (tissue masses in the back of your mouth) are large compared to the opening into your windpipe.
- You're overweight. The extra soft fat tissue can thicken the wall of the windpipe. This causes the inside opening to narrow and makes it harder to keep open.
- The shape of your head and neck (bony structure) may cause a smaller airway size in the mouth and throat area.
- The aging process limits the ability of brain signals to keep your throat muscles stiff during sleep. This makes it more likely that the airway will narrow or collapse.

Not enough air flows into your lungs when your airways are fully or partly blocked during sleep. This can cause loud snoring and a drop in your blood oxygen levels.

When the oxygen drops to dangerous levels, it triggers your brain to disturb your sleep. This helps tighten the upper airway muscles and open your windpipe. Normal breaths then start again, often with a loud snort or choking sound.

The frequent drops in oxygen levels and reduced sleep quality trigger the release of stress hormones. These compounds raise your heart rate and increase your risk for high blood pressure, heart attack, stroke, and irregular heartbeats. The hormones also raise the risk for or worsen heart failure.

Untreated sleep apnea also can lead to changes in how your body uses energy. These changes increase your risk for obesity and diabetes.

Who Is at Risk for Sleep Apnea?

It's estimated that more than twelve million American adults have obstructive sleep apnea. More than half of the people who have this condition are overweight.

Sleep apnea is more common in men. One out of twenty-five middle-aged men and one out of fifty middle-aged women have sleep apnea.

Sleep apnea becomes more common as you get older. At least one out of ten people over the age of sixty-five has sleep apnea. Women are much more likely to develop sleep apnea after menopause.

African Americans, Hispanics, and Pacific Islanders are more likely to develop sleep apnea than Caucasians.

If someone in your family has sleep apnea, you're more likely to develop it.

People who have small airways in their noses, throats, or mouths also are more likely to have sleep apnea. Smaller airways may be due to the shape of these structures or allergies or other medical conditions that cause congestion in these areas.

Small children often have enlarged tonsil tissues in the throat. This can make them prone to developing sleep apnea.

Other risk factors for sleep apnea include smoking, high blood pressure, and risk factors for stroke or heart failure.

What Are the Signs and Symptoms of Sleep Apnea?

Major Signs and Symptoms

One of the most common signs of obstructive sleep apnea is loud and chronic (ongoing) snoring. Pauses may occur in the snoring. Choking or gasping may follow the pauses.

The snoring usually is loudest when you sleep on your back; it may be less noisy when you turn on your side. Snoring may not happen every night. Over time, the snoring may happen more often and get louder.

You're asleep when the snoring or gasping occurs. You will likely not know that you're having problems breathing or be able to judge how severe the problem is. Your family members or bed partner will often notice these problems before you do.

Not everyone who snores has sleep apnea.

Another common sign of sleep apnea is fighting sleepiness during the day, at work, or while driving. You may find yourself rapidly falling asleep during the quiet moments of the day when you're not active.

Other Signs and Symptoms

Others signs and symptoms of sleep apnea may include the following:

- Morning headaches
- Memory or learning problems and not being able to concentrate
- Feeling irritable, depressed, or having mood swings or personality changes

- Urination at night
- A dry throat when you wake up

In children, sleep apnea can cause hyperactivity, poor school performance, and aggressiveness. Children who have sleep apnea also may have unusual sleeping positions, bedwetting, and may breathe through their mouths instead of their noses during the day.

How Is Sleep Apnea Diagnosed?

Doctors diagnose sleep apnea based on your medical and family histories, a physical exam, and results from sleep studies. Usually, your primary care doctor evaluates your symptoms first. He or she then decides whether you need to see a sleep specialist.

These specialists are doctors who diagnose and treat people with sleep problems. Such doctors include lung, nerve, or ear, nose, and throat specialists. Other types of doctors also can be sleep specialists.

Medical and Family Histories

Your doctor will ask you and your family questions about how you sleep and how you function during the day. To help your doctor, consider keeping a sleep diary for one to two weeks. Write down how much you sleep each night, as well as how sleepy you feel at various times during the day.

Your doctor also will want to know how loudly and often you snore or make gasping or choking sounds during sleep. Often you're not aware of such symptoms and must ask a family member or bed partner to report them.

If you're a parent of a child who may have sleep apnea, tell your child's doctor about your child's signs and symptoms.

Let your doctor know if anyone in your family has been diagnosed with sleep apnea or has had symptoms of the disorder.

Many people aren't aware of their symptoms and aren't diagnosed.

Physical Exam

Your doctor will check your mouth, nose, and throat for extra or large tissues. The tonsils often are enlarged in children with sleep apnea. A physical exam and medical history may be all that's needed to diagnose sleep apnea in children.

Adults with the condition may have an enlarged uvula or soft palate. The uvula is the tissue that hangs from the middle of the back of your mouth. The soft palate is the roof of your mouth in the back of your throat.

Sleep Studies

A sleep study is the most accurate test for diagnosing sleep apnea. It captures what happens with your breathing while you sleep.

A sleep study is often done in a sleep center or sleep lab, which may be part of a hospital. You may stay overnight in the sleep center.

Polysomnogram

A polysomnogram, or PSG, is the most common study for diagnosing sleep apnea. This test records the following:

- Brain activity
- Eye movement and other muscle activity
- Breathing and heart rate
- How much air moves in and out of your lungs while you're sleeping
- The amount of oxygen in your blood

A PSG is painless. You will go to sleep as usual, except you will have sensors on your scalp, face, chest, limbs, and finger. The staff at the sleep center will use the sensors to check on you throughout the night.

A sleep specialist reviews the results of your PSG to see whether you have sleep apnea and how severe it is. He or she will use the results to plan your treatment.

How Is Sleep Apnea Treated?

Goals of Treatment

The goals of treating obstructive sleep apnea are to:

- restore regular breathing during sleep;
- relieve symptoms such as loud snoring and daytime sleepiness.

Treatment may help other medical problems linked to sleep apnea, such as high blood pressure. Treatment also can reduce your risk for heart disease, stroke, and diabetes.

Specific Types of Treatment

Lifestyle changes, mouthpieces, breathing devices, and/or surgery are used to treat sleep apnea. Currently, there are no medicines to treat sleep apnea.

Lifestyle changes and/or mouthpieces may be enough to relieve mild sleep apnea. People who have moderate or severe sleep apnea also will need breathing devices or surgery.

Lifestyle changes: If you have mild sleep apnea, some changes in daily activities or habits may be all that you need. Avoid alcohol and medicines that make you sleepy. They make it harder for your throat to stay open while you sleep. Lose weight if you're overweight or obese. Even a little weight loss can improve your symptoms. Sleep on your side instead of your back to help keep your throat open. You can sleep with special pillows or shirts that prevent you from sleeping on your back. Keep your nasal passages open at night with nose sprays or allergy medicines, if needed. Talk to your doctor about whether these treatments might help you. Stop smoking.

Mouthpiece: A mouthpiece, sometimes called an oral appliance, may help some people who have mild sleep apnea. Your doctor also may recommend a mouthpiece if you snore loudly but don't have sleep apnea.

A dentist or orthodontist can make a custom-fit plastic mouthpiece for treating sleep apnea. (An orthodontist specializes in correcting teeth or jaw problems.) The mouthpiece will adjust your lower jaw and your tongue to help keep your airways open while you sleep.

If you use a mouthpiece, it's important that you check with your doctor about discomfort or pain while using the device. You may need periodic office visits so your doctor can adjust your mouthpiece to fit better.

Breathing devices: Continuous positive airway pressure (CPAP) is the most common treatment for moderate to severe sleep apnea in adults. A CPAP machine uses a mask that fits over your mouth and nose, or just over your nose. The machine gently blows air into your throat.

The air presses on the wall of your airway. The air pressure is adjusted so that it's just enough to stop the airways from becoming narrowed or blocked during sleep.

Treating sleep apnea may help you stop snoring. But stopping snoring doesn't mean that you no longer have sleep apnea or can stop using CPAP. Sleep apnea will return if CPAP is stopped or not used correctly.

Usually, a technician will come to your home to bring the CPAP equipment. The technician will set up the CPAP machine and adjust it based on your doctor's orders. After the initial setup, you may need to have the CPAP adjusted on occasion for the best results.

CPAP treatment may cause side effects in some people. These side effects include a dry or stuffy nose, irritated skin on your face, sore eyes, and headaches. If your CPAP isn't properly adjusted, you may get stomach bloating and discomfort while wearing the mask.

If you're having trouble with CPAP side effects, work with your sleep specialist, his or her nursing staff, and the CPAP technician. Together, you can take steps to reduce these side effects. These steps include adjusting the CPAP settings or the size/fit of the mask, or adding moisture to the air as it flows through the mask. A nasal spray may relieve a dry, stuffy, or runny nose.

There are many different kinds of CPAP machines and masks. Be sure to tell your doctor if you're not happy with the type you're using. He or she may suggest switching to a different kind that may work better for you.

People who have severe sleep apnea symptoms generally feel much better once they begin treatment with CPAP.

Surgery: Some people who have sleep apnea may benefit from surgery. The type of surgery and how well it works depend on the cause of the sleep apnea.

Surgery is done to widen breathing passages. It usually involves removing, shrinking, or stiffening excess tissue in the mouth and throat or resetting the lower jaw.

Surgery to shrink or stiffen excess tissue in the mouth or throat is done in a doctor's office or a hospital. Shrinking tissue may involve small shots or other treatments to the tissue. A series of such treatments may be needed to shrink the excess tissue. To stiffen excess tissue, the doctor makes a small cut in the tissue and inserts a small piece of stiff plastic.

Surgery to remove excess tissue is only done in a hospital. You're given medicine that makes you sleep during the surgery. After surgery, you may have throat pain that lasts for one to two weeks.

Surgery to remove the tonsils, if they're blocking the airway, may be very helpful for some children. Your child's doctor may suggest waiting some time to see whether these tissues shrink on their own. This is common as small children grow.

Living with Sleep Apnea

Obstructive sleep apnea can be very serious. However, following an effective treatment plan can often improve your quality of life quite a bit.

Treatment can improve your sleep and relieve daytime tiredness. It also may make you less likely to develop high blood pressure, heart disease, and other health problems linked to sleep apnea.

Treatment may improve your overall health and happiness as well as your quality of sleep (and possibly your family's quality of sleep).

Ongoing Health Care Needs

Follow up with your doctor regularly to make sure your treatment is working. Tell him or her if the treatment is causing side effects that you can't handle.

This ongoing care is especially important if you're getting continuous positive airway pressure (CPAP) treatment. It may take a while before you adjust to using CPAP.

If you aren't comfortable with your CPAP device or it doesn't seem to be working, let your doctor know. You may need to switch to a different device or mask. Or, you may need treatment to relieve CPAP side effects.

Try not to gain weight. Weight gain can worsen sleep apnea and require adjustments to your CPAP device. In contrast, weight loss may relieve your sleep apnea.

Until your sleep apnea is properly treated, know the dangers of driving or operating heavy machinery while sleepy.

If you're having any type of surgery that requires medicine to put you to sleep, let your surgeon and doctors know you have sleep apnea. They might have to take extra steps to make sure your airway stays open during the surgery.

How Can Family Members Help?

Often, people with sleep apnea don't know they have it. They're not aware that their breathing stops and starts many times while they're sleeping. Family members or bed partners usually are the first to notice signs of sleep apnea.

Family members can do many things to help a loved one who has sleep apnea:

- Let the person know if he or she snores loudly during sleep or has breathing stops and starts.

- Encourage the person to get medical help.
- Help the person follow the doctor's treatment plan, including CPAP.
- Provide emotional support.

Chapter 44

Urologic Concerns

Chapter Contents

Section 44.1

Kidney Stones

"Kidney Stones," by Bernard Fallon, M.D. Reprinted with permission of the University of Iowa Department of Urology, © 2006.

Kidney stones are a major health problem, affecting up to 10 percent of all Americans at some time in their lives. Men are affected three times as often as women, and most frequent stone formers have their first stone in their twenties. Kidney stones are more common during hot weather, but can occur at any time of the year.

A kidney stone is a collection of mineral salts and protein that collect to form a solid crystalline mass. They can start as tiny stones that pass in the urine unnoticed, or they may grow to a size that cannot be passed and become symptomatic. Most kidney stones are composed of calcium-containing crystals, but some are due to metabolic disturbances, which may cause stone composed of uric acid, or chronic urinary tract infections, which may cause stone made of phosphate.

If a stone grows large enough it can get caught in the kidney or the ureter (the tube that drains the kidney into the bladder). Once it gets caught, the stone may partially or completely block the flow of urine. This blockage causes pain that is usually felt in the middle of the back or side and may radiate toward the groin. Sometimes the pain can be so severe as to cause nausea and vomiting. Fevers and chills may accompany a stone that is associated with infection. If a stone that is blocking urine flow is left untreated it can cause damage to the kidney or ureter.

If your symptoms sound like you may have a stone your doctor may perform a full history and physical examination, check laboratory tests on your blood and urine, and order x-rays. The x-ray tests often include a plain film and/or computed tomography (CT) scan of your abdomen. Other tests that may be considered include intravenous pyelography (IVP) or an ultrasound of your kidneys to detect blockage.

If your stone is relatively small (5 mm or less, or less than one-fifth of an inch), your doctor may decide to treat your symptoms with pain medications and allow the stone to pass on its own. Your doctor may ask you to urinate into a strainer so that if you pass a stone, it can be caught and analyzed, which will give important information as to why you formed the stone. Most stones that are 5 mm or less (less than one-fifth of an inch) will pass on their own, usually within a few days, sometimes a few weeks. Smaller stones pass more quickly.

If the stone is large, or continues to cause problems or appears infected, your doctor may refer you to a urologist, who may elect to perform a procedure during which a small tube is placed in your ureter via a scope. This tube can serve to allow the urine to pass, which alleviates pain, and may allow the ureter to dilate, letting the stone pass as well.

Until the advent of more modern techniques in the early 1980s, most stones were treated with open surgery. Now, the majority of stones can be treated without open surgery or with minimally invasive endoscopic techniques (see "Lithotripsy" section). Many of these procedures are same-day surgery, allowing you to return home the same day.

Preventing future stones from forming is a very important part of stone management, and cooperation with your doctor's advice is vital to staying stone-free. Many stones can be prevented by maintaining adequate oral fluid intake, especially water or citrus juices like lemonade. Your doctor may ask you to collect your urine for a twenty-four-hour period so that more information can be gained about why you are forming stones. After reviewing the results with you, your doctor may re-emphasize adequate oral fluid intake, or he/she may prescribe a medication to correct any abnormalities found during the twenty-four-hour collection.

Decreasing dietary protein and salt intake in the diet also helps to reduce the likeliness of recurrent stones. Calcium is found in most stones (about 80 percent), but it is not necessary to restrict dietary calcium unless you ingest an unusually large amount.

Treatment with Lithotripsy

Lithotripsy is a treatment for kidney stones which has been in wide use since 1982. Lithotripsy works without open surgery. Kidney stones can be broken up with shock waves, and then the stone fragments pass out of the body in the urine.

Lithotripsy is generally performed on an outpatient basis, often using sedation, but most frequently under a general anesthetic. The process uses a device called a lithotriptor. Because all the energy is generated by a machine outside the body and no incisions are made, the process is called extracorporeal shock wave lithotripsy (ESWL). This treatment can be used to break stones located in the kidney or in the ureter. Stones that are larger than 1.5 centimeters (one-half inch) may be too large to fully break up with one treatment, and might be better treated by some other method, including open surgery. ESWL can be used in adults and in children, but care must be used to avoid injuring adjacent organs, such as the lungs, in children.

Lithotriptors generate shock waves by various mechanisms but all fragment stones based on the same principles. Shock waves travel easily through the soft tissues of the body with minimal damage to surrounding structures, but are focused on the kidney stones. The stones absorb the energy from these waves and break up. Small stone fragments are then passed in the urine. The treatment is rarely painful, but passing the stone fragments may be.

Depending on the location and size of the stone, as well as the number of fragments produced, your doctor may or may not place a stent in your ureter (the tube that connects the kidney to the bladder to drain urine). A stent is a small plastic tube that allows the kidney to drain into the bladder and the stones to pass around the tube. The stent is located entirely on the inside and will have to be removed in the clinic at a later time, using a scope passed into the bladder. Removal of the stent is done without anesthesia, and is slightly uncomfortable, but takes only about one minute.

Kidney stones are crystalline masses that form from minerals and proteins in the urine. Stones come in various sizes and compositions. Certain types of stones will respond to this treatment better than others. Most kidney stones are very small, less than one-quarter of an inch, and pass without the need for lithotripsy or any other treatment.

If you have kidney stones that are too large to pass, lithotripsy may make removal fairly simple. Your recovery time will be much shorter than with surgery. However, this procedure does not alter the reasons that the stones formed. To prevent future stones, follow the therapy and dietary changes that your healthcare provider suggests. The most important suggestion will be a large fluid intake, which results in a lot of urine output and dilution of the chemicals which may produce stones.

Section 44.2

Urethral Stricture

The urethra is the tube that carries urine from the bladder (through the penis in males) to the outside of the body. A urethral stricture can occur anywhere in the urethra. A urethral stricture is a scarred or hardened area that causes narrowing of the caliber of the urethra. The stricture eventually reduces or obstructs the flow of urine out of the bladder, making it difficult to urinate. The bladder therefore must work harder to push the urine through the narrowed area of the urethra (the stricture).

There are many causes of urethral strictures:

- Trauma to the urethra or penis (blunt or penetrating urogenital trauma)
- Urethral injury associated with traumatic pelvic fractures (motor vehicle accidents, falls, industrial injuries, etc.)
- Straddle injury or direct trauma to the perineum
- Recurrent urinary tract infections
- Sexually transmitted diseases
- Lichen sclerosis (balanitis xerotica obliterans or BXO)
- Congenital abnormalities of the urethra or penis
- Catheterization or instrumentation of the urethra
- Surgical procedures
    - Prior treatment for urethral diseases, such as urethral stricture or urethral cancer
    - Prior reconstructive surgery for congenital abnormalities of the urethra or penis (hypospadias, chordee, epispadias)

    - Prior gender reassignment surgery
    - Prior urologic surgery
- Unknown causes of urethral scarring (idiopathic)

If a urethral stricture is not treated appropriately, the increased strain on the bladder can damage and weaken the bladder muscle. This can lead to a number of serious health problems such as urinary retention (inability to pass urine), urinary incontinence (leakage of urine), inflammation or infection of the urinary tract, reflux (urine backs up into the kidneys), and kidney failure.

Symptoms and Signs

Symptoms and signs of a urethral stricture may include a weak or slow urine stream, hesitation or trouble starting urination, taking a long time to urinate and empty the bladder, sense of incomplete emptying, dribbling, urgency, irritation or burning during urination, urinary frequency during the day and at night, or urinary retention. Sometimes one may intermittently or continuously leak urine because the bladder is full beyond its capacity and overflow incontinence occurs. Sometimes a urethral stricture is diagnosed when a healthcare provider cannot insert a catheter through the urethra into the bladder.

Evaluation

Evaluation of men with urethral injury or with a known or suspected urethral stricture may include a combination of:

- physical examination;
- urinalysis, urine culture, urine cytology (examination of the urine for signs of infection, blood, and other abnormalities);
- uroflowmetry (mechanical measurement of urine output and flow rate):
- ultrasound postvoid residual (measures the residual urine in the bladder after one tries to empty completely);
- radiologic imaging (x-rays to identify anatomy of the urethra, bladder, and urinary tract):
    - retrograde urethrogram (RUG);
    - cystogram;

- voiding cystourethrogram (VCUG);
- ultrasound (US);

- fiberoptic urethroscopy and cystoscopy (visual inspection of the interior of the urethra and bladder using a flexible instrument (cystoscope) that is inserted into the urethra using local anesthesia);
- laboratory studies (blood tests)—blood urea nitrogen (BUN), creatinine, others.

It is very important to have an accurate diagnosis and evaluation of the length and location of a urethral stricture. Once a urethral stricture is diagnosed, your urologist will determine any further evaluation that is needed. Options for treatment will be presented and discussed with you. Several treatment options are available for men with urethral strictures. Some urethral strictures can be managed using a single procedure. If a stricture returns after one or more treatments, it is called a recurrent stricture. Without appropriate treatment, a stricture will recur almost 100 percent of the time. Strategies for prevention of a recurrent stricture will also be discussed with you.

Temporary Management

Temporary management options for urethral strictures include:

- **Catheterization:** A thin, flexible, plastic tube (catheter) is inserted into the urethra to temporarily drain urine from the bladder.
- **Suprapubic catheter:** A thin, flexible, plastic tube (catheter) is inserted into the bladder through the abdomen to temporarily drain urine.

Treatment Options

Treatment options for urethral stricture disease include:

- **Dilation:** A balloon catheter or dilators(plastic or metal) are inserted into the urethra to gradually stretch (dilate) the strictured area in the urethra.
- **Obturation:** A thin, flexible, plastic tube (catheter) is inserted into the urethra on a regular basis to keep the stricture open.

- **Urethrotomy (endoscopic internal urethrotomy or incision):**
  - A minimally invasive procedure where an incision is made in the scar tissue in the urethra to open the stricture.
  - This is done through a fiberoptic cystoscope (endoscope) placed in the urethra with anesthesia.
- **Urethroplasty or open urethral reconstruction:**
  - Anastomotic urethroplasty (the narrowed section of the urethra is surgically opened or removed, and the urethra is repaired with a tissue graft or flap).
  - Substitution urethroplasty (buccal mucosa graft [BMG], genital or other full-thickness skin grafts, or vascularized preputial or genital skin flaps).
  - One, two, or multiple-staged reconstructive procedures.
- **Perineal urethrostomy:** A surgical procedure that creates a permanent and wider opening in the urethra in the perineum (the space between the anus and the scrotum).

Long-Term Follow-Up

After the urethral stricture has been treated, frequent follow-up exams will be needed during the first year and then periodically thereafter to ensure that the stricture does not recur.

Section 44.3

Urinary Incontinence

Excerpted from "Urinary Incontinence in Men," National Institute of Diabetes and Digestive and Kidney Diseases, National Institutes of Health, NIH Publication No. 07-5280, June 2007.

Urinary incontinence (UI) is the accidental leakage of urine. At different ages, males and females have different risks for developing UI. In childhood, girls usually develop bladder control at an earlier age than boys, and bedwetting—or nocturnal enuresis—is less common in girls than in boys. However, adult women are far more likely than adult men to experience UI because of anatomical differences in the pelvic region and the changes induced by pregnancy and childbirth. Nevertheless, many men do suffer from incontinence. Its prevalence increases with age, but UI is not an inevitable part of aging.

UI is a treatable problem. To find a treatment that addresses the root of the problem, you need to talk with your health care provider. The three forms of UI are as follows:

- Stress incontinence, which is the involuntary loss of urine during actions—such as coughing, sneezing, and lifting—that put abdominal pressure on the bladder.
- Urge incontinence, which is the involuntary loss of urine following an overwhelming urge to urinate that cannot be halted.
- Overflow incontinence, which is the constant dribbling of urine usually associated with urinating frequently and in small amounts.

What Causes UI in Men?

For the urinary system to do its job, muscles and nerves must work together to hold urine in the bladder and then release it at the right time.

Nerve Problems

Any disease, condition, or injury that damages nerves can lead to urination problems. Nerve problems can occur at any age.

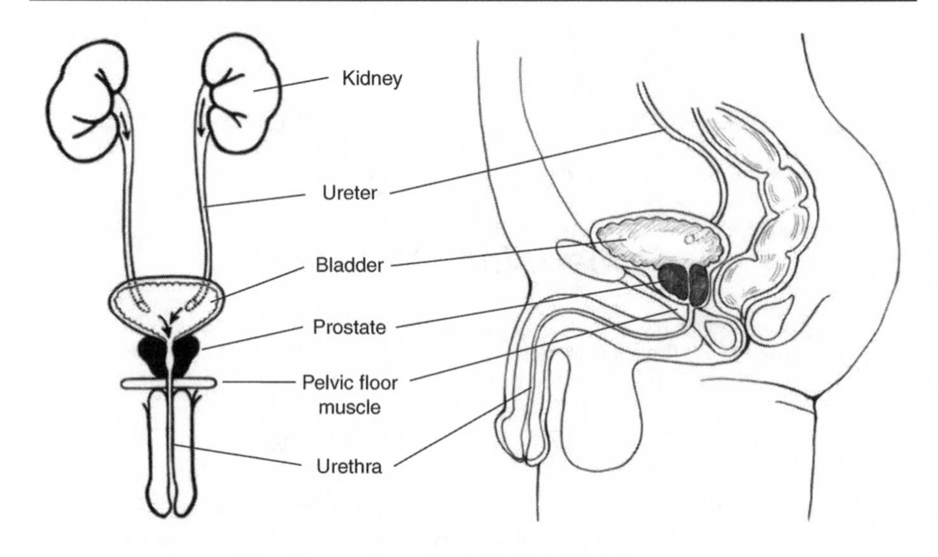

Figure 44.1. *Male urinary tract, front and side views.*

Men who have had diabetes for many years may develop nerve damage that affects their bladder control.

Stroke, Parkinson disease, and multiple sclerosis all affect the brain and nervous system, so they can also cause bladder emptying problems.

Overactive bladder is a condition in which the bladder squeezes at the wrong time. The condition may be caused by nerve problems, or it may occur without any clear cause. A person with overactive bladder may have any two or all three of the following symptoms:

- **Urinary frequency:** Urination eight or more times a day or two or more times at night
- **Urinary urgency:** The sudden, strong need to urinate immediately
- **Urge incontinence:** Urine leakage that follows a sudden, strong urge to urinate

Spinal cord injury may affect bladder emptying by interrupting the nerve signals required for bladder control.

Prostate Problems

The prostate is a male gland about the size and shape of a walnut. It surrounds the urethra just below the bladder, where it adds fluid to semen before ejaculation. Any of the following problems with the prostate can cause urinary incontinence:

- **Benign prostatic hyperplasia (BPH):** The prostate gland commonly becomes enlarged as a man ages. This condition is called benign prostatic hyperplasia (BPH) or benign prostatic hypertrophy. As the prostate enlarges, it may squeeze the urethra and affect the flow of the urinary stream. The lower urinary tract symptoms (LUTS) associated with the development of BPH rarely occur before age forty, but more than half of men in their sixties and up to 90 percent in their seventies and eighties have some LUTS. The symptoms vary, but the most common ones involve changes or problems with urination, such as a hesitant, interrupted, weak stream; urgency and leaking or dribbling; more frequent urination, especially at night; and urge incontinence. Problems with urination do not necessarily signal blockage caused by an enlarged prostate. Women don't usually have urinary hesitancy and a weak stream or dribbling.
- **Radical prostatectomy:** The surgical removal of the entire prostate gland—called radical prostatectomy—is one treatment for prostate cancer. In some cases, the surgery may lead to erection problems and UI.
- **External beam radiation:** This procedure is another treatment method for prostate cancer. The treatment may result in either temporary or permanent bladder problems.

Prostate Symptom Scores

If your prostate could be involved in your incontinence, your healthcare provider may ask you a series of standardized questions, either the International Prostate Symptom Score or the American Urological Association (AUA) Symptom Scale. Some of the questions you will be asked for the AUA Symptom Scale will be the following:

- Over the past month or so, how often have you had to urinate again in less than two hours?
- Over the past month or so, from the time you went to bed at night until the time you got up in the morning, how many times did you typically get up to urinate?
- Over the past month or so, how often have you had a sensation of not emptying your bladder completely after you finished urinating?

- Over the past month or so, how often have you had a weak urinary stream?
- Over the past month or so, how often have you had to push or strain to begin urinating?

Your answers to these questions may help identify the problem or determine which tests are needed. Your symptom score evaluation can be used as a baseline to see how effective later treatments are at relieving those symptoms.

How Is UI Diagnosed?

Medical history: The first step in solving a urinary problem is talking with your healthcare provider. Your general medical history, including any major illnesses or surgeries, and details about your continence problem and when it started will help your doctor determine the cause. You should talk about how much fluid you drink a day and whether you use alcohol or caffeine. You should also talk about the medicines you take, both prescription and nonprescription, because they might be part of the problem.

Voiding diary: You may be asked to keep a voiding diary, which is a record of fluid intake and trips to the bathroom, plus any episodes of leakage. Studying the diary will give your healthcare provider a better idea of your problem and help direct additional tests.

Physical examination: A physical exam will check for prostate enlargement or nerve damage. In a digital rectal exam, the doctor inserts a gloved finger into the rectum and feels the part of the prostate next to it. This exam gives the doctor a general idea of the size and condition of the gland. To check for nerve damage, the doctor may ask about tingling sensations or feelings of numbness and may check for changes in sensation, muscle tone, and reflexes.

EEG and EMG: Your doctor might recommend other tests, including an electroencephalogram (EEG), a test where wires are taped to the forehead to sense dysfunction in the brain. In an electromyogram (EMG), the wires are taped to the lower abdomen to measure nerve activity in muscles and muscular activity that may be related to loss of bladder control.

Ultrasound: For an ultrasound, or sonography, a technician holds a device, called a transducer, that sends harmless sound waves into the body and catches them as they bounce back off the organs inside to create a picture on a monitor. In abdominal ultrasound, the technician slides the transducer over the surface of your abdomen for images of the bladder and kidneys. In transrectal ultrasound, the technician uses a wand inserted in the rectum for images of the prostate.

Urodynamic testing: Urodynamic testing focuses on the bladder's ability to store urine and empty steadily and completely, and on your sphincter control mechanism. It can also show whether the bladder is having abnormal contractions that cause leakage. The testing involves measuring pressure in the bladder as it is filled with fluid through a small catheter. This test can help identify limited bladder capacity, bladder overactivity or underactivity, weak sphincter muscles, or urinary obstruction. If the test is performed with EMG surface pads, it can also detect abnormal nerve signals and uncontrolled bladder contractions.

How Is UI Treated?

No single treatment works for everyone. Your treatment will depend on the type and severity of your problem, your lifestyle, and your preferences, starting with the simpler treatment options. Many men regain urinary control by changing a few habits and doing exercises to strengthen the muscles that hold urine in the bladder. If these behavioral treatments do not work, you may choose to try medicines or a continence device—either an artificial sphincter or a catheter. For some men, surgery is the best choice.

Behavioral treatments: For some men, avoiding incontinence is as simple as limiting fluids at certain times of the day or planning regular trips to the bathroom—a therapy called timed voiding or bladder training. As you gain control, you can extend the time between trips. Bladder training also includes Kegel exercises to strengthen the pelvic muscles, which help hold urine in the bladder. Extensive studies have not yet conclusively shown that Kegel exercises are effective in reducing incontinence in men, but many clinicians find them to be an important element in therapy for men.

How Do You Do Kegel Exercises?

The first step is to find the right muscles. Imagine that you are trying to stop yourself from passing gas. Squeeze the muscles you would use. If you sense a "pulling" feeling, those are the right muscles for pelvic exercises.

Do not squeeze other muscles at the same time or hold your breath. Also, be careful not to tighten your stomach, leg, or buttock muscles. Squeezing the wrong muscles can put more pressure on your bladder control muscles. Squeeze just the pelvic muscles.

Pull in the pelvic muscles and hold for a count of 3. Then relax for a count of 3. Repeat, but do not overdo it. Work up to three sets of ten repeats. Start doing your pelvic muscle exercises lying down. This position is the easiest for doing Kegel exercises because the muscles then do not need to work against gravity. When your muscles get stronger, do your exercises sitting or standing. Working against gravity is like adding more weight.

Be patient. Do not give up. It takes just five minutes, three times a day. Your bladder control may not improve for three to six weeks, although most people notice an improvement after a few weeks.

Medicines

Medicines can affect bladder control in different ways. Some medicines help prevent incontinence by blocking abnormal nerve signals that make the bladder contract at the wrong time, while others slow the production of urine. Still others relax the bladder or shrink the prostate. Before prescribing a medicine to treat incontinence, your doctor may consider changing a prescription you already take. For example, diuretics are often prescribed to treat high blood pressure because they reduce fluid in the body by increasing urine production. Some men may find that switching from a diuretic to another kind of blood pressure medicine takes care of their incontinence.

If changing medicines is not an option, your doctor may choose from the following types of drugs for incontinence:

- **Alpha-blockers:** Terazosin (Hytrin®), doxazosin (Cardura®), tamsulosin (Flomax®), and alfuzosin (Uroxatral®) are used to treat problems caused by prostate enlargement and bladder outlet obstruction. They act by relaxing the smooth muscle of the prostate and bladder neck, allowing normal urine flow and preventing abnormal bladder contractions that can lead to urge incontinence.
- **5-alpha reductase inhibitors:** Finasteride (Proscar®) and dutasteride (Avodart®) work by inhibiting the production of the male hormone DHT, which is thought to be responsible for

prostate enlargement. These 5-alpha reductase inhibitors may help to relieve voiding problems by shrinking an enlarged prostate.

- **Imipramine:** Marketed as Tofranil®, this drug belongs to a class of drugs called tricyclic antidepressants. It relaxes muscles and blocks nerve signals that might cause bladder spasms.
- **Antispasmodics:** Propantheline (Pro-Banthine®), tolterodine (Detrol LA®), oxybutynin (Ditropan XL®), darifenacin (Enablex®), trospium chloride (Sanctura®), and solifenacin succinate (VESIcare®) belong to a class of drugs that work by relaxing the bladder muscle and relieving spasms. Their most common side effect is dry mouth, although large doses may cause blurred vision, constipation, a fast heartbeat, headache, and flushing.

Surgical Treatments

Surgical treatments can help men with incontinence that results from nerve-damaging events, such as spinal cord injury or radical prostatectomy.

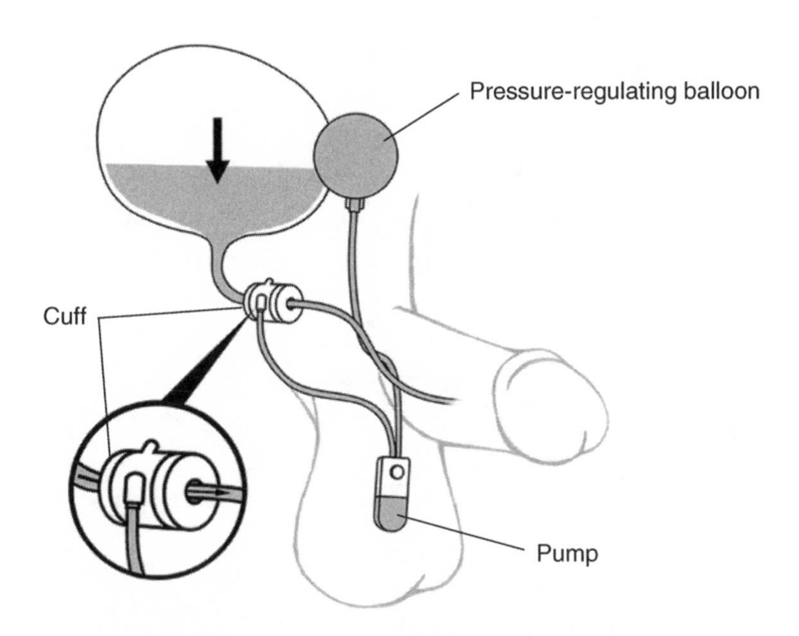

Figure 44.2. *Artificial sphincter*

Artificial sphincter: Some men may eliminate urine leakage with an artificial sphincter, an implanted device that keeps the urethra closed until you are ready to urinate. This device can help people who have incontinence because of weak sphincter muscles or because of nerve damage that interferes with sphincter muscle function. It does not solve incontinence caused by uncontrolled bladder contractions. Surgery to place the artificial sphincter requires general or spinal anesthesia. The device has three parts: a cuff that fits around the urethra, a small balloon reservoir placed in the abdomen, and a pump placed in the scrotum. The cuff is filled with liquid that makes it fit tightly around the urethra to prevent urine from leaking. When it is time to urinate, you squeeze the pump with your fingers to deflate the cuff so that the liquid moves to the balloon reservoir and urine can flow through the urethra. When your bladder is empty, the cuff automatically refills in the next two to five minutes to keep the urethra tightly closed.

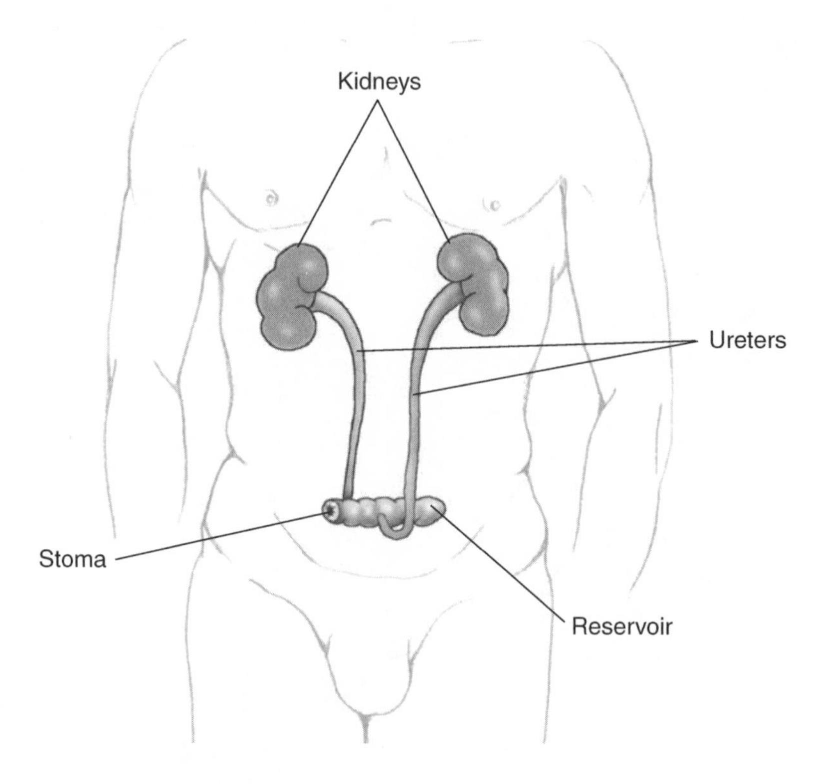

Figure 44.3. *Urinary diversion*

Male sling: Surgery can improve some types of urinary incontinence in men. In a sling procedure, the surgeon creates a support for the urethra by wrapping a strip of material around the urethra and attaching the ends of the strip to the pelvic bone. The sling keeps constant pressure on the urethra so that it does not open until the patient consciously releases the urine.

Urinary diversion: If the bladder must be removed or all bladder function is lost because of nerve damage, you may consider surgery to create a urinary diversion. In this procedure, the surgeon creates a reservoir by removing a piece of the small intestine and directing the ureters to the reservoir. The surgeon also creates a stoma, an opening on the lower abdomen where the urine can be drained through a catheter or into a bag.

Chapter 45

"Women's" Concerns: Men Are at Risk, Too

Chapter Contents

Section 45.1

Body Image Issues

Reprinted from "Body Image Issues," National Women's Health Information Center, July 17, 2008.

Did you know that men, like women, can struggle with body image issues? Some men secretly live with an eating disorder or body dysmorphic disorder—conditions that not only can harm your health, but also interfere with daily living. People with body image disorders often isolate themselves from others and can suffer from depression and other mental health problems.

Eating Disorders

Eating disorders involve extreme emotions, attitudes, and behaviors surrounding weight and food issues. Many more women than men have anorexia and bulimia. But binge eating disorder affects men and women equally. With binge eating disorder, people overeat well beyond the point of feeling full. Sometimes, people try to make up for their binges by dieting or not eating. Body weight ranges from normal to severely obese.

Body Dysmorphic Disorder

People with body dysmorphic disorder have extreme concern over a real or imagined "flaw" in appearance. Men and women are affected equally, but focus concern on different parts of the body. Men tend to be preoccupied by their skin, hair, nose, and genitals. People with this condition often feel "ugly" and can be self-conscious around others.

Obsession with food or how you look is no way to live. If you have body image issues, don't let shame or embarrassment keep you from seeking help. Medicines and counseling can help people with eating disorders and body image disorders.

Section 45.2

Gynecomastia: A Breast Disorder in Men

Excerpted from "Gynecomastia,"

Definition

Gynecomastia is the development of abnormally large breasts in males.

Considerations

The condition may occur in one or both breasts and begins as a small lump beneath the nipple, which may be tender. The breasts often enlarge unevenly. Gynecomastia during puberty is not uncommon and usually goes away over a period of months.

In newborns, breast development may be associated with milk flow (galactorrhea). This condition usually lasts for a couple of weeks, but in rare cases may last until the child is two years old.

Causes

The most common cause of gynecomastia is puberty.

Other causes include:

- chronic liver disease;
- exposure to anabolic steroid hormones;
- exposure to estrogen hormone;
- genetic disorders;
- kidney failure;
- marijuana use;
- side effects of some medications;
- testosterone (male hormone) deficiency.

Rare causes include:

- genetic defects;
- overactive thyroid;
- tumors.

Home Care

Apply cold compresses and use analgesics as your health care provider recommends if swollen breasts are also tender.

When to Contact a Medical Professional

Call your health care provider if the breasts have developed abnormally or if there is swelling or pain in one or both breasts.

Note: Gynecomastia in children who have not yet reached puberty should always be checked by a health care provider.

What to Expect at Your Office Visit

Your health care provider will take a medical history and perform a physical examination.

Medical history questions may include:

- Is one or both breasts involved?
- What is the age and gender of the patient?
- What medications is the person taking?
- How long has gynecomastia been present?
- Is the gynecomastia staying the same, getting better, or getting worse?
- What other symptoms are present?

Testing may not be necessary, but the following tests may be done to rule out certain diseases:

- blood hormone level tests;
- breast ultrasound;
- liver and kidney function studies;
- mammogram.

Intervention

If an underlying condition is found, it is treated. Gynecomastia during puberty usually goes away on its own; however, persistent, extreme, or uneven breast enlargement may be embarrassing for an adolescent boy. Breast reduction surgery may be recommended.

After Seeing Your Health Care Provider

If your health care provider made a diagnosis related to gynecomastia, you may want to note that diagnosis in your personal medical record.

Section 45.3

Osteoporosis in Men

Reprinted from "Osteoporosis in Men," National Institute of Arthritis, Musculoskeletal and Skin Diseases, National Institutes of Health, August 2008.

Osteoporosis is a disease that causes the skeleton to weaken and the bones to break. It poses a significant threat to more than two million men in the United States. After age fifty, 6 percent of all men will experience a hip fracture and 5 percent will have a vertebral fracture as a result of osteoporosis.

Despite these compelling figures, a majority of American men view osteoporosis solely as a "woman's disease," according to a 1996 Gallup Poll. Moreover, among men whose lifestyle habits put them at increased risk, few recognize the disease as a significant threat to their mobility and independence.

Osteoporosis is called a "silent disease" because it progresses without symptoms until a fracture occurs. It develops less often in men than in women because men have larger skeletons, their bone loss starts later and progresses more slowly, and they have no period of rapid hormonal change and bone loss. However, in the last few years the problem of osteoporosis in men has been recognized as an important public health issue, particularly in light of estimates that the number of men above the age of seventy will continue to increase as life expectancy continues to rise.

Clearly, more information is needed about the causes and treatment of osteoporosis in men, and researchers are beginning to turn their attention to this long-neglected group.

For example, in 1999, the National Institutes of Health launched a major research effort that will attempt to answer some of the many remaining questions. The seven-year, multisite study will follow more than five thousand men ages sixty-five and older to determine how much the risk of fracture in men is related to bone mass and structure, biochemistry, lifestyle, tendency to fall, and other factors.

The results of such studies will help doctors to better understand how to prevent, manage, and treat osteoporosis in men.

What Causes Osteoporosis?

Bone is constantly changing—that is, old bone is removed and replaced by new bone. During childhood, more bone is produced than removed, so the skeleton grows in both size and strength. For most people, bone mass peaks during the third decade of life. By this age, men typically have accumulated more bone mass than women. After this point, the amount of bone in the skeleton typically begins to decline slowly as removal of old bone exceeds formation of new bone.

Men in their fifties do not experience the rapid loss of bone mass that women do in the years following menopause. By age sixty-five or seventy, however, men and women are losing bone mass at the same rate, and the absorption of calcium, an essential nutrient for bone health throughout life, decreases in both sexes. Excessive bone loss causes bone to become fragile and more likely to fracture.

Fractures resulting from osteoporosis most commonly occur in the hip, spine, and wrist, and can be permanently disabling. Hip fractures are especially dangerous. Perhaps because such fractures tend to occur at older ages in men than in women, men who sustain hip fractures are more likely than women to die from complications.

Primary and Secondary Osteoporosis

There are two main types of osteoporosis: primary and secondary. In cases of primary osteoporosis, either the condition is caused by age-related bone loss (sometimes called senile osteoporosis) or the cause is unknown (idiopathic osteoporosis). The term "idiopathic osteoporosis" is used only for men less than seventy years old; in older men, age-related bone loss is assumed to be the cause.

The majority of men with osteoporosis have at least one (sometimes more than one) secondary cause. In cases of secondary osteoporosis, the loss of bone mass is caused by certain lifestyle behaviors, diseases, or medications. The most common causes of secondary osteoporosis in men include exposure to glucocorticoid medications, hypogonadism (low levels of testosterone), alcohol abuse, smoking, gastrointestinal disease, hypercalciuria, and immobilization.

Causes of Secondary Osteoporosis in Men

- Glucocorticoid medications
- Other immunosuppressive drugs
- Hypogonadism (low testosterone levels)
- Excessive alcohol consumption
- Smoking
- Chronic obstructive pulmonary disease and asthma
- Cystic fibrosis
- Gastrointestinal disease
- Hypercalciuria
- Anticonvulsant medications
- Thyrotoxicosis
- Hyperparathyroidism
- Immobilization
- Osteogenesis imperfecta
- Homocystinuria
- Neoplastic disease
- Ankylosing spondylitis and rheumatoid arthritis
- Systemic mastocytosis

Glucocorticoid medications: Glucocorticoids are steroid medications used to treat diseases such as asthma and rheumatoid arthritis. Bone loss is a very common side effect of these medications. The bone loss these medications cause may be due to their direct effect on bone, muscle weakness or immobility, reduced intestinal absorption of calcium, a decrease in testosterone levels, or, most likely, a combination of these factors.

When glucocorticoid medications are used on an ongoing basis, bone mass often decreases quickly and continuously, with most of the bone loss in the ribs and vertebrae. Therefore, people taking these medications should talk to their doctor about having a bone mineral density (BMD) test. Men should also be tested to monitor testosterone levels, as glucocorticoids often reduce testosterone in the blood.

A treatment plan to minimize loss of bone during long-term glucocorticoid therapy may include using the minimal effective dose, and discontinuing the drug or administering it through the skin, if possible. Adequate calcium and vitamin D intake is important, as these nutrients help reduce the impact of glucocorticoids on the bones. Other possible treatments include testosterone replacement and osteoporosis medication. Alendronate and risedronate are two bisphosphonate medications approved by the U.S. Food and Drug Administration (FDA) for use by men and women with glucocorticoid-induced osteoporosis.

Hypogonadism: Hypogonadism refers to abnormally low levels of sex hormones. It is well known that loss of estrogen causes osteoporosis in women. In men, reduced levels of sex hormones may also cause osteoporosis.

While it is natural for testosterone levels to decrease with age, there should not be a sudden drop in this hormone that is comparable to the drop in estrogen experienced by women at menopause. However, medications like glucocorticoids, cancer treatments (especially for prostate cancer), and many other factors can affect testosterone levels. Testosterone replacement therapy may be helpful in preventing or slowing bone loss. Its success depends on factors such as age and how long testosterone levels have been reduced. Also, it is not yet clear how long any beneficial effect of testosterone replacement will last. Therefore, doctors usually treat the osteoporosis directly, using medications approved for this purpose.

Recent research suggests that estrogen deficiency may also be a cause of osteoporosis in men. For example, estrogen levels are low in men with hypogonadism and may play a part in bone loss. Osteoporosis has been found in some men who have rare disorders involving estrogen. Therefore, the role of estrogen in men is under active investigation.

Alcohol abuse: There is a wealth of evidence that alcohol abuse may decrease bone density and lead to an increase in fractures. Low bone mass is common in men who seek medical help for alcohol abuse.

In cases where bone loss is linked to alcohol abuse, the first goal of treatment is to help the patient stop—or at least reduce—his consumption of alcohol. More research is needed to determine whether bone lost to alcohol abuse will rebuild once drinking stops, or even whether further damage will be prevented. It is clear, though, that alcohol abuse causes many other health and social problems, so quitting is ideal. A treatment plan may also include a balanced diet with lots of calcium- and vitamin D-rich foods, a program of physical exercise, and smoking cessation.

Smoking: Bone loss is more rapid, and rates of hip and vertebral fracture are higher, among men who smoke, although more research is needed to determine exactly how smoking damages bone. Tobacco, nicotine, and other chemicals found in cigarettes may be directly toxic to bone, or they may inhibit absorption of calcium and other nutrients needed for bone health. Quitting is the ideal approach, as smoking is harmful in so many ways. As with alcohol, it is not known whether quitting smoking leads to reduced rates of bone loss or to a gain in bone mass.

Gastrointestinal disorders: Several nutrients—including amino acids, calcium, magnesium, phosphorous, and vitamins D and K—are important for bone health. Diseases of the stomach and intestines can lead to bone disease when they impair absorption of these nutrients. In such cases, treatment for bone loss may include taking supplements to replenish these nutrients.

Hypercalciuria: Hypercalciuria is a disorder that causes too much calcium to be lost through the urine, which makes the calcium unavailable for building bone. Patients with hypercalciuria should talk to their doctor about having a BMD test and, if bone density is low, discuss treatment options.

Immobilization: Weight-bearing exercise is essential for maintaining healthy bones. Without it, bone density may decline rapidly. Prolonged bed rest (following fractures, surgery, spinal cord injuries, or illness) or immobilization of some part of the body often results in significant bone loss. It is crucial to resume weight-bearing exercise (such as walking, jogging, dancing, and lifting weights) as soon as possible after a period of prolonged bed rest. If this is not possible, you should work with your doctor to minimize other risk factors for osteoporosis.

How Is Osteoporosis Diagnosed in Men?

Osteoporosis can be effectively treated if it is detected before significant bone loss has occurred. A medical workup to diagnose osteoporosis will include a complete medical history, x-rays, and urine and blood tests. The doctor may also order a BMD (bone mineral density) test. This test can identify osteoporosis, determine your risk for fractures (broken bones), and measure your response to osteoporosis treatment. The most widely recognized bone mineral density test is called a dual-energy x-ray absorptiometry or DXA test. It is painless: a bit like having an x-ray, but with much less exposure to radiation. It can measure bone density at your hip and spine.

It is increasingly common for women to be diagnosed with osteoporosis or low bone mass using a BMD test, often at midlife when doctors begin to watch for signs of bone loss. In men, however, the diagnosis is often not made until a fracture occurs or a man complains of back pain and sees his doctor. This makes it especially important for men to inform their doctors about risk factors for developing osteoporosis, loss of height or change in posture, a fracture, or sudden back pain.

What Are the Risk Factors for Men?

Several risk factors have been linked to osteoporosis in men:

- Chronic diseases that affect the kidneys, lungs, stomach, and intestines or alters hormone levels.
- Regular use of certain medications, such as glucocorticoids.
- Undiagnosed low levels of the sex hormone testosterone.
- Unhealthy lifestyle habits: smoking, excessive alcohol use, low calcium intake, inadequate physical exercise.
- Age—the older you are, the greater your risk.
- Race—Caucasian men appear to be at particularly high risk, but all men can develop this disease.

Some doctors may be unsure how to interpret the results of a BMD test in men, because it is not known whether the World Health Organization guidelines used to diagnose osteoporosis or low bone mass in women are also appropriate for men. Although controversial, the International Society for Clinical Densitometry recommends using separate guidelines when interpreting BMD test results in men.

What Treatments Are Available?

Once a man has been diagnosed with osteoporosis, his doctor may prescribe one of the medications approved by the FDA for this disease. Alendronate and risedronate have been approved to treat the disease in men, postmenopausal women, and in men and women with glucocorticoid-induced osteoporosis. Teriparatide is approved to treat osteoporosis in men and women who are at increased risk of fracture.

The treatment plan will also likely include the nutrition, exercise, and lifestyle guidelines for preventing bone loss listed at the end of this section.

If bone loss is due to glucocorticoid use, the doctor may prescribe a bisphosphonate (e.g., alendronate or risedronate), monitor bone density and testosterone levels, and suggest using the minimum effective dose of glucocorticoid. The doctor may also suggest discontinuing the drug when practical, and/or administering it topically (through the skin).

Other possible prevention or treatment approaches include calcium and/or vitamin D supplements and regular physical activity.

If osteoporosis is the result of another condition (such as testosterone deficiency) or exposure to certain other medications, the doctor may design a treatment plan to address the underlying cause.

How Can Osteoporosis Be Prevented?

There have been fewer research studies on osteoporosis in men than in women. However, experts agree that all people should take the following steps to preserve their bone health:

- Avoid smoking, reduce alcohol intake, and increase your level of physical activity.
- Ensure a daily calcium intake that is adequate for your age.
- Ensure an adequate intake of vitamin D. Normally, the body makes enough vitamin D from exposure to as little as ten minutes of sunlight a day. If exposure to sunlight is inadequate, dietary vitamin D intake should be between 200 and 600 IU (International Units) per day (See Table 45.1). In one quart of fortified milk and most multivitamins there are 400 IU of vitamin D.
- Engage in a regular regimen of weight-bearing exercises in which bones and muscles work against gravity. This might include walking, jogging, racquet sports, stair climbing, team

sports, lifting weights, and using resistance machines. A doctor should evaluate the exercise program of anyone already diagnosed with osteoporosis to determine if twisting motions and impact activities, such as those used in golf, tennis, or basketball, need to be curtailed.

- Discuss with your doctor the use of medications that are known to cause bone loss, such as glucocorticoids.
- Recognize and seek treatment for any underlying medical conditions that affect bone health.

Table 45.1. Recommendations for Calcium and Vitamin D Intake

Age	Calcium (mg)	Vitamin D (IU)
19–30	1,000	200
31–50	1,000	200
51–70	1,200	400
70+	1,200	600
Upper limit	2,500	2,000

Source: National Academy of Sciences, 1997

Part Five

Additional Help and Information

Chapter 46

Glossary of Terms Related to Men's Health

abnormality: A growth or area of tissue that is not normal. An abnormality may be cancer or likely to become cancer.[1]

acute: Acute often means urgent. An acute disease happens suddenly. It lasts a short time. Acute is the opposite of chronic, or long lasting.[4]

adjuvant therapy: Treatment given after the main treatment to help cure a disease.[1]

allergy: An abnormally high sensitivity to certain substances, such as pollens or foods. Common signs of allergies may include sneezing, itching, and skin rashes.[2]

anesthesia: A drug administered for medical purposes that causes a partial or total loss of feeling.[2]

aneurysm: A weak or thin spot on an artery wall that has stretched or ballooned out from the wall and filled with blood, or damage to an artery leading to pooling of blood between the layers of the blood vessel walls.[3]

The terms in this glossary were excerpted from "Lung Cancer Glossary," National Cancer Institute, July 8, 2008 [marked 1]; "Real Men Wear Gowns Glossary," Agency for Healthcare Research and Quality, accessed August 28, 2008 [marked 2]; "Stroke: Hope through Research," National Institute of Neurological Disorders and Stroke, National Institutes of Health, NIH Publication No. 99-2222, August 20, 2008 [marked 3]; and "Urologic Diseases Dictionary," National Institute of Diabetes and Digestive and Kidney Diseases, National Institutes of Health, September 2004 [marked 4].

antibiotic: A drug, such as penicillin or streptomycin, that can destroy or prevent the growth of bacteria. Antibiotics are widely used to prevent and treat infectious diseases.[2]

antibodies: Proteins in the body made by the immune system that fight infection and disease.[1]

anticoagulants: A drug therapy used to prevent the formation of blood clots that can become lodged in cerebral arteries and cause strokes.[3]

aphasia: The inability to understand or create speech, writing, or language in general due to damage to the speech centers of the brain.[3]

apraxia: A movement disorder characterized by the inability to perform skilled or purposeful voluntary movements, generally caused by damage to the areas of the brain responsible for voluntary movement.[3]

arteriography: An x-ray of the carotid artery taken when a special dye is injected into the artery.[3]

atherosclerosis: A blood vessel disease characterized by deposits of lipid material on the inside of the walls of large- to medium-sized arteries which make the artery walls thick, hard, brittle, and prone to breaking.[3]

atrial fibrillation: Irregular beating of the left atrium, or left upper chamber, of the heart.[3]

balloon dilation: A treatment for benign prostatic hyperplasia or prostate enlargement. A tiny balloon is inflated inside the urethra to make it wider so urine can flow more freely from the bladder.[4]

benign prostatic hyperplasia (BPH): An enlarged prostate not caused by cancer. BPH can cause problems with urination because the prostate squeezes the urethra at the opening of the bladder.[4]

biological therapy: Treatment to boost the immune system's power to fight infections and other diseases. It can also be used to lessen side effects of some treatments. Also called immunotherapy, biotherapy, or biological response modifier (BRM) therapy.[1]

biopsy: To remove cells or tissues from the body for testing and examination under a microscope.[1]

bronchi: The large airways connecting the windpipe to the lungs. The single form is bronchus.[1]

bronchoscopy: A way to look at the inside of the windpipe, the bronchi, and/or the lungs using a lighted tube. The tube is inserted through the patient's nose or mouth. Bronchoscopy may be used to find cancer or as part of some treatments.[1]

carcinogen: Something that causes cancer.[1]

carotid artery: An artery, located on either side of the neck, that supplies the brain with blood.[3]

carotid endarterectomy: Surgery used to remove fatty deposits from the carotid arteries.[3]

CAT scan: A set of detailed pictures of areas inside the body, taken from different angles. The pictures are made by a computer linked to an x-ray machine. Other names for a CAT scan are computerized axial tomography, computed tomography (CT scan), and computerized tomography.[1]

catheter: A tube that is inserted through the urethra to the bladder to drain urine.[4]

cerebral blood flow (CBF): The flow of blood through the arteries that lead to the brain, called the cerebrovascular system.[3]

cerebrospinal fluid (CSF): Clear fluid that bathes the brain and spinal cord.[3]

cerebrovascular disease: A reduction in the supply of blood to the brain either by narrowing of the arteries through the buildup of plaque on the inside walls of the arteries, called stenosis, or through blockage of an artery due to a blood clot.[3]

chemoprevention: Using things such as drugs or vitamins to try to prevent or slow down cancer. Chemoprevention may be used to help keep someone from ever getting cancer. It is also used to help keep some cancers from coming back.[1]

chemotherapy: Using drugs to treat cancer.[1]

cholesterol: A waxy substance, produced naturally by the liver and also found in foods, that circulates in the blood and helps maintain tissues and cell membranes. Excess cholesterol in the body can contribute to atherosclerosis and high blood pressure.[3]

chronic: Lasting a long time. Chronic diseases develop slowly. Chronic kidney disease may develop over many years and lead to end-stage renal disease.[4]

clinical trial: A kind of research study where patients volunteer to test new ways of screening for, preventing, finding, or treating a disease. Also called a clinical study.[1]

cystinuria: A condition in which urine contains high levels of the amino acid cystine. If cystine does not dissolve in the urine, it can build up to form kidney stones.[4]

cystitis: Inflammation of the bladder, causing pain and a burning feeling in the pelvis or urethra.[4]

cystocele: Fallen bladder. When the bladder falls or sags from its normal position down to the pelvic floor, it can cause either urinary leakage or urinary retention.[4]

diabetes mellitus: A condition characterized by high blood glucose (sugar) resulting from the body's inability to use glucose efficiently. In type 1 diabetes, the pancreas makes little or no insulin; in type 2 diabetes, the body is resistant to the effects of available insulin.[4]

diagnosis: The act of identifying or determining the nature and cause of a disease or injury through evaluating the patient's history, an examination, and a review of laboratory data.[2]

dysphagia: Trouble swallowing.[1]

dyspnea: Shortness of breath.[1]

edema: The swelling of a cell that results from the influx of large amounts of water or fluid into the cell.[3]

elective surgery: A surgery that is optional, not required.[2]

embolic stroke: A stroke caused by an embolus.[3]

embolus: A free-roaming clot that usually forms in the heart.[3]

emphysema: A disease that affects the tiny air sacs in the lungs. Emphysema makes it harder to breathe. People who smoke have a greater chance of getting emphysema.[1]

enuresis: Urinary incontinence not caused by a physical disorder.[4]

erectile dysfunction: The inability to get or maintain an erection for satisfactory sexual intercourse. Also called impotence.[4]

erection: Enlargement and hardening of the penis caused by increased blood flow into the penis and decreased blood flow out of it as a result of sexual excitement.[4]

extracorporeal shockwave lithotripsy (ESWL): A nonsurgical procedure using shock waves to break up kidney stones.[4]

first line therapy: The first course of treatment used against a disease.[1]

functional magnetic resonance imaging (fMRI): A type of imaging that measures increases in blood flow within the brain.[3]

gene: The basic unit of heredity. Genes decide eye color and other traits. Genes also play a role in how high a person's risk is for certain diseases.[1]

gene therapy: Treatment that changes a gene. Gene therapy is used to help the body fight cancer. It also can be used to make cancer cells more sensitive to treatment.[1]

genitals: Sex organs, including the penis and testicles in men and the vagina and vulva in women.[4]

health history: A regularly updated record of a person's past and present health status.[2]

hematuria: Blood in the urine, which can be a sign of a kidney stone or other urinary problem.[4]

hemiparesis: Weakness on one side of the body.[3]

hemiplegia: Complete paralysis on one side of the body.[3]

hemorrhagic stroke: Sudden bleeding into or around the brain.[3]

high-density lipoprotein (HDL): Also known as the good cholesterol; a compound consisting of a lipid and a protein that carries a small percentage of the total cholesterol in the blood and deposits it in the liver.[3]

hormone: A natural chemical produced in one part of the body and released into the blood to trigger or regulate particular functions of the body.[4]

hydronephrosis: Swelling at the top of the ureter, usually because something is blocking the urine from flowing into or out of the bladder.[4]

hypercalciuria: Abnormally large amounts of calcium in the urine.[4]

hyperoxaluria: Unusually large amounts of oxalate in the urine, leading to kidney stones.[4]

hypertension (high blood pressure): Characterized by persistently high arterial blood pressure defined as a measurement greater than or equal to 140 mm/Hg systolic pressure over 90 mm/Hg diastolic pressure.[3]

hypospadias: A birth defect in which the opening of the urethra, called the urinary meatus, is on the underside of the penis instead of at the tip.[4]

immune system: The complex group of organs and cells that defends the body against infections and other diseases.[1]

immunosuppressant: A drug given to suppress the natural responses of the body's immune system. Immunosuppressants are given to transplant patients to prevent organ rejection and to patients with autoimmune diseases like lupus.[4]

impotence: See erectile dysfunction.[4]

incontinence: Loss of bladder or bowel control; the accidental loss of urine or feces.[4]

ischemia: A loss of blood flow to tissue, caused by an obstruction of the blood vessel, usually in the form of plaque stenosis or a blood clot.[3]

ischemic stroke: Ischemia in the tissues of the brain.[3]

kidney: A bean-shaped organ that filters waste products from the body and forms urine that is passed into the bladder. Human beings are born with two kidneys, one on each side of the lower back.[1]

kidney stone: A stone that develops from crystals that form in urine and build up on the inner surfaces of the kidney, in the renal pelvis, or in the ureters.[4]

larynx: Voice box. The larynx is part of the breathing system and is found in the throat.[1]

lithotripsy: A method of breaking up kidney stones using shock waves or other means.[4]

lobe: A part of an organ, such as the lung.[1]

lobectomy: Surgery to remove a lobe of an organ.[1]

low-density lipoprotein (LDL): Also known as the bad cholesterol; a compound consisting of a lipid and a protein that carries the majority of the total cholesterol in the blood and deposits the excess along the inside of arterial walls.[3]

lymph nodes: Small glands that help the body fight infection and disease. They filter a fluid called lymph and contain white blood cells.[1]

magnetic resonance imaging (MRI) scan: A type of imaging involving the use of magnetic fields to detect subtle changes in the water content of tissues.[3]

medical record: A file that contains a patient's medical history and care.[2]

mesothelioma: A tumor in the lining of the chest or abdomen (stomach area).[1]

metastasis: When cancer spreads to other parts of the body.[1]

necrosis: A form of cell death resulting from anoxia, trauma, or any other form of irreversible damage to the cell; involves the release of toxic cellular material into the intercellular space, poisoning surrounding cells.[3]

neoadjuvant therapy: Treatment given before the main treatment to help cure a disease.[1]

nephrotic syndrome: A collection of symptoms that indicate kidney damage. Symptoms include high levels of protein in the urine, lack of protein in the blood, and high blood cholesterol.[4]

neuron: The main functional cell of the brain and nervous system, consisting of a cell body, an axon, and dendrites.[3]

neuroprotective agents: Medications that protect the brain from secondary injury caused by stroke.[3]

neutropenia: An abnormal decrease in a type of white blood cells. The body needs white blood cells to fight disease and infection.[1]

outpatient surgery: A procedure in which the patient is not required to stay overnight in a hospital; also called same-day surgery.[2]

oxalate: A chemical that combines with calcium in urine to form the most common type of kidney stone (calcium oxalate stone).[4]

pancreas: A large gland that helps digest food and also makes some important hormones.[1]

pelvis: The bowl-shaped bone that supports the spine and holds up the digestive, urinary, and reproductive organs. The legs connect to the body at the pelvis.[4]

penis: The male organ used for urination and sex.[4]

peripheral neuropathy: Numbness, tingling, burning, or weakness that usually begins in the hands or feet. Some anticancer drugs can cause this problem.[1]

Peyronie disease: A plaque (hardened area) that forms on the penis, preventing that area from stretching. During erection, the penis bends in the direction of the plaque, or the plaque may lead to indentation and shortening of the penis.[4]

plaque: Fatty cholesterol deposits found along the inside of artery walls that lead to atherosclerosis and stenosis of the arteries.[3]

pleural effusion: When too much fluid collects between the lining of the lung and the lining of the inside wall of the chest.[1]

pneumonectomy: Surgery to remove a lung.[1]

preventive medical test: Tests designed to rule out or avoid disease. For example, screening for high blood pressure and treating it before it causes serious health problems is an example of a preventive medical test. [2]

prognosis: A prediction of the probable outcome of a disease.[2]

prostate: In men, a walnut-shaped gland that surrounds the urethra at the neck of the bladder. The prostate supplies fluid that goes into semen.[4]

prostate cancer: Cancer that begins in the prostate.[1]

prostate-specific antigen (PSA): A protein made only by the prostate gland. High levels of PSA in the blood may be a sign of prostate cancer.[4]

prostatitis: Inflammation of the prostate gland. Chronic prostatitis means the prostate gets inflamed over and over again. The most common form of prostatitis is not associated with any known infecting organism.[4]

proteinuria: A condition in which the urine contains large amounts of protein, a sign that the kidneys are not functioning properly.[4]

radiation: The emission of energy in waves or particles. Often used to treat cancer cells.[1]

recurrence: When cancer comes back after a period when no cancer could be found.[1]

resection: Surgery to remove tissue, an organ, or part of an organ.[1]

side effect: An effect of a drug, chemical, or other medicine that is in addition to its intended effect, especially an effect that is harmful or unpleasant.[2]

specialist: A doctor who devotes attention to a particular class of diseases or patients.[2]

stage: How much cancer is in the body and how far it has spread.[1]

stenosis: Narrowing of an artery due to the buildup of plaque on the inside wall of the artery.[3]

stress urinary incontinence: Leakage of urine caused by actions—such as coughing, laughing, sneezing, running, or lifting—that place pressure on the bladder from inside the body. Stress urinary incontinence can result from either a cystocele (fallen bladder) or weak sphincter muscles.[4]

subarachnoid hemorrhage: Bleeding within the meninges, or outer membranes, of the brain into the clear fluid that surrounds the brain.[3]

symptom: Something that indicates the presence of a disorder or disease.[2]

thrombolytics: Drugs used to treat an ongoing, acute ischemic stroke by dissolving the blood clot causing the stroke and thereby restoring blood flow through the artery.[3]

thrombosis: The formation of a blood clot in one of the cerebral arteries of the head or neck that stays attached to the artery wall until it grows large enough to block blood flow.[3]

thrombotic stroke: A stroke caused by thrombosis.[3]

total serum cholesterol: A combined measurement of a person's high-density lipoprotein (HDL) and low-density lipoprotein (LDL).[3]

transcranial magnetic stimulation (TMS): A small magnetic current delivered to an area of the brain to promote plasticity and healing.[3]

transient ischemic attack (TIA): A short-lived stroke that lasts from a few minutes up to twenty-four hours; often called a mini-stroke.[3]

ultrasound: A technique that bounces safe, painless sound waves off organs to create an image of their structure.

ureters: Tubes that carry urine from the kidneys to the bladder.[4]

urethra: The tube that carries urine from the bladder to the outside of the body.[4]

urethritis: Inflammation of the urethra.[4]

urge urinary incontinence: Urinary leakage when the bladder contracts unexpectedly by itself.[4]

urinalysis: A test of a urine sample that can reveal many problems of the urinary tract and other body systems.[4]

urinary frequency: Urination eight or more times a day.[4]

urinary tract infection (UTI): An illness caused by harmful bacteria growing in the urinary tract.[4]

urinary tract: The system that takes wastes from the blood and carries them out of the body in the form of urine. The urinary tract includes the kidneys, ureters, bladder, and urethra.[4]

urinary urgency: Inability to delay urination.[4]

urine: Liquid waste product filtered from the blood by the kidneys, stored in the bladder, and expelled from the body through the urethra by the act of voiding or urinating.[4]

vaccine: A substance meant to help the immune system respond to and resist disease.[1]

vasodilators: Medications that increase blood flow to the brain by expanding or dilating blood vessels.[3]

Chapter 47

Directory of Agencies That Provide Information about Men's Health

General

American Academy of Family Physicians
P.O. Box 11210
Shawnee Mission, KS 66207-1210
Toll-Free: 800-274-2237
Phone: 913-906-6000
Fax: 913-906-6075
Website: http://www.aafp.org

Centers for Disease Control and Prevention
1600 Clifton Road, NE
Atlanta, GA 30333
Toll-Free: 800-311-3435
Phone: 404-639-3311
Website: http://www.cdc.gov

Men's Health Network
P.O. Box 75972
Washington, DC 20013
Website:
www.menshealthnetwork.org
E-mail:
info@menshealthnetwork.org

National Heart, Lung, and Blood Institute
P.O. Box 30105
Bethesda, MD 20824-0105
Phone: 301-592-8573
Website: www.nhlbi.nih.gov

The information in this chapter was compiled from various sources deemed accurate. All contact information was verified and updated in March 2009. Inclusion does not imply endorsement. This list is intended to serve as a starting point for information gathering; it is not comprehensive.

National Institute of Neurological Disorders and Stroke
NIH Neurological Institute
P.O. Box 5801
Bethesda, MD 20824
Toll-Free: 800-352-9424
Phone: 301-496-5751
TTY: 301-468-5981
Website: http://www.ninds.nih.gov

National Kidney and Urologic Diseases Information Clearinghouse
3 Information Way
Bethesda, MD 20892-3580
Toll-Free: 800-891-5390
Fax: 703-738-4929
TTY: 866-569-1162
Website:
www.kidney.niddk.nih.gov
E-mail:
nkudic@info.niddk.nih.gov

National Women's Health Information Center
Toll-Free: 800-994-9662
TDD: 888-220-5446
Website: http://
www.4woman.gov

NIH Senior Health
Website: http://
www.nihseniorhealth.gov

U.S. Food and Drug Administration
10903 New Hampshire Ave.
Silver Spring, MD 20903
Toll-Free: 888-INFO-FDA
(888-463-6332)
Website: http://www.fda.gov

Alzheimer Disease

Alzheimer's Association
225 N. Michigan Ave., Fl. 17
Chicago, IL 60601-7633
Toll-Free: 800-272-3900
Phone: 312-335-8700
Fax: 866-699-1246
TDD: 312-335-5886
Website: http://www.alz.org
E-mail: info@alz.org

Alzheimer's Disease Education and Referral Center
P.O. Box 8250
Silver Spring, MD 20907
Toll-Free: 800-438-4380
Fax: 301-495-3334
Website: http://www.nia.nih.gov/
alzheimers

National Institute on Aging
Building 31, Room 5C27
31 Center Drive, MSC 2292
Bethesda, MD 20892
Phone: 301-496-1752
Fax: 301-496-1072
TTY: 800-222-4225
Website: http://www.nia.nih.gov

Cancer

American Cancer Society
Website: http://www.cancer.org

Cancer Information Service
National Cancer Institute (NCI)
NCI Public Inquiries Office
6116 Executive Boulevard
MSC 8322
Room 3036A
Bethesda, MD 20892-8322
Toll-Free: 800-4CANCER (800-422-6237)
TTY: 800-332-8615
Website: http://www.cancer.gov
E-mail: cancergovstaff@mail.nih.gov

Cardiovascular Disorders

American Heart Association
National Center
7272 Greenville Avenue
Dallas, TX 75231
Toll-Free: 800-AHA-USA-1 (800-242-8721)
Website: http://www.americanheart.org

American Stroke Association
National Center
7272 Greenville Avenue
Dallas TX 75231
Toll-Free: 888-4-STROKE (888-478-7653)
Website: http://www.strokeassociation.org

Sudden Cardiac Arrest Association
1133 Connecticut Avenue, NW
11th Floor
Washington, DC 20036
Toll-Free: 866-972-SCAA (7222)
Website: www.suddencardiacarrest.org
E-mail: info@suddencardiacarrest.org

Diabetes

American Diabetes Association (ADA)
Attn: National Call Center
1701 North Beauregard Street
Alexandria, VA 22311
Toll-Free: 800-DIABETES (342-2383)
Website: www.diabetes.org

National Diabetes Education Program
1 Information Way
Bethesda, MD 20814-9692
Toll-Free: 800-438-5383
Website: http://www.ndep.nih.gov

Human Immunodeficiency Virus/Acquired Immunodeficiency Syndrome (HIV/AIDS)

AIDSinfo
P.O. Box 6303
Rockville, MD 20849-6303
Toll-Free: 800-HIV-0440 (800-448-0440)
Phone: 301-519-0459
Fax: 301-519-6616
TTY: 888-480-3739
Website: http://aidsinfo.nih.gov
E-mail: ContactUs@aidsinfo.nih.gov

Kidney and Urologic Disorders

American Association of Kidney Patients
3505 East Frontage Road
Suite 315
Tampa, FL 33607
Toll-Free: 800-749-2257
Phone: 813-636-8100
Fax: 813-636-8122
Website: http://www.aakp.org
E-mail: info@aakp.org

American Kidney Fund
6110 Executive Boulevard
Suite 1010
Rockville, MD 20852
Toll-Free: 800-638-8299
Phone: 301-881-3052
Fax: 301-881-0898
Website: http://www.kidneyfund.org
E-mail: helpline@kidneyfund.org

American Urological Association (AUA)
1000 Corporate Boulevard
Linthicum, MD 21090
Toll-Free: 866-RING-AUA (746-4282)
Phone: 410-689-3700
Fax: 410-689-3800
Website: www.auanet.org or www.urologyhealth.org
E-mail: aua@auanet.org

National Association for Continence
P.O. Box 1019
Charleston, SC 29402-1019
Toll-Free: 800-BLADDER (252-3337)
Phone: 843-377-0900
Website: http://www.nafc.org
E-mail: memberservices@nafc.org

National Kidney and Urologic Diseases
Information Clearinghouse
3 Information Way
Bethesda, MD 20892-3580
Toll-Free: 800-891-5390
Fax: 703-738-4929
TTY: 866-569-1162
Website: http://www.kidney.niddk.nih.gov
E-mail: nkudic@info.niddk.nih.gov

National Kidney Foundation, Inc.
30 East 33rd Street
New York, NY 10016
Toll-Free: 800-622-9010
Phone: 212-889-2210
Website: http://www.kidney.org

Mental Health Concerns

National Institute of Mental Health (NIMH)
6001 Executive Boulevard, Room 8184, MSC 9663
Bethesda, MD 20892-9663
Toll-Free: 866-615-6464
Phone: 301-443-4513
Fax: 301-443-4279
TTY: 866-415-8051 or 301-443-8431
Website: http://www.nimh.nih.gov
E-mail: nimhinfo@nih.gov

Substance Abuse and Mental Health Services Administration
Health Information Network
P.O. Box 2345
Rockville, MD 20847-2345
Toll-Free: 877-SAMHSA-7 (877-726-4727)
Fax: 240-221-4292
TTY: 800-487-4889
Website: http://www.samhsa.gov
E-mail: SHIN@samhsa.hhs.gov

Muscular Dystrophy

Muscular Dystrophy Association
3300 East Sunrise Drive
Tucson, AZ 85718-3208
Toll-Free: 800-344-4863
Phone: 520-529-2000
Fax: 520-529-5300
Website: http://www.mda.org
E-mail: mda@mdausa.org

National Institute of Arthritis and Musculoskeletal and Skin Diseases (NIAMS)
National Institutes of Health, DHHS
31 Center Dr., Rm. 4C02
MSC 2350
Bethesda, MD 20892-2350
Toll-Free: 877-22-NIAMS (226-4267)
Phone: 301-496-8190
Website: http://www.niams.nih.gov
E-mail: NIAMSinfo@mail.nih.gov

Parent Project Muscular Dystrophy (PPMD)
158 Linwood Plaza, Suite 220
Fort Lee, NJ 07024
Toll-Free: 800-714-KIDS (5437)
Phone: 201-944-9985
Fax: 201-944-9987
Website: http://www.parentprojectmd.org
E-mail: info@parentprojectmd.org

Nutrition

American Dietetic Association
120 South Riverside Plaza, Suite 2000
Chicago, IL 60606-6995
Toll-Free: 800-877-1600
Website: http://www.eatright.org

Food and Nutrition Information Center
U.S. Department of Agriculture
Agricultural Research Service, National Agricultural Library
10301 Baltimore Avenue
Room 105
Beltsville, MD 20705-2351
Phone: 301-504-5719
Website: http://www.nal.usda.gov/fnic

Physical Fitness

President's Council on Physical Fitness and Sports
Department W
200 Independence Avenue, SW, Room 738-H
Washington, DC 20201-0004
Phone: 202-690-9000
Website: http://www.fitness.gov

Prostate Disorders

American Urological Association (AUA)
1000 Corporate Boulevard
Linthicum, MD 21090
Toll-Free: 866-RING-AUA (746-4282)
Phone: 410-689-3700
Fax: 410-689-3800
Website: www.auanet.org or www.urologyhealth.org
E-mail: aua@auanet.org

Prostatitis Foundation
1063 30th Street, Box 8
Smithshire, IL 61478
Toll-Free: 888-891-4200
Fax: 309-325-7184
Website: http://www.prostatitis.org
E-mail: mcapstone@aol.com

Us Too! International, Inc.
(Prostate Cancer Survivors)
5003 Fairview Avenue
Downers Grove, IL 60515
Toll-Free: 800-80-US-TOO (808-7866)
Phone: 630-795-1002
Website: www.ustoo.org

Sexual Dysfunction

American Association of Sex Educators, Counselors, and Therapists (AASECT)
P.O. Box 1960
Ashland, VA 23005-1960
Phone: 804-752-0026
Fax: 804-752-0056
Website: www.aasect.org

Society for Sex Therapy and Research
409 12th St., S.W., PO Box 96920
Washington, DC 20090-6920
Phone: 202-863-1644
Website: http://www.sstarnet.org/

Stroke

American Stroke Association: A Division of American Heart Association
7272 Greenville Avenue
Dallas, TX 75231-4596
Toll-Free: 888-4STROKE (478-7653)
Fax: 214-706-5231
Website: http://www.strokeassociation.org
E-mail: strokeassociation@heart.org

Brain Attack Coalition
31 Center Drive
Room 8A07
Bethesda, MD 20892-2540
Phone: 301-496-5751
Fax: 301-402-2186
Website: http://www.stroke-site.org

National Stroke Association
9707 East Easter Lane, Suite B
Centennial, CO 80112-3747
Toll-Free: 800-STROKES (787-6537)
Phone: 303-649-9299
Fax: 303-649-1328
Website: http://www.stroke.org
E-mail: info@stroke.org

Index

Index

Page numbers followed by 'n' indicate a footnote. Page numbers in *italics* indicate a table or illustration.

A

B

D

E

F

G

H

I

J

K

L

M

O

P

Q

R

S

T

U

V

W

X

Y

Z

Health Reference Series

Complete Catalog

List price $93 per volume. School and library price $84 per volume.

Adolescent Health Sourcebook, 2nd Edition

Basic Consumer Health Information about the Physical, Mental, and Emotional Growth and Development of Adolescents, Including Medical Care, Nutritional and Physical Activity Requirements, Puberty, Sexual Activity, Acne, Tanning, Body Piercing, Common Physical Illnesses and Disorders, Eating Disorders, Attention Deficit Hyperactivity Disorder, Depression, Bullying, Hazing, and Adolescent Injuries Related to Sports, Driving, and Work

Along with Substance Abuse Information about Nicotine, Alcohol, and Drug Use, a Glossary, and Directory of Additional Resources

Edited by Joyce Brennfleck Shannon. 655 pages. 2007. 978-0-7808-0943-7.

"A particularly good resource for both parents and teens. The concise presentation of the material in brief and well-organized chapters creates an easy volume to browse."

—*School Library Journal, Jun '07*

"I don't believe there are any other books written in such easy to understand language that encompass such a breadth of topics. This is a complete revision of the book and is an excellent resource for parents and teens."

—*Doody's Review Service, 2007*

Adult Health Concerns Sourcebook

Basic Consumer Health Information about Medical and Mental Concerns of Adults, Including Facts about Choosing Healthcare Providers, Navigating Insurance Options, Maintaining Wellness, Preventing Cancer, Heart Disease, Stroke, Diabetes, and Osteoporosis, and Understanding Aging-Related Health Concerns, Including Menopause, Cognitive Changes, and Changes in the Coronary and Vascular Systems

Along with Tips on Caring for Aging Parents and Dealing with Health-Related Work and Travel Issues, a Glossary, and a Directory of Resources for Additional Help and Information

Edited by Sandra J. Judd. 648 pages. 2008. 978-0-7808-0999-4.

"Provides a thorough list of topics that are important to adult health and for caregivers."

—*CHOICE, Nov '08*

"Written in easy-to-understand language . . . the content is well-organized and is intended to aid adults in making health care-related decisions."

—*AORN Journal, Dec '08*

AIDS Sourcebook, 4th Edition

Basic Consumer Health Information about Human Immunodeficiency Virus (HIV) and Acquired Immunodeficiency Syndrome (AIDS), Featuring Updated Statistics and Facts about Risks, Prevention, Screening, Diagnosis, Treatments, Side Effects, and Complications, and Including a Section about the Impact of HIV/AIDS on the Health of Women, Children, and Adolescents

Along with Tips on Managing Life with AIDS, Reports on Current Research Initiatives and Clinical Trials, a Glossary of Related Terms, and Resource Directories for Further Help and Information

Edited by Ivy L. Alexander. 680 pages. 2008. 978-0-7808-0997-0.

SEE ALSO *Contagious Diseases Sourcebook, 2nd Edition*

Alcoholism Sourcebook, 2nd Edition

Basic Consumer Health Information about Alcohol Use, Abuse, and Dependence, Featuring Facts about the Physical, Mental, and Social Health Effects of Alcohol Addiction, Including Alcoholic Liver Disease, Pancreatic Disease, Cardiovascular Disease, Neurological Disorders, and the Effects of Drinking during Pregnancy

Along with Information about Alcohol Treatment, Medications, and Recovery Programs, in Addition to Tips for Reducing the Prevalence of Underage Drinking, Statistics about Alcohol Use, a Glossary of Related Terms, and Directories of Resources for More Help and Information

Edited by Amy L. Sutton. 625 pages. 2007. 978-0-7808-0942-0.

"A comprehensive look at the adverse effects of alcohol on people of all ages . . . It serves to whet the reader's appetite to continue learning using other resources. It is practical, easy to read, and enlightening, and is the first book a lay person should consult to learn about alcoholism."

—*Doody's Review Service, 2007*

"Should be a basic acquisition for any serious public or college-level library including health reference titles for general-interest readers."

—*California Bookwatch, Feb '07*

SEE ALSO *Drug Abuse Sourcebook, 2nd Edition*

Allergies Sourcebook, 3rd Edition

Basic Consumer Health Information about Allergic Disorders, Such as Anaphylaxis, Hives, Eczema, Rhinitis, Sinusitis, and Conjunctivitis, and Their Triggers, Including Pollen, Mold, Dust Mites, Animal Dander, Insects, Chemicals, Food, Food Additives, and Medications

Along with Advice about the Diagnosis and Treatment of Allergy Symptoms, a Glossary of Related Terms, a Directory of Resources for Help and Information, and Suggestions for Additional Reading

Edited by Amy L. Sutton. 588 pages. 2007. 978-0-7808-0950-5.

SEE ALSO *Asthma Sourcebook, 2nd Edition*

Alzheimer Disease Sourcebook, 4th Edition

Basic Consumer Health Information about Alzheimer Disease, Other Dementias, and Related Disorders, Including Multi-Infarct Dementia, Dementia with Lewy Bodies, Frontotemporal Dementia (Pick Disease), Wernicke-Korsakoff Syndrome (Alcohol-Related Dementia), AIDS Dementia Complex, Huntington Disease, Creutzfeldt-Jacob Disease, and Delirium

Along with Information about Coping with Memory Loss and Forgetfulness, Maintaining Skills, and Long-Term Planning for People with Dementia, and Suggestions Addressing Common Caregiver Concerns, Updated Information about Current Research Efforts, a Glossary of Related Terms, and Directories of Sources for Additional Help and Information

Edited by Karen Bellenir. 603 pages. 2008. 978-0-7808-1001-3.

"An invaluable resource for persons who have received a diagnosis, for caregivers, and for family members dealing with this insidious disease. It is recommended for public, community college, and ready-reference sections in academic libraries."

—*ARBAonline, Jul '08*

SEE ALSO *Brain Disorders Sourcebook, 2nd Edition*

Arthritis Sourcebook, 2nd Edition

Basic Consumer Health Information about Osteoarthritis, Rheumatoid Arthritis, Other Rheumatic Disorders, Infectious Forms of Arthritis, and Diseases with Symptoms Linked to Arthritis, Featuring Facts about Diagnosis, Pain Management, and Surgical Therapies

Along with Coping Strategies, Research Updates, a Glossary, and Resources for Additional Help and Information

Edited by Amy L. Sutton. 567 pages. 2004. 978-0-7808-0667-2.

"This easy-to-read volume is recommended for consumer health collections within public or academic libraries."

—*E-Streams, May '05*

"As expected, this updated edition continues the excellent reputation of this series in providing sound, usable health information. . . . Highly recommended."

—*American Reference Books Annual, 2005*

Asthma Sourcebook, 2nd Edition

Basic Consumer Health Information about the Causes, Symptoms, Diagnosis, and Treatment of Asthma in Infants, Children, Teenagers, and Adults, Including Facts about Different Types of Asthma, Common Co-Occurring Conditions, Asthma Management Plans, Triggers, Medications, and Medication Delivery Devices

Along with Asthma Statistics, Research Updates, a Glossary, a Directory of Asthma-Related Resources, and More

Edited by Karen Bellenir. 581 pages. 2006. 978-0-7808-0866-9.

Attention Deficit Disorder Sourcebook

Basic Consumer Health Information about Attention Deficit/Hyperactivity Disorder in Children and Adults, Including Facts about Causes, Symptoms, Diagnostic Criteria, and Treatment Options Such as Medications, Behavior Therapy, Coaching, and Homeopathy

Along with Reports on Current Research Initiatives, Legal Issues, and Government Regulations, and Featuring a Glossary of Related Terms, Internet Resources, and a List of Additional Reading Material

Edited by Dawn D. Matthews. 447 pages. 2002. 978-0-7808-0624-5.

"Recommended reference source."

—*Booklist, Jan '03*

SEE ALSO *Learning Disabilities Sourcebook, 3rd Edition*

Autism and Pervasive Developmental Disorders Sourcebook

Basic Consumer Health Information about Autism Spectrum and Pervasive Developmental Disorders, Such as Classical Autism, Asperger Syndrome, Rett Syndrome, and Childhood Disintegrative Disorder, Including Information about Related Genetic Disorders and Medical Problems and Facts about Causes, Screening Methods, Diagnostic Criteria, Treatments and Interventions, and Family and Education Issues

Along with a Glossary of Related Terms, Tips for Evaluating the Validity of Health Claims, and a Directory of Resources for Additional Help and Information

Edited by Sandra J. Judd. 603 pages. 2007. 978-0-7808-0953-6.

"Recommended for public libraries"

—*SciTech Book News, Mar '08*

SEE ALSO *Learning Disabilities Sourcebook, 3rd Edition*

Back and Neck Disorders Sourcebook, 2nd Edition

Basic Consumer Health Information about Spinal Pain, Spinal Cord Injuries, and Related Disorders, Such as Degenerative Disk Disease, Osteoarthritis, Scoliosis, Sciatica, Spina Bifida, and Spinal Stenosis, and Featuring Facts about Maintaining Spinal Health, Self-Care, Pain Management, Rehabilitative Care, Chiropractic Care, Spinal Surgeries, and Complementary Therapies

Along with Suggestions for Preventing Back and Neck Pain, a Glossary of Related Terms, and a Directory of Resources

Edited by Amy L. Sutton. 607 pages. 2004. 978-0-7808-0738-9.

"Recommended. ...An easy to use, comprehensive medical reference book."

—*E-Streams, Sep '05*

"For anyone who has back or neck problems, this book is ideal. Its easy-to-understand language and variety of topics makes this sourcebook a worthwhile read. The price...is reasonable for the amount of information contained in the book"

—*Occupational Therapy in Health Care, 2007*

Blood and Circulatory Disorders Sourcebook, 2nd Edition

Basic Consumer Health Information about the Blood and Circulatory System and Related Disorders, Such as Anemia and Other Hemoglobin Diseases, Cancer of the Blood and Associated Bone Marrow Disorders, Clotting and Bleeding Problems, and Conditions That Affect the Veins, Blood Vessels, and Arteries, Including Facts about the Donation and Transplantation of Bone Marrow, Stem Cells, and Blood and Tips for Keeping the Blood and Circulatory System Healthy

Along with a Glossary of Related Terms and Resources for Additional Help and Information

Edited by Amy L. Sutton. 634 pages. 2005. 978-0-7808-0746-4.

"Highly recommended pick for basic consumer health reference holdings at all levels."

—*The Bookwatch, Aug '05*

Brain Disorders Sourcebook, 2nd Edition

Basic Consumer Health Information about Acquired and Traumatic Brain Injuries, Infections of the Brain, Epilepsy and Seizure Disorders, Cerebral Palsy, and Degenerative Neurological Disorders, Including Amyotrophic Lateral Sclerosis (ALS), Dementias, Multiple Sclerosis, and More

Along with Information on the Brain's Structure and Function, Treatment and Rehabilitation Options, Reports on Current Research Initiatives, a Glossary of Terms Related to Brain Disorders and Injuries, and a Directory of Sources for Further Help and Information

Edited by Sandra J. Judd. 600 pages. 2005. 978-0-7808-0744-0.

"This easy-to-read volume provides up-to-date health information... Recommended for consumer health collections within public or academic libraries."

—*E-Streams, Feb '06*

SEE ALSO *Alzheimer Disease Sourcebook, 4th Edition*

Breast Cancer Sourcebook, 3rd Edition

Basic Consumer Health Information about Breast Health and Breast Cancer, Including Facts about Environmental, Genetic, and Other Risk Factors, Prevention Efforts, Screening and Diagnostic Methods, Surgical Treatment Options and Other Care Choices, Complementary and Alternative Therapies, and Post-Treatment Concerns

Along with Statistical Data, News about Research Advances, a Glossary of Related Terms, and Directories of Resources for Additional Information and Support

Edited by Karen Bellenir. 606 pages. 2009. 978-0-7808-1030-3.

SEE ALSO *Cancer Sourcebook for Women, 3rd Edition, Women's Health Concerns Sourcebook, 3rd Edition*

Breastfeeding Sourcebook

Basic Consumer Health Information about the Benefits of Breastmilk, Preparing to Breastfeed, Breastfeeding as a Baby Grows, Nutrition, and More, Including Information on Special Situations and Concerns Such as Mastitis, Illness, Medications, Allergies, Multiple Births, Prematurity, Special Needs, and Adoption

Along with a Glossary and Resources for Additional Help and Information

Edited by Jenni Lynn Colson. 367 pages. 2002. 978-0-7808-0332-9.

SEE ALSO *Pregnancy and Birth Sourcebook, 2nd Edition*

Burns Sourcebook

Basic Consumer Health Information about Various Types of Burns and Scalds, Including Flame, Heat, Cold, Electrical, Chemical, and Sun Burns

Along with Information on Short-Term and Long-Term Treatments, Tissue Reconstruction, Plastic Surgery, Prevention Suggestions, and First Aid

Edited by Allan R. Cook. 604 pages. 1999. 978-0-7808-0204-9.

"This is an exceptional addition to the series and is highly recommended for all consumer health collections, hospital libraries, and academic medical centers."

—*E-Streams, Mar '00*

"This key reference guide is an invaluable addition to all health care and public libraries in confronting this ongoing health issue."

—*American Reference Books Annual, 2000*

SEE ALSO *Dermatological Disorders Sourcebook, 2nd Edition*

Cancer Sourcebook, 5th Edition

Basic Consumer Health Information about Major Forms and Stages of Cancer, Featuring Facts about Head and Neck Cancers, Lung Cancers, Gastrointestinal Cancers, Genitourinary Cancers, Lymphomas, Blood Cell Cancers, Endocrine Cancers, Skin Cancers, Bone Cancers, Metastatic Cancers, and More

Along with Facts about Cancer Treatments, Cancer Risks and Prevention, a Glossary of Related Terms, Statistical Data, and a Directory of Resources for Additional Information

Edited by Karen Bellenir. 1105 pages. 2007. 978-0-7808-0947-5.

"The 5th, updated edition of *Cancer Sourcebook* should be in every public and health lending library collection... An unparalleled discussion essential for any health collections considering an all-in-one basic general reference."

—*California Bookwatch, Aug '07*

SEE ALSO *Breast Cancer Sourcebook, 3rd Edition, Cancer Sourcebook for Women, 3rd Edition, Cancer Survivorship Sourcebook, Leukemia Sourcebook*

Cancer Sourcebook for Women, 3rd Edition

Basic Consumer Health Information about Leading Causes of Cancer in Women, Featuring Facts about Gynecologic Cancers and Related Concerns, Such as Breast Cancer, Cervical Cancer, Endometrial Cancer, Uterine Sarcoma, Vaginal Cancer, Vulvar Cancer, and Common Non-Cancerous Gynecologic Conditions, in Addition to Facts about Lung Cancer, Colorectal Cancer, and Thyroid Cancer in Women

Along with Information about Cancer Risk Factors, Screening and Prevention, Treatment Options, and Tips on Coping with Life after Cancer Treatment, a Glossary of Cancer Terms, and a Directory of Resources for Additional Help and Information

Edited by Amy L. Sutton. 687 pages. 2006. 978-0-7808-0867-6.

"This excellent book provides the general public with information compiled in a way that will help them to gain the knowledge they need. 4 Stars!"

—*Doody's Review Service, Dec '06*

"An indispensable reference for health consumers and cancer patients. Recommended for public libraries and academic libraries with a medical department."

—*E-Streams, Sep '08*

Cancer Survivorship Sourcebook

Basic Consumer Health Information about the Physical, Educational, Emotional, Social, and Financial Needs of Cancer Patients from Diagnosis, through Cancer Treatment, and Beyond, Including Facts about Researching Specific Types of Cancer and Learning about Clinical Trials and Treatment Options, and Featuring Tips for Coping with the Side Effects of Cancer Treatments and Adjusting to Life after Cancer Treatment Concludes

Along with Suggestions for Caregivers, Friends, and Family Members of Cancer Patients, a Glossary of Cancer Care Terms, and Directories of Related Resources

Edited by Karen Bellenir. 633 pages. 2007. 978-0-7808-0985-7.

"Well organized and comprehensive in coverage, the book speaks to issues encountered both during and after cancer treatment. Recommended for consumer health and public libraries."

—*Library Journal, Aug 1 '07*

"*Cancer Survivorship Sourcebook* will be useful to anyone who has a friend or loved one with a cancer diagnosis."

—*American Reference Books Annual, 2008*

SEE ALSO *Cancer Sourcebook, 5th Edition*

Cardiovascular Diseases and Disorders Sourcebook, 3rd Edition

Basic Consumer Health Information about Heart and Vascular Diseases and Disorders, Such as Angina, Heart Attacks, Arrhythmias, Cardiomyopathy, Valve Disease, Atherosclerosis, and Aneurysms, with Information about Managing Cardiovascular Risk Factors and Maintaining Heart Health, Medications and Procedures Used to Treat Cardiovascular Disorders, and Concerns of Special Significance to Women

Along with Reports on Current Research Initiatives, a Glossary of Related Medical Terms, and a Directory of Sources for Further Help and Information

Edited by Sandra J. Judd. 687 pages. 2005. 978-0-7808-0739-6.

"This updated sourcebook is still the best first stop for comprehensive introductory information on cardiovascular diseases."

—*American Reference Books Annual, 2006*

"Recommended for public libraries and libraries supporting health care professionals."

—*E-Streams, Sep '05*

Caregiving Sourcebook

Basic Consumer Health Information for Caregivers, Including a Profile of Caregivers, Caregiving Responsibilities and Concerns, Tips for Specific Conditions, Care Environments, and the Effects of Caregiving

Along with Facts about Legal Issues, Financial Information, and Future Planning, a Glossary, and a Listing of Additional Resources

Edited by Joyce Brennfleck Shannon. 583 pages. 2001. 978-0-7808-0331-2.

"Essential for most collections."

—*Library Journal, Apr 1 '02*

"An ideal addition to the reference collection of any public library. Health sciences information professionals may also want to acquire the *Caregiving Sourcebook* for their hospital or academic library for use as a ready reference tool by health care workers interested in aging and caregiving."

—*E-Streams, Jan '02*

Child Abuse Sourcebook, 2nd Edition

Basic Consumer Health Information about the Physical, Sexual, and Emotional Abuse of Children, Neglect, Münchhausen Syndrome by Proxy (MSBP), and Shaken Baby Syndrome, and Featuring Facts about Withholding Medical Care, Corporal Punishment, Child Maltreatment in Youth Sports, and Parental Substance Abuse

Along with Information about Child Protective Services, Foster Care, Adoption, Parenting Challenges, Abuse Prevention Programs, and Intervention, Treatment, and Recovery Guidelines, a Glossary of Related Terms, and Resources for Additional Help and Information

Edited by Joyce Brennfleck Shannon. 600 pages. 2009. 978-0-7808-1037-2.

SEE ALSO *Domestic Violence Sourcebook, 3rd Edition*

Childhood Diseases and Disorders Sourcebook, 2nd Edition

Basic Consumer Health Information about the Physical, Mental, and Developmental Health of Pre-Adolescent Children, Including Facts about Infectious Diseases, Asthma, Allergies, Diabetes, and Other Acute and Chronic Conditions Affecting the Gastrointestinal Tract, Ears, Nose, Throat, Liver, Kidneys, Heart, Blood, Brain, Muscles, Bones, and Skin

Along with Reports on Recommended Childhood Vaccinations, Wellness Guidelines, a Glossary of Related Medical Terms, and a List of Resources for Parents

Edited by Sandra J. Judd. 694 pages. 2009. 978-0-7808-1031-0.

SEE ALSO *Healthy Children Sourcebook*

Colds, Flu and Other Common Ailments Sourcebook

Basic Consumer Health Information about Common Ailments and Injuries, Including Colds, Coughs, the Flu, Sinus Problems, Headaches, Fever, Nausea and Vomiting, Menstrual Cramps, Diarrhea, Constipation, Hemorrhoids, Back Pain, Dandruff, Dry and Itchy Skin, Cuts, Scrapes, Sprains, Bruises, and More

Along with Information about Prevention, Self-Care, Choosing a Doctor, Over-the-Counter Medications, Folk Remedies, and Alternative Therapies, and Including a Glossary of Important Terms and a Directory of Resources for Further Help and Information

Edited by Chad T. Kimball. 622 pages. 2001. 978-0-7808-0435-7.

"A good starting point for research on common illnesses. It will be a useful addition to public and consumer health library collections."

—*American Reference Books Annual, 2002*

"Will prove valuable to any library seeking to maintain a current, comprehensive reference collection of health resources. . . Excellent reference."

—*The Bookwatch, Aug '01*

Communication Disorders Sourcebook

Basic Information about Deafness and Hearing Loss, Speech and Language Disorders, Voice Disorders, Balance and Vestibular Disorders, and Disorders of Smell, Taste, and Touch

Edited by Linda M. Ross. 533 pages. 1996. 978-0-7808-0077-9.

"This is skillfully edited and is a welcome resource for the layperson. It should be found in every public and medical library."

—*Booklist Health Sciences Supplement, Oct '97*

Complementary and Alternative Medicine Sourcebook, 3rd Edition

Basic Consumer Health Information about Complementary and Alternative Medical Therapies, Including Acupuncture, Ayurveda, Traditional Chinese Medicine, Herbal Medicine, Homeopathy, Naturopathy, Biofeedback, Hypnotherapy, Yoga, Art Therapy, Aromatherapy, Clinical Nutrition, Vitamin and Mineral Supplements, Chiropractic, Massage, Reflexology, Crystal Therapy, Therapeutic Touch, and More

Along with Facts about Alternative and Complementary Treatments for Specific Conditions Such as Cancer, Diabetes, Osteoarthritis, Chronic Pain, Menopause, Gastrointestinal Disorders, Headaches, and Mental Illness, a Glossary, and a Resource List for Additional Help and Information

Edited by Sandra J. Judd. 630 pages. 2006. 978-0-7808-0864-5.

"A 'must' reference for any serious healthcare collection. Public library holdings, too, will welcome it as a popular reference."

—*California Bookwatch, Oct '06*

"Both basic and informative at the same time... a useful resource for health care professionals as well as consumers interested in learning more information about CAM therapies."

—*AORN Journal, Jan '08*

"A quality, indexed, referenced guideline for many alternative practices that are quite popular around the world...It is neatly organized to find facts quickly, is peer-reviewed, and stays current with the most recent advances."

—*Journal of Dental Hygiene, Jul '07*

Congenital Disorders Sourcebook, 2nd Edition

Basic Consumer Health Information about Nonhereditary Birth Defects and Disorders Related to Prematurity, Gestational Injuries, Congenital Infections, and Birth Complications, Including Heart Defects, Hydrocephalus, Spina Bifida, Cleft Lip and Palate, Cerebral Palsy, and More

Along with Facts about the Prevention of Birth Defects, Fetal Surgery and Other Treatment Options, Research Initiatives, a Glossary of Related Terms, and Resources for Additional Information and Support

Edited by Sandra J. Judd. 619 pages. 2007. 978-0-7808-0945-1.

"Congenital Disorders Sourcebook provides an excellent, non-technical overview of many aspects of pregnancy with the focus on congenital disorders."

—*American Reference Books Annual, 2008*

"An excellent readable reference aimed at the lay public for difficult to understand medical problems. An excellent starting point for the interested parent or family member who may then be motivated to seek more information."

—*Doody's Review Service, 2007*

SEE ALSO *Pregnancy and Birth Sourcebook, 2nd Edition*

Contagious Diseases Sourcebook, 2nd Edition

Basic Consumer Health Information about Diseases Spread from Person to Person through Direct Physical Contact, Airborne Transmissions, Sexual Contact, or Contact with Blood or Other Body Fluids, Including Pneumococcal, Staphylococcal, and Streptococcal Diseases, Colds, Influenza, Lice, Measles, Mumps, Tuberculosis, and Others

Along with Facts about Self-Care and Over-the-Counter Medications, Antibiotics and Drug Resistance, Disease Prevention, Vaccines, and Bioterrorism, a Glossary, and a Directory of Resources for More Information

Edited by Joyce Brennfleck Shannon. 600 pages. 2009. 978-0-7808-1075-4.

SEE ALSO *AIDS Sourcebook, 4th Edition, Hepatitis Sourcebook*

Cosmetic and Reconstructive Surgery Sourcebook, 2nd Edition

Basic Consumer Information about Plastic Surgery and Non-Surgical Appearance-Enhancing Procedures, Including Facts about Botulinum Toxin, Collagen Replacement, Dermabrasion,

Chemical Peels, Eyelid Surgery, Nose Reshaping, Lip Augmentation, Liposuction, Breast Enlargement and Reduction, Tummy Tucking, and Other Skin, Hair, Facial, and Body Shaping Procedures

Along with Information about Reconstructive Procedures for Congenital Disorders, Disfiguring Diseases, Burns, and Traumatic Injuries, a Glossary of Related Terms, and a Directory of Additional Resources

Edited by Karen Bellenir. 483 pages. 2007. 978-0-7808-0951-2.

"A practical guide for health care consumers and health care workers. . . . This easy-to-read reference guide would be useful for novice and veteran health care consumers, surgical technology students, nursing students, and perioperative nurses new to plastic and reconstructive surgery. It also may be helpful for medical-surgical nurses as a guide for patient teaching in their practices."

—*AORN Journal, Aug '08*

SEE ALSO *Surgery Sourcebook, 2nd Edition*

Death and Dying Sourcebook, 2nd Edition

Basic Consumer Health Information about End-of-Life Care and Related Perspectives and Ethical Issues, Including End-of-Life Symptoms and Treatments, Pain Management, Quality-of-Life Concerns, the Use of Life Support, Patients' Rights and Privacy Issues, Advance Directives, Physician-Assisted Suicide, Caregiving, Organ and Tissue Donation, Autopsies, Funeral Arrangements, and Grief

Along with Statistical Data, Information about the Leading Causes of Death, a Glossary, and Directories of Support Groups and Other Resources

Edited by Joyce Brennfleck Shannon. 626 pages. 2006. 978-0-7808-0871-3.

Dental Care and Oral Health Sourcebook, 3rd Edition

Basic Consumer Health Information about Dental Care and Oral Health Throughout the Lifespan, Including Facts about Cavities, Bad Breath, Cold and Canker Sores, Dry Mouth, Toothaches, Gum Disease, Malocclusion, Temporomandibular Joint and Muscle Disorders, Oral Cancers, and Dental Emergencies

Along with Information about Mouth Hygiene, Crowns, Bridges, Implants, and Fillings, Surgical, Orthodontic, and Cosmetic Dental Procedures, Pain Management, Health Conditions that Impact Oral Care, a Glossary of Related Terms, and a Directory of Additional Resources

Edited by Amy L. Sutton. 619 pages. 2008. 978-0-7808-1032-7.

Depression Sourcebook, 2nd Edition

Basic Consumer Health Information about Unipolar Depression, Bipolar Disorder, Dysthymia, Seasonal Affective Disorder, Postpartum Depression, and Other Depressive Disorders, Including Facts about Populations at Special Risk, Coexisting Medical Conditions, Symptoms, Treatment Options, and Suicide Prevention

Along with Statistical Data, a Glossary of Related Terms, and a Directory of Resources for Additional Help and Information

Edited by Sandra J. Judd. 646 pages. 2008. 978-0-7808-1003-7.

"Recommended for public libraries."

—*ARBAonline, Nov '08*

SEE ALSO *Mental Health Disorders Sourcebook, 4th Edition*

Dermatological Disorders Sourcebook, 2nd Edition

Basic Consumer Health Information about Conditions and Disorders Affecting the Skin, Hair, and Nails, Such as Acne, Rosacea, Rashes, Dermatitis, Pigmentation Disorders, Birthmarks, Skin Cancer, Skin Injuries, Psoriasis, Scleroderma, and Hair Loss, Including Facts about Medications and Treatments for Dermatological Disorders and Tips for Maintaining Healthy Skin, Hair, and Nails

Along with Information about How Aging Affects the Skin, a Glossary of Related Terms, and a Directory of Resources for Additional Help and Information

Edited by Amy L. Sutton. 617 pages. 2006. 978-0-7808-0795-2.

"Helpfully brings together. . . sources in one convenient place, saving the user hours of research time."
—*American Reference Books Annual, 2006*

SEE ALSO *Burns Sourcebook*

Diabetes Sourcebook, 4th Edition

Basic Consumer Health Information about Type 1 and Type 2 Diabetes Mellitus, Gestational Diabetes, Monogenic Forms of Diabetes, and Insulin Resistance, with Guidelines for Lifestyle Modifications and the Medical Management of Diabetes, Including Facts about Insulin, Insulin Delivery Devices, Oral Diabetes Medications, Self-Monitoring of Blood Glucose, Meal Planning, Physical Activity Recommendations, Foot Care, and Treatment Options for People with Kidney Failure

Along with a Section about Diabetes Complications and Co-Occurring Conditions, a Glossary of Related Terms, and Directories of Resources for Additional Help and Information

Edited by Karen Bellenir. 627 pages. 2008. 978-0-7808-1005-1.

"Completely and comprehensively covering almost everything a student or physician would need to know.... well worth the investment."
—*Internet Bookwatch, Dec '08*

SEE ALSO *Endocrine and Metabolic Disorders Sourcebook, 2nd Edition*

Diet and Nutrition Sourcebook, 3rd Edition

Basic Consumer Health Information about Dietary Guidelines and the Food Guidance System, Recommended Daily Nutrient Intakes, Serving Proportions, Weight Control, Vitamins and Supplements, Nutrition Issues for Different Life Stages and Lifestyles, and the Needs of People with Specific Medical Concerns, Including Cancer, Celiac Disease, Diabetes, Eating Disorders, Food Allergies, and Cardiovascular Disease

Along with Facts about Federal Nutrition Support Programs, a Glossary of Nutrition and Dietary Terms, and Directories of Additional Resources for More Information about Nutrition

Edited by Joyce Brennfleck Shannon. 605 pages. 2006. 978-0-7808-0800-3.

"A valuable resource tool for any individual."
—*Journal of Dental Hygiene, Apr '07*

"From different recommended eating habits to reduce disease and common ailments to nutrition advice for those with specific conditions, *Diet and Nutrition Sourcebook* is especially important because so much is changing in this area, and so rapidly."
—*California Bookwatch, Jun '06*

SEE ALSO *Digestive Diseases and Disorders Sourcebook, Eating Disorders Sourcebook, 2nd Edition, Gastrointestinal Diseases and Disorders Sourcebook, 2nd Edition, Vegetarian Sourcebook*

Digestive Diseases and Disorders Sourcebook

Basic Consumer Health Information about Diseases and Disorders that Impact the Upper and Lower Digestive System, Including Celiac Disease, Constipation, Crohn's Disease, Cyclic Vomiting Syndrome, Diarrhea, Diverticulosis and Diverticulitis, Gallstones, Heartburn, Hemorrhoids, Hernias, Indigestion (Dyspepsia), Irritable Bowel Syndrome, Lactose Intolerance, Ulcers, and More

Along with Information about Medications and Other Treatments, Tips for Maintaining a Healthy Digestive Tract, a Glossary, and Directory of Digestive Diseases Organizations

Edited by Karen Bellenir. 323 pages. 2000. 978-0-7808-0327-5.

"An excellent addition to all public or patient-research libraries."
—*American Reference Books Annual, 2001*

"Recommended reference source."
—*Booklist, May '00*

SEE ALSO *Diet and Nutrition Sourcebook, 3rd Edition, Gastrointestinal Diseases and Disorders Sourcebook, 2nd Edition*

Disabilities Sourcebook

Basic Consumer Health Information about Physical and Psychiatric Disabilities, Including Descriptions of Major Causes of Disability, Assistive and Adaptive Aids, Workplace Issues, and Accessibility Concerns

Along with Information about the Americans with Disabilities Act, a Glossary, and Resources for Additional Help and Information

Edited by Dawn D. Matthews. 602 pages. 2000. 978-0-7808-0389-3.

"A must for libraries with a consumer health section."

—*American Reference Books Annual, 2002*

"A much needed addition to the Omnigraphics *Health Reference Series*. A current reference work to provide people with disabilities, their families, caregivers or those who work with them, a broad range of information in one volume, has not been available until now. . . . It is recommended for all public and academic library reference collections."

—*E-Streams, May '01*

"An excellent source book in easy-to-read format covering many current topics; highly recommended for all libraries."

—*CHOICE, Jan '01*

Disease Management Sourcebook

Basic Consumer Health Information about Coping with Chronic and Serious Illnesses, Navigating the Health Care System, Communicating with Health Care Providers, Assessing Health Care Quality, and Making Informed Health Care Decisions, Including Facts about Second Opinions, Hospitalization, Surgery, and Medications

Along with a Section about Children with Chronic Conditions, Information about Legal, Financial, and Insurance Issues, a Glossary of Related Terms, and Directories of Additional Resources

Edited by Joyce Brennfleck Shannon. 621 pages. 2008. 978-0-7808-1002-0.

"Consumers need to know how to manage their health care the same way they manage anything else in their lives. The text is very readable and is written for the layperson and consumer. The cost is not prohibitive. This book should be in all collections of health care libraries and public libraries."

—*ARBAonline, Jul '08*

"The information is very current, and the selection of font and layout make the book easy to read. A hardback that will stand up to much usage, this is an excellent resource for consumers. . . . Recommended. General readers."

—*CHOICE, Nov '08*

"Intended for lay readers, this resource clarifies the many confusing and overwhelming details associated with chronic disease care. Meticulous and clearly explained, the book even includes diagrams intended to ease comprehension of over-the-counter medication labels. An essential guide to navigating the health-care rapids."

—*Library Journal, Aug '08*

Domestic Violence Sourcebook, 3rd Edition

Basic Consumer Health Information about Warning Signs, Risk Factors, and Health Consequences of Intimate Partner Violence, Sexual Violence and Rape, Stalking, Human Trafficking, Child Maltreatment, Teen Dating Violence, and Elder Abuse

Along with Facts about Victims and Perpetrators, Strategies for Violence Prevention, and Emergency Interventions, Safety Plans, and Financial and Legal Tips for Victims, a Glossary of Related Terms, and Directories of Resources for Additional Information and Support

Edited by Joyce Brennfleck Shannon. 600 pages. 2009. 978-0-7808-1038-9.

SEE ALSO *Child Abuse Sourcebook, 2nd Edition*

Drug Abuse Sourcebook, 2nd Edition

Basic Consumer Health Information about Illicit Substances of Abuse and the Misuse of Prescription and Over-the-Counter Medications, Including Depressants, Hallucinogens, Inhalants, Marijuana, Stimulants, and Anabolic Steroids

Along with Facts about Related Health Risks, Treatment Programs, Prevention Programs, a Glossary of Abuse and Addiction Terms, a Glossary of Drug-Related Street Terms, and a Directory of Resources for More Information

Edited by Catherine Ginther. 581 pages. 2004. 978-0-7808-0740-2.

"Commendable for organizing useful, normally scattered government and association-produced data into a logical sequence."

—*American Reference Books Annual, 2006*

"An excellent library reference."
—*The Bookwatch, May '05*

SEE ALSO *Alcoholism Sourcebook, 2nd Edition*

Ear, Nose, and Throat Disorders Sourcebook, 2nd Edition

Basic Consumer Health Information about Disorders of the Ears, Hearing Loss, Vestibular Disorders, Nasal and Sinus Problems, Throat and Vocal Cord Disorders, and Otolaryngologic Cancers, Including Facts about Ear Infections and Injuries, Genetic and Congenital Deafness, Sensorineural Hearing Disorders, Tinnitus, Vertigo, Ménière Disease, Rhinitis, Sinusitis, Snoring, Sore Throats, Hoarseness, and More

Along with Reports on Current Research Initiatives, a Glossary of Related Medical Terms, and a Directory of Sources for Further Help and Information

Edited by Sandra J. Judd. 631 pages. 2007. 978-0-7808-0872-0.

"A resource book for the general public that provides comprehensive coverage of basic up-to-date medical information about the causes, symptoms, diagnosis, and treatment of diseases and disorders that affect the ears, nose, sinuses, throat, and voice. . . . The majority of information is presented in question and answer format, much like questions a patient might ask of a health care provider. An extensive index facilitates the reader's ability to easily access information on any specific topic."
—*Journal of Dental Hygiene, Oct '07*

"A handy compilation of information on common and some not so common ailments of the ears, nose, and throat."
—*Doody's Review Service, 2007*

Eating Disorders Sourcebook, 2nd Edition

Basic Consumer Health Information about Anorexia Nervosa, Bulimia, Binge Eating, Compulsive Exercise, Female Athlete Triad, and Other Eating Disorders, Including Facts about Body Image and Other Cultural and Age-Related Risk Factors, Prevention Efforts, Adverse Health Effects, Treatment Options, and the Recovery Process

Along with Guidelines for Healthy Weight Control, a Glossary, and Directories of Additional Resources

Edited by Joyce Brennfleck Shannon. 557 pages. 2007. 978-0-7808-0948-2.

"Recommended for the reference collection of large public libraries."
—*American Reference Books Annual, 2008*

"A basic health reference any health or general library needs."
—*Internet Bookwatch, Jun '07*

SEE ALSO *Diet and Nutrition Sourcebook, 3rd Edition, Mental Health Disorders Sourcebook, 4th Edition*

Emergency Medical Services Sourcebook

Basic Consumer Health Information about Preventing, Preparing for, and Managing Emergency Situations, When and Who to Call for Help, What to Expect in the Emergency Room, the Emergency Medical Team, Patient Issues, and Current Topics in Emergency Medicine

Along with Statistical Data, a Glossary, and Sources of Additional Help and Information

Edited by Jenni Lynn Colson. 472 pages. 2002. 978-0-7808-0420-3.

"Handy and convenient for home, public, school, and college libraries. Recommended."
—*CHOICE, Apr '03*

"This reference can provide the consumer with answers to most questions about emergency care in the United States, or it will direct them to a resource where the answer can be found."
—*American Reference Books Annual, 2003*

SEE ALSO *Injury and Trauma Sourcebook*

Endocrine and Metabolic Disorders Sourcebook, 2nd Edition

Basic Consumer Health Information about Hormonal and Metabolic Disorders that Affect the Body's Growth, Development, and Functioning, Including Disorders of the Pancreas, Ovaries and Testes, and Pituitary, Thyroid, Parathyroid, and Adrenal Glands, with Facts about Growth Disorders, Addison Disease, Cushing Syndrome, Conn Syndrome, Diabetic Disorders, Multiple Endocrine Neoplasia, Inborn Errors of Metabolism, and More

Along with Information about Endocrine Functioning, Diagnostic and Screening Tests, a Glossary of Related Terms, and Directories of Additional Resources

Edited by Joyce Brennfleck Shannon. 597 pages. 2007. 978-0-7808-0952-9.

SEE ALSO *Diabetes Sourcebook, 4th Edition*

Environmental Health Sourcebook, 2nd Edition

Basic Consumer Health Information about the Environment and Its Effect on Human Health, Including the Effects of Air Pollution, Water Pollution, Hazardous Chemicals, Food Hazards, Radiation Hazards, Biological Agents, Household Hazards, Such as Radon, Asbestos, Carbon Monoxide, and Mold, and Information about Associated Diseases and Disorders, Including Cancer, Allergies, Respiratory Problems, and Skin Disorders

Along with Information about Environmental Concerns for Specific Populations, a Glossary of Related Terms, and Resources for Further Help and Information

Edited by Dawn D. Matthews. 650 pages. 2003. 978-0-7808-0632-0.

"Recommended for teenage and adult students and readers, and for public and academic libraries, as well as any library focusing on consumer health."

—*E-Streams, May '04*

"This recently updated edition continues the level of quality and the reputation of the numerous other volumes in Omnigraphics' *Health Reference Series*."

—*American Reference Books Annual, 2004*

Ethnic Diseases Sourcebook

Basic Consumer Health Information for Ethnic and Racial Minority Groups in the United States, Including General Health Indicators and Behaviors, Ethnic Diseases, Genetic Testing, the Impact of Chronic Diseases, Women's Health, Mental Health Issues, and Preventive Health Care Services

Along with a Glossary and a Listing of Additional Resources

Edited by Joyce Brennfleck Shannon. 648 pages. 2001. 978-0-7808-0336-7.

"Not many books have been written on this topic to date, and the *Ethnic Diseases Sourcebook* is a strong addition to the list. It will be an important introductory resource for health consumers, students, health care personnel, and social scientists. It is recommended for public, academic, and large hospital libraries."

—*American Reference Books Annual, 2002*

"Will prove valuable to any library seeking to maintain a current, comprehensive reference collection of health resources. . . . An excellent source of health information about genetic disorders which affect particular ethnic and racial minorities in the U.S."

—*The Bookwatch, Aug '01*

Eye Care Sourcebook, 3rd Edition

Basic Consumer Health Information about Eye Care and Eye Disorders, Including Facts about the Diagnosis, Prevention, and Treatment of Refractive Disorders, Cataracts, Glaucoma, Macular Degeneration, and Problems Affecting the Cornea, Retina, and Lacrimal Glands

Along with Advice about Preventing Eye Injuries and Tips for Living with Low Vision or Blindness, a Glossary of Related Terms, and Directories of Resources for More Help and Information

Edited by Amy L. Sutton. 646 pages. 2008. 978-0-7808-1000-6.

Family Planning Sourcebook

Basic Consumer Health Information about Planning for Pregnancy and Contraception, Including Traditional Methods, Barrier Methods, Hormonal Methods, Permanent Methods, Future Methods, Emergency Contraception, and Birth Control Choices for Women at Each Stage of Life

Along with Statistics, a Glossary, and Sources of Additional Information

Edited by Amy Marcaccio Keyzer. 503 pages. 2001. 978-0-7808-0379-4.

"Recommended for public, health, and undergraduate libraries as part of the circulating collection."

—*E-Streams, Mar '02*

"Will prove valuable to any library seeking to maintain a current, comprehensive reference collection of health resources. . . . Excellent reference."

—*The Bookwatch, Aug '01*

SEE ALSO *Pregnancy and Birth Sourcebook, 2nd Edition*

Fitness and Exercise Sourcebook, 3rd Edition

Basic Consumer Health Information about the Physical and Mental Benefits of Fitness, Including Cardiorespiratory Endurance, Muscular Strength, Muscular Endurance, and Flexibility, with Facts about Sports Nutrition and Exercise-Related Injuries and Tips about Physical Activity and Exercises for People of All Ages and for People with Health Concerns

Along with Advice on Selecting and Using Exercise Equipment, Maintaining Exercise Motivation, a Glossary of Related Terms, and a Directory of Resources for More Help and Information

Edited by Amy L. Sutton. 635 pages. 2007. 978-0-7808-0946-8.

"Updates the consumer information on the physical and mental benefits of physical activity throughout the lifespan offered in earlier editions. . . . Recommended. All readers; all levels."

—*CHOICE, Oct '07*

"An exceptionally well-rounded coverage perfect for any concerned about developing and understanding a fitness program."

—*California Bookwatch, Jun '07*

SEE ALSO *Sports Injuries Sourcebook, 3rd Edition*

Food Safety Sourcebook

Basic Consumer Health Information about the Safe Handling of Meat, Poultry, Seafood, Eggs, Fruit Juices, and Other Food Items, and Facts about Pesticides, Drinking Water, Food Safety Overseas, and the Onset, Duration, and Symptoms of Foodborne Illnesses, Including Types of Pathogenic Bacteria, Parasitic Protozoa, Worms, Viruses, and Natural Toxins

Along with the Role of the Consumer, the Food Handler, and the Government in Food Safety; a Glossary, and Resources for Additional Help and Information

Edited by Dawn D. Matthews. 327 pages. 1999. 978-0-7808-0326-8.

"Recommended reference source."

—*Booklist, May '00*

"This book takes the complex issues of food safety and foodborne pathogens and presents them in an easily understood manner. [It does] an excellent job of covering a large and often confusing topic."

— *American Reference Books Annual, 2000*

Forensic Medicine Sourcebook

Basic Consumer Information for the Layperson about Forensic Medicine, Including Crime Scene Investigation, Evidence Collection and Analysis, Expert Testimony, Computer-Aided Criminal Identification, Digital Imaging in the Courtroom, DNA Profiling, Accident Reconstruction, Autopsies, Ballistics, Drugs and Explosives Detection, Latent Fingerprints, Product Tampering, and Questioned Document Examination

Along with Statistical Data, a Glossary of Forensics Terminology, and Listings of Sources for Further Help and Information

Edited by Annemarie S. Muth. 574 pages. 1999. 978-0-7808-0232-2.

"Given the expected widespread interest in its content and its easy to read style, this book is recommended for most public and all college and university libraries."

—*E-Streams, Feb '01*

"A wealth of information, useful statistics, references are up-to-date and extremely complete. This wonderful collection of data will help students who are interested in a career in any type of forensic field. It is a great resource for attorneys who need information about types of expert witnesses needed in a particular case. It also offers useful information for fiction and nonfiction writers whose work involves a crime. A fascinating compilation. All levels."

—*CHOICE, Jan '00*

"There are several items that make this book attractive to consumers who are seeking certain forensic data. . . . This is a useful current

source for those seeking general forensic medical answers."
—*American Reference Books Annual, 2000*

Gastrointestinal Diseases and Disorders Sourcebook, 2nd Edition

Basic Consumer Health Information about the Upper and Lower Gastrointestinal (GI) Tract, Including the Esophagus, Stomach, Intestines, Rectum, Liver, and Pancreas, with Facts about Gastroesophageal Reflux Disease, Gastritis, Hernias, Ulcers, Celiac Disease, Diverticulitis, Irritable Bowel Syndrome, Hemorrhoids, Gastrointestinal Cancers, and Other Diseases and Disorders Related to the Digestive Process

Along with Information about Commonly Used Diagnostic and Surgical Procedures, Statistics, Reports on Current Research Initiatives and Clinical Trials, a Glossary, and Resources for Additional Help and Information

Edited by Sandra J. Judd. 654 pages. 2006. 978-0-7808-0798-3.

"The text is designed for the general reader seeking information on prevention, disease warning signs, diagnostic and therapeutic questions. . . . It is an excellent resource for the general reader to conveniently locate credible, coordinated and indexed information. . . . The sourcebook will prove very helpful for patients, caregivers and should be available in every physician waiting room."
—*Doody's Review Service, 2006*

SEE ALSO *Diet and Nutrition Sourcebook, 3rd Edition, Digestive Diseases and Disorders Sourcebook*

Genetic Disorders Sourcebook, 4th Edition

Basic Consumer Health Information about Hereditary Diseases and Disorders, Including Facts about the Human Genome, Genetic Inheritance Patterns, Disorders Associated with Specific Genes, Such as Sickle Cell Disease, Hemophilia, and Cystic Fibrosis, Chromosome Disorders, Such as Down Syndrome, Fragile X Syndrome, and Turner Syndrome, and Complex Diseases and Disorders Resulting from the Interaction of Environmental and Genetic Factors, Such as Allergies, Cancer, and Obesity

Along with Facts about Genetic Testing, Suggestions for Parents of Children with Special Needs, Reports on Current Research Initiatives, a Glossary of Genetic Terminology, and Resources for Additional Help and Information

Edited by Sandra J. Judd. 600 pages. 2009. 978-0-7808-1076-1.

Head Trauma Sourcebook

Basic Information for the Layperson about Open-Head and Closed-Head Injuries, Treatment Advances, Recovery, and Rehabilitation

Along with Reports on Current Research Initiatives

Edited by Karen Bellenir. 414 pages. 1997. 978-0-7808-0208-7.

Headache Sourcebook

Basic Consumer Health Information about Migraine, Tension, Cluster, Rebound and Other Types of Headaches, with Facts about the Cause and Prevention of Headaches, the Effects of Stress and the Environment, Headaches during Pregnancy and Menopause, and Childhood Headaches

Along with a Glossary and Other Resources for Additional Help and Information

Edited by Dawn D. Matthews. 342 pages. 2002. 978-0-7808-0337-4.

"Highly recommended for academic and medical reference collections."
—*Library Bookwatch, Sep '02*

SEE ALSO *Pain Sourcebook, 3rd Edition*

Healthy Aging Sourcebook

Basic Consumer Health Information about Maintaining Health through the Aging Process, Including Advice on Nutrition, Exercise, and Sleep, Help in Making Decisions about Midlife Issues and Retirement, and Guidance Concerning Practical and Informed Choices in Health Consumerism

Along with Data Concerning the Theories of Aging, Different Experiences in Aging by Minority Groups, and Facts about Aging Now and Aging in the Future; and Featuring a Glossary, a Guide to Consumer Help, Additional Suggested Reading, and Practical Resource Directory

Edited by Jenifer Swanson. 537 pages. 1999. 978-0-7808-0390-9.

"Recommended reference source."

—*Booklist, Feb '00*

SEE ALSO *Physical and Mental Issues in Aging Sourcebook*

Healthy Children Sourcebook

Basic Consumer Health Information about the Physical and Mental Development of Children between the Ages of 3 and 12, Including Routine Health Care, Preventative Health Services, Safety and First Aid, Healthy Sleep, Dental Care, Nutrition, and Fitness, and Featuring Parenting Tips on Such Topics as Bedwetting, Choosing Day Care, Monitoring TV and Other Media, and Establishing a Foundation for Substance Abuse Prevention

Along with a Glossary of Commonly Used Pediatric Terms and Resources for Additional Help and Information.

Edited by Chad T. Kimball. 624 pages. 2003. 978-0-7808-0247-6.

"Should be required reading for parents and teachers."

—*E-Streams, Jun '04*

"It is hard to imagine that any other single resource exists that would provide such a comprehensive guide of timely information on health promotion and disease prevention for children aged 3 to 12."

—*American Reference Books Annual, 2004*

"This easy-to-read volume is a tremendous resource."

—*AORN Journal, May '05*

SEE ALSO *Childhood Diseases and Disorders Sourcebook, 2nd Edition*

Healthy Heart Sourcebook for Women

Basic Consumer Health Information about Cardiac Issues Specific to Women, Including Facts about Major Risk Factors and Prevention, Treatment and Control Strategies, and Important Dietary Issues

Along with a Special Section Regarding the Pros and Cons of Hormone Replacement Therapy and Its Impact on Heart Health, and Additional Help, Including Recipes, a Glossary, and a Directory of Resources

Edited by Dawn D. Matthews. 321 pages. 2000. 978-0-7808-0329-9.

"A good reference source and recommended for all public, academic, medical, and hospital libraries."

—*Medical Reference Services Quarterly, Summer '01*

"Contains very important information about coronary artery disease that all women should know. The information is current and presented in an easy-to-read format. The book will make a good addition to any library."

—*American Medical Writers Association Journal, Summer '00*

SEE ALSO *Cardiovascular Diseases and Disorders Sourcebook, 3rd Edition, Women's Health Concerns Sourcebook, 3rd Edition*

Hepatitis Sourcebook

Basic Consumer Health Information about Hepatitis A, Hepatitis B, Hepatitis C, and Other Forms of Hepatitis, Including Autoimmune Hepatitis, Alcoholic Hepatitis, Nonalcoholic Steatohepatitis, and Toxic Hepatitis, with Facts about Risk Factors, Screening Methods, Diagnostic Tests, and Treatment Options

Along with Information on Liver Health, Tips for People Living with Chronic Hepatitis, Reports on Current Research Initiatives, a Glossary of Terms Related to Hepatitis, and a Directory of Sources for Further Help and Information

Edited by Sandra J. Judd. 570 pages. 2006. 978-0-7808-0749-5.

"The breadth of information found in this one book would not be readily found in another source. Highly recommended."

—*American Reference Books Annual, 2006*

SEE ALSO *Contagious Diseases Sourcebook*

Household Safety Sourcebook

Basic Consumer Health Information about Household Safety, Including Information about Poisons, Chemicals, Fire, and Water Hazards in the Home

Along with Advice about the Safe Use of Home Maintenance Equipment, Choosing Toys and Nursery Furniture, Holiday and Recreation Safety, a Glossary, and Resources for Further Help and Information

Edited by Dawn D. Matthews. 587 pages. 2002. 978-0-7808-0338-1.

"As a sourcebook on household safety this book meets its mark. It is encyclopedic in scope and covers a wide range of safety issues that are commonly seen in the home."

—E-Streams, Jul '02

Hypertension Sourcebook

Basic Consumer Health Information about the Causes, Diagnosis, and Treatment of High Blood Pressure, with Facts about Consequences, Complications, and Co-Occurring Disorders, Such as Coronary Heart Disease, Diabetes, Stroke, Kidney Disease, and Hypertensive Retinopathy, and Issues in Blood Pressure Control, Including Dietary Choices, Stress Management, and Medications

Along with Reports on Current Research Initiatives and Clinical Trials, a Glossary, and Resources for Additional Help and Information

Edited by Dawn D. Matthews and Karen Bellenir. 588 pages. 2004. 978-0-7808-0674-0.

"Academic, public, and medical libraries will want to add the *Hypertension Sourcebook* to their collections."

—E-Streams, Aug '05

"The strength of this source is the wide range of information given about hypertension."

—American Reference Books Annual, 2005

SEE ALSO *Stroke Sourcebook, 2nd Edition*

Immune System Disorders Sourcebook, 2nd Edition

Basic Consumer Health Information about Disorders of the Immune System, Including Immune System Function and Response, Diagnosis of Immune Disorders, Information about Inherited Immune Disease, Acquired Immune Disease, and Autoimmune Diseases, Including Primary Immune Deficiency, Acquired Immunodeficiency Syndrome (AIDS), Lupus, Multiple Sclerosis, Type 1 Diabetes, Rheumatoid Arthritis, and Graves' Disease

Along with Treatments, Tips for Coping with Immune Disorders, a Glossary, and a Directory of Additional Resources

Edited by Joyce Brennfleck Shannon. 643 pages. 2005. 978-0-7808-0748-8.

"Highly recommended for academic and public libraries."

—American Reference Books Annual, 2006

"The updated second edition is a 'must' for any consumer health library seeking a solid resource covering the treatments, symptoms, and options for immune disorder sufferers. . . . An excellent guide."

—MBR Bookwatch, Jan '06

SEE ALSO *AIDS Sourcebook, 4th Edition, Arthritis Sourcebook, 2nd Edition*

Infant and Toddler Health Sourcebook

Basic Consumer Health Information about the Physical and Mental Development of Newborns, Infants, and Toddlers, Including Neonatal Concerns, Nutrition Recommendations, Immunization Schedules, Common Pediatric Disorders, Assessments and Milestones, Safety Tips, and Advice for Parents and Other Caregivers

Along with a Glossary of Terms and Resource Listings for Additional Help

Edited by Jenifer Swanson. 570 pages. 2000. 978-0-7808-0246-9.

"As a reference for the general public, this would be useful in any library."

—E-Streams, May '01

"Recommended reference source."

—Booklist, Feb '01

Infectious Diseases Sourcebook

Basic Consumer Health Information about Non-Contagious Bacterial, Viral, Prion, Fungal, and Parasitic Diseases Spread by Food and Water, Insects and Animals, or Environmental Contact, Including Botulism, E. Coli, Encephalitis, Legionnaires' Disease, Lyme Disease, Malaria, Plague, Rabies, Salmonella, Tetanus, and Others, and Facts about Newly Emerging Diseases, Such as Hantavirus, Mad Cow Disease, Monkeypox, and West Nile Virus

Along with Information about Preventing Disease Transmission, the Threat of Bioterrorism, and Current Research Initiatives, with a Glossary and Directory of Resources for More Information

Edited by Karen Bellenir. 610 pages. 2004. 978-0-7808-0675-7.

"This reference continues the excellent tradition of the *Health Reference Series* in consolidating a wealth of information on a selected topic into a format that is easy to use and accessible to the general public."

—*American Reference Books Annual, 2005*

"Recommended for public and academic libraries."

—*E-Streams, Jan '05*

Injury and Trauma Sourcebook

Basic Consumer Health Information about the Impact of Injury, the Diagnosis and Treatment of Common and Traumatic Injuries, Emergency Care, and Specific Injuries Related to Home, Community, Workplace, Transportation, and Recreation

Along with Guidelines for Injury Prevention, a Glossary, and a Directory of Additional Resources

Edited by Joyce Brennfleck Shannon. 675 pages. 2002. 978-0-7808-0421-0.

"Practitioners should be aware of guides such as this in order to facilitate their use by patients and their families."

—*Doody's Health Sciences Book Review Journal, Sep-Oct '02*

"Recommended reference source."

—*Booklist, Sep '02*

"Highly recommended for academic and medical reference collections."

—*Library Bookwatch, Sep '02*

SEE ALSO *Emergency Medical Services Sourcebook, Sports Injuries Sourcebook, 3rd Edition*

Learning Disabilities Sourcebook, 3rd Edition

Basic Consumer Health Information about Dyslexia, Auditory and Visual Processing Disorders, Communication Disorders, Dyscalculia, Dysgraphia, and Other Conditions That Impede Learning, Including Attention Deficit/Hyperactivity Disorder, Autism Spectrum Disorders, Hearing and Visual Impairments, Chromosome-Based Disorders, and Brain Injury

Along with Facts about Brain Function, Assessment, Therapy and Remediation, Accommodations, Assistive Technology, Legal Protections, and Tips about Family Life, School Transitions, and Employment Strategies, a Glossary of Related Terms, and Directories of Additional Resources

Edited by Joyce Brennfleck Shannon. 613 pages. 2009. 978-0-7808-1039-6.

SEE ALSO *Attention Deficit Disorder Sourcebook, Autism and Pervasive Developmental Disorders Sourcebook*

Leukemia Sourcebook

Basic Consumer Health Information about Adult and Childhood Leukemias, Including Acute Lymphocytic Leukemia (ALL), Chronic Lymphocytic Leukemia (CLL), Acute Myelogenous Leukemia (AML), Chronic Myelogenous Leukemia (CML), and Hairy Cell Leukemia, and Treatments Such as Chemotherapy, Radiation Therapy, Peripheral Blood Stem Cell and Marrow Transplantation, and Immunotherapy

Along with Tips for Life During and After Treatment, a Glossary, and Directories of Additional Resources

Edited by Joyce Brennfleck Shannon. 564 pages. 2003. 978-0-7808-0627-6.

"Unlike other medical books for the layperson, . . . the language does not talk down to the reader. . . . This volume is highly recommended for all libraries."

—*American Reference Books Annual, 2004*

"A fine title which ranges from diagnosis to alternative treatments, staging, and tips for life during and after diagnosis."

—*The Bookwatch, Dec '03*

SEE ALSO *Cancer Sourcebook, 5th Edition*

Liver Disorders Sourcebook

Basic Consumer Health Information about the Liver and How It Works; Liver Diseases, Including Cancer, Cirrhosis, Hepatitis, and Toxic and Drug Related Diseases; Tips for Maintaining a Healthy Liver; Laboratory Tests, Radiology Tests, and Facts about Liver Transplantation

Along with a Section on Support Groups, a Glossary, and Resource Listings

Edited by Joyce Brennfleck Shannon. 580 pages. 2000. 978-0-7808-0383-1.

"This title is recommended for health sciences and public libraries with consumer health collections."

—*E-Streams, Oct '00*

"Recommended reference source."

—*Booklist, Jun '00*

SEE ALSO *Gastrointestinal Diseases and Disorders Sourcebook, 2nd Edition, Hepatitis Sourcebook*

Lung Disorders Sourcebook

Basic Consumer Health Information about Emphysema, Pneumonia, Tuberculosis, Asthma, Cystic Fibrosis, and Other Lung Disorders, Including Facts about Diagnostic Procedures, Treatment Strategies, Disease Prevention Efforts, and Such Risk Factors as Smoking, Air Pollution, and Exposure to Asbestos, Radon, and Other Agents

Along with a Glossary and Resources for Additional Help and Information

Edited by Dawn D. Matthews. 657 pages. 2002. 978-0-7808-0339-8.

"Highly recommended for academic and medical reference collections."

—*Library Bookwatch, Sep '02*

SEE ALSO *Respiratory Disorders Sourcebook, 2nd Edition*

Medical Tests Sourcebook, 3rd Edition

Basic Consumer Health Information about X-Rays, Blood Tests, Stool and Urine Tests, Biopsies, Mammography, Endoscopic Procedures, Ultrasound Exams, Computed Tomography, Magnetic Resonance Imaging (MRI), Nuclear Medicine, Genetic Testing, Home-Use Tests, and More

Along with Facts about Preventive Care and Screening Test Guidelines, Screening and Assessment Tests Associated with Such Specific Concerns as Cancer, Heart Disease, Allergies, Diabetes, Thyroid Disfunction, and Infertility, a Glossary of Related Terms, and a Directory of Resources for Additional Help and Information

Edited by Karen Bellenir. 627 pages. 2008. 978-0-7808-1040-2

"This volume has a wide scope that makes it useful . . . Can be a valuable reference guide."

—*ARBAonline, Nov '08*

Men's Health Concerns Sourcebook, 3rd Edition

Basic Consumer Health Information about Wellness in Men and Gender-Related Differences in Health, With Facts about Heart Disease, Cancer, Traumatic Injury, and Other Leading Causes of Death in Men, Reproductive Concerns, Sexual Dysfunction, Disorders of the Prostate, Penis, and Testes, Sex-Linked Genetic Disorders, and Other Medical and Mental Concerns of Men

Along with Statistical Data, a Glossary of Related Terms, and a Directory of Resources for Additional Information

Edited by Sandra J. Judd. 600 pages. 2009. 978-0-7808-1033-4.

SEE ALSO *Prostate and Urological Disorders Sourcebook*

Mental Health Disorders Sourcebook, 4th Edition

Basic Consumer Health Information about the Causes and Symptoms of Mental Health Problems, Including Depression, Bipolar Disorder, Anxiety Disorders, Posttraumatic Stress Disorder, Obsessive-Compulsive Disorder, Eating Disorders, Addictions, and Personality and Psychotic Disorders

Along with Information about Medications and Treatments, Mental Health Concerns in Children, Adolescents, and Adults, Tips on Living with Mental Health Disorders, a Glossary of Related Terms, and a Directory of Resources for Additional Help and Information

Edited by Amy L. Sutton. 600 pages. 2009. 978-0-7808-1041-9.

SEE ALSO *Depression Sourcebook, 2nd Edition, Stress-Related Disorders Sourcebook, 2nd Edition*

Mental Retardation Sourcebook

Basic Consumer Health Information about Mental Retardation and Its Causes, Including

Down Syndrome, Fetal Alcohol Syndrome, Fragile X Syndrome, Genetic Conditions, Injury, and Environmental Sources

Along with Preventive Strategies, Parenting Issues, Educational Implications, Health Care Needs, Employment and Economic Matters, Legal Issues, a Glossary, and a Resource Listing for Additional Help and Information

Edited by Joyce Brennfleck Shannon. 627 pages. 2000. 978-0-7808-0377-0.

"Public libraries will find the book useful for reference and as a beginning research point for students, parents, and caregivers."

—*American Reference Books Annual, 2001*

"The strength of this work is that it compiles many basic fact sheets and addresses for further information in one volume. It is intended and suitable for the general public."

—*E-Streams, Nov '00*

"An invaluable overview."

—*Reviewer's Bookwatch, Jul '00*

Movement Disorders Sourcebook, 2nd Edition

Basic Consumer Health Information about the Symptoms and Causes of Movement Disorders, Including Parkinson Disease, Amyotrophic Lateral Sclerosis, Cerebral Palsy, Muscular Dystrophy, Multiple Sclerosis, Myasthenia, Myoclonus, Spina Bifida, Dystonia, Essential Tremor, Choreatic Disorders, Huntington Disease, Tourette Syndrome, and Other Disorders That Cause Slowed, Absent, or Excessive Movements

Along with Information about Surgical and Nonsurgical Interventions, Physical Therapies, Strategies for Independent Living, a Glossary of Related Terms, and a Directory of Resources for Additional Help and Information

Edited by Amy L. Sutton. 600 pages. 2009. 978-0-7808-1034-1.

SEE ALSO *Multiple Sclerosis Sourcebook, Muscular Dystrophy Sourcebook*

Multiple Sclerosis Sourcebook

Basic Consumer Health Information about Multiple Sclerosis (MS) and Its Effects on Mobility, Vision, Bladder Function, Speech, Swallowing, and Cognition, Including Facts about Risk Factors, Causes, Diagnostic Procedures, Pain Management, Drug Treatments, and Physical and Occupational Therapies

Along with Guidelines for Nutrition and Exercise, Tips on Choosing Assistive Equipment, Information about Disability, Work, Financial, and Legal Issues, a Glossary of Related Terms, and a Directory of Additional Resources

Edited by Joyce Brennfleck Shannon. 553 pages. 2007. 978-0-7808-0998-7.

SEE ALSO *Movement Disorders Sourcebook, 2nd Edition*

Muscular Dystrophy Sourcebook

Basic Consumer Health Information about Congenital, Childhood-Onset, and Adult-Onset Forms of Muscular Dystrophy, Such as Duchenne, Becker, Emery-Dreifuss, Distal, Limb-Girdle, Facioscapulohumeral (FSHD), Myotonic, and Ophthalmoplegic Muscular Dystrophies, Including Facts about Diagnostic Tests, Medical and Physical Therapies, Management of Co-Occurring Conditions, and Parenting Guidelines

Along with Practical Tips for Home Care, a Glossary, and Directories of Additional Resources

Edited by Joyce Brennfleck Shannon. 552 pages. 2004. 978-0-7808-0676-4.

"This book is highly recommended for public and academic libraries as well as health care offices that support the information needs of patients and their families."

—*E-Streams, Apr '05*

"Excellent reference."

—*The Bookwatch, Jan '05*

SEE ALSO *Movement Disorders Sourcebook, 2nd Edition*

Obesity Sourcebook

Basic Consumer Health Information about Diseases and Other Problems Associated with Obesity, and Including Facts about Risk Factors, Prevention Issues, and Management Approaches

Along with Statistical and Demographic Data, Information about Special Populations,

Research Updates, a Glossary, and Source Listings for Further Help and Information

Edited by Wilma Caldwell and Chad T. Kimball. 360 pages. 2001. 978-0-7808-0333-6.

"The book synthesizes the reliable medical literature on obesity into one easy-to-read and useful resource for the general public."

—*American Reference Books Annual, 2002*

"Well suited for the health reference collection of a public library or an academic health science library that serves the general population."

—*E-Streams, Sep '01*

Osteoporosis Sourcebook

Basic Consumer Health Information about Primary and Secondary Osteoporosis and Juvenile Osteoporosis and Related Conditions, Including Fibrous Dysplasia, Gaucher Disease, Hyperthyroidism, Hypophosphatasia, Myeloma, Osteopetrosis, Osteogenesis Imperfecta, and Paget's Disease

Along with Information about Risk Factors, Treatments, Traditional and Non-Traditional Pain Management, a Glossary of Related Terms, and a Directory of Resources

Edited by Allan R. Cook. 568 pages. 2001. 978-0-7808-0239-1.

"This resource is recommended as a great reference source for public, health, and academic libraries, and is another triumph for the editors of Omnigraphics."

—*American Reference Books Annual, 2002*

"Will prove valuable to any library seeking to maintain a current, comprehensive reference collection of health resources. . . . From prevention to treatment and associated conditions, this provides an excellent survey."

—*The Bookwatch, Aug '01*

SEE ALSO *Healthy Aging Sourcebook, Women's Health Concerns Sourcebook, 3rd Edition*

Pain Sourcebook, 3rd Edition

Basic Consumer Health Information about Acute and Chronic Pain, Including Nerve Pain, Bone Pain, Muscle Pain, Cancer Pain, and Disorders Characterized by Pain, Such as Arthritis, Temporomandibular Muscle and Joint (TMJ) Disorder, Carpal Tunnel Syndrome, Headaches, Heartburn, Sciatica, and Shingles, and Facts about Diagnostic Tests and Treatment Options for Pain, Including Over-the-Counter and Prescription Drugs, Physical Rehabilitation, Injection and Infusion Therapies, Implantable Technologies, and Complementary Medicine

Along with Tips for Living with Pain, a Glossary of Related Terms, and a Directory of Additional Resources

Edited by Joyce Brennfleck Shannon. 644 pages. 2008. 978-0-7808-1006-8.

"Excellent for ready-reference users and can be used for beginning students in health fields . . . appropriate for the consumer health collection in both public and academic libraries."

—*ARBAonline, Nov '08*

Pediatric Cancer Sourcebook

Basic Consumer Health Information about Leukemias, Brain Tumors, Sarcomas, Lymphomas, and Other Cancers in Infants, Children, and Adolescents, Including Descriptions of Cancers, Treatments, and Coping Strategies

Along with Suggestions for Parents, Caregivers, and Concerned Relatives, a Glossary of Cancer Terms, and Resource Listings

Edited by Edward J. Prucha. 575 pages. 1999. 978-0-7808-0245-2.

"An excellent source of information. Recommended for public, hospital, and health science libraries with consumer health collections."

—*E-Streams, Jun '00*

"A valuable addition to all libraries specializing in health services and many public libraries."

—*American Reference Books Annual, 2000*

SEE ALSO *Childhood Diseases and Disorders Sourcebook, 2nd Edition, Healthy Children Sourcebook*

Physical and Mental Issues in Aging Sourcebook

Basic Consumer Health Information on Physical and Mental Disorders Associated with the Aging Process, Including Concerns about Cardiovascular Disease, Pulmonary Disease, Oral Health, Digestive Disorders, Musculoskeletal and Skin Disorders, Metabolic

Changes, Sexual and Reproductive Issues, and Changes in Vision, Hearing, and Other Senses

Along with Data about Longevity and Causes of Death, Information on Acute and Chronic Pain, Descriptions of Mental Concerns, a Glossary of Terms, and Resource Listings for Additional Help

Edited by Jenifer Swanson. 660 pages. 1999. 978-0-7808-0233-9.

"This is a treasure of health information for the layperson."
—*CHOICE Health Sciences Supplement, May '00*

"Recommended for public libraries."
—*American Reference Books Annual, 2000*

SEE ALSO *Healthy Aging Sourcebook*

Podiatry Sourcebook, 2nd Edition

Basic Consumer Health Information about Disorders, Diseases, and Deformities that Affect the Foot and Ankle, Including Sprains, Corns, Calluses, Bunions, Plantar Warts, Plantar Fasciitis, Neuromas, Clubfoot, Flat Feet, Achilles Tendonitis, and Much More

Along with Information about Selecting a Foot Care Specialist, Foot Fitness, Shoes and Socks, Diagnostic Tests and Corrective Procedures, Financial Assistance for Corrective Devices, a Glossary of Related Terms, and a Directory of Resources for Additional Help and Information

Edited by Ivy L. Alexander. 516 pages. 2007. 978-0-7808-0944-4.

"An excellent resource. . . . Although there have been various types of 'foot books' published in the past, none are as comprehensive as this one. 5 Stars (out of 5)!"
—*Doody's Review Service, 2007*

"Perfect for both health libraries and general-interest lending collections."
—*Internet Bookwatch, Jul '07*

Pregnancy and Birth Sourcebook, 3rd Edition

Basic Consumer Health Information about Pregnancy and Fetal Development, Including Facts about Fertility and Conception, Physical and Emotional Changes during Pregnancy, Prenatal Care and Diagnostic Tests, High-Risk Pregnancies and Complications, Labor, Delivery, and the Postpartum Period

Along with Tips on Maintaining Health and Wellness during Pregnancy and Caring for Newborn Infants, a Glossary of Related Terms, and Directories of Resources for Additional Help and Information

Edited by Amy L. Sutton. 600 pages. 2009. 978-0-7808-1074-7.

SEE ALSO *Breastfeeding Sourcebook, Congenital Disorders Sourcebook, 2nd Edition, Family Planning Sourcebook, Women's Health Concerns Sourcebook, 3rd Edition*

Prostate and Urological Disorders Sourcebook

Basic Consumer Health Information about Urogenital and Sexual Disorders in Men, Including Prostate and Other Andrological Cancers, Prostatitis, Benign Prostatic Hyperplasia, Testicular and Penile Trauma, Cryptorchidism, Peyronie Disease, Erectile Dysfunction, and Male Factor Infertility, and Facts about Commonly Used Tests and Procedures, Such as Prostatectomy, Vasectomy, Vasectomy Reversal, Penile Implants, and Semen Analysis

Along with a Glossary of Andrological Terms and a Directory of Resources for Additional Information

Edited by Karen Bellenir. 604 pages. 2006. 978-0-7808-0797-6.

"Certain to be a popular pick among library reference holdings. . . . No prior knowledge is assumed for any of the conditions or terms herein, making it a most accessible general-interest reference."
—*California Bookwatch, Apr '06*

SEE ALSO *Men's Health Concerns Sourcebook, 3rd Edition, Urinary Tract and Kidney Diseases and Disorders Sourcebook, 2nd Edition*

Prostate Cancer Sourcebook

Basic Consumer Health Information about Prostate Cancer, Including Information about the Associated Risk Factors, Detection, Diagnosis, and Treatment of Prostate Cancer

Along with Information on Non-Malignant Prostate Conditions, and Featuring a Section

Listing Support and Treatment Centers and a Glossary of Related Terms

Edited by Dawn D. Matthews. 340 pages. 2001. 978-0-7808-0324-4.

"Recommended reference source."
—*Booklist, Jan '02*

"A valuable resource for health care consumers seeking information on the subject. . . . All text is written in a clear, easy-to-understand language that avoids technical jargon. Any library that collects consumer health resources would strengthen their collection with the addition of the *Prostate Cancer Sourcebook*."
—*American Reference Books Annual, 2002*

SEE ALSO *Cancer Sourcebook, 5th Edition, Men's Health Concerns Sourcebook, 3rd Edition*

Rehabilitation Sourcebook

Basic Consumer Health Information about Rehabilitation for People Recovering from Heart Surgery, Spinal Cord Injury, Stroke, Orthopedic Impairments, Amputation, Pulmonary Impairments, Traumatic Injury, and More, Including Physical Therapy, Occupational Therapy, Speech/Language Therapy, Massage Therapy, Dance Therapy, Art Therapy, and Recreational Therapy

Along with Information on Assistive and Adaptive Devices, a Glossary, and Resources for Additional Help and Information

Edited by Dawn D. Matthews. 519 pages. 2000. 978-0-7808-0236-0.

"This is an excellent resource for public library reference and health collections."
—*American Reference Books Annual, 2001*

"Recommended reference source."
—*Booklist, May '00*

Respiratory Disorders Sourcebook, 2nd Edition

Basic Consumer Health Information about Infectious, Inflammatory, and Chronic Conditions Affecting the Lungs and Respiratory System, Including Pneumonia, Bronchitis, Influenza, Tuberculosis, Sarcoidosis, Asthma, Cystic Fibrosis, Chronic Obstructive Pulmonary Disease, Lung Abscesses, Pulmonary Embolism, Occupational Lung Diseases, and Other Bacterial, Viral, and Fungal Infections

Along with Facts about the Structure and Function of the Lungs and Airways, Methods of Diagnosing Respiratory Disorders, and Treatment and Rehabilitation Options, a Glossary of Related Terms, and a Directory of Resources for Additional Help and Information

Edited by Sandra L. Judd. 638 pages. 2008. 978-0-7808-1007-5.

"A great addition for public and school libraries because it provides concise health information . . . readers can start with this reference source and get satisfactory answers before proceeding to other medical reference tools for more in depth information . . . A good guide for health education on lung disorders."
—*ARBAonline, Nov '08*

SEE ALSO *Lung Disorders Sourcebook*

Sexually Transmitted Diseases Sourcebook, 4th Edition

Basic Consumer Health Information about Chlamydial Infections, Gonorrhea, Hepatitis, Herpes, HIV/AIDS, Human Papillomavirus, Pubic Lice, Scabies, Syphilis, Trichomoniasis, Vaginal Infections, and Other Sexually Transmitted Diseases, Including Facts about Risk Factors, Symptoms, Diagnosis, Treatment, and the Prevention of Sexually Transmitted Infections

Along with Updates on Current Research Initiatives, a Glossary of Related Terms, and Resources for Additional Help and Information

Edited by Laura Larsen. 600 pages. 2009. 978-0-7808-1073-0.

SEE ALSO *AIDS Sourcebook, 4th Edition, Contagious Diseases Sourcebook, 2nd Edition, Men's Health Concerns Sourcebook, 3rd Edition, Women's Health Concerns Sourcebook, 3rd Edition*

Sleep Disorders Sourcebook, 2nd Edition

Basic Consumer Health Information about Sleep and Sleep Disorders, Including Insomnia, Sleep Apnea, Restless Legs Syndrome, Narcolepsy, Parasomnias, and Other Health Problems That Affect Sleep, Plus Facts about Diagnostic Procedures, Treatment Strategies,

Sleep Medications, and Tips for Improving Sleep Quality

Along with a Glossary of Related Terms and Resources for Additional Help and Information

Edited by Amy L. Sutton. 567 pages. 2005. 978-0-7808-0743-3.

"This book will be useful for just about everybody, especially the 40 million Americans with sleep disorders."

—*American Reference Books Annual, 2006*

"A welcome addition to public libraries and consumer health libraries."

—*Medical Reference Services Quarterly, Summer '06*

Smoking Concerns Sourcebook

Basic Consumer Health Information about Nicotine Addiction and Smoking Cessation, Featuring Facts about the Health Effects of Tobacco Use, Including Lung and Other Cancers, Heart Disease, Stroke, and Respiratory Disorders, Such as Emphysema and Chronic Bronchitis

Along with Information about Smoking Prevention Programs, Suggestions for Achieving and Maintaining a Smoke-Free Lifestyle, Statistics about Tobacco Use, Reports on Current Research Initiatives, a Glossary of Related Terms, and Directories of Resources for Additional Help and Information

Edited by Karen Bellenir. 595 pages. 2004. 978-0-7808-0323-7.

"Provides everything needed for the student or general reader seeking practical details on the effects of tobacco use."

—*The Bookwatch, Mar '05*

"Public libraries and consumer health care libraries will find this work useful."

—*American Reference Books Annual, 2005*

SEE ALSO *Respiratory Disorders Sourcebook, 2nd Edition*

Sports Injuries Sourcebook, 3rd Edition

Basic Consumer Health Information about Sprains and Strains, Fractures, Growth Plate Injuries, Overtraining Injuries, and Injuries to the Head, Face, Shoulders, Elbows, Hands, Spinal Column, Knees, Ankles, and Feet, and with Facts about Heat-Related Illness, Steroids and Sport Supplements, Protective Equipment, Diagnostic Procedures, Treatment Options, and Rehabilitation

Along with a Glossary of Related Terms and a Directory of Resources for Additional Help and Information

Edited by Sandra J. Judd. 623 pages. 2007. 978-0-7808-0949-9.

SEE ALSO *Fitness and Exercise Sourcebook, 3rd Edition*

Stress-Related Disorders Sourcebook, 2nd Edition

Basic Consumer Health Information about Stress and Stress-Related Disorders, Including Types of Stress, Sources of Acute and Chronic Stress, the Impact of Stress on the Body's Systems, and Mental and Emotional Health Problems Associated with Stress, Such as Depression, Anxiety Disorders, Substance Abuse, Posttraumatic Stress Disorder, and Suicide

Along with Advice about Getting Help for Stress-Related Disorders, Information about Stress Management Techniques, a Glossary of Stress-Related Terms, and a Directory of Resources for Additional Help and Information

Edited by Amy L. Sutton. 608 pages. 2007. 978-0-7808-0996-3.

"Accessible to the lay reader. Highly recommended for medical and psychiatric collections."

—*Library Journal, Mar '08*

"Well-written for a general readership, the 2nd Edition of *Stress-Related Disorders Sourcebook* is a useful addition to the health reference literature."

—*American Reference Books Annual, 2008*

SEE ALSO *Mental Health Disorders Sourcebook, 4th Edition*

Stroke Sourcebook, 2nd Edition

Basic Consumer Health Information about Stroke, Including Ischemic, Hemorrhagic, and Mini Strokes, as Well as Risk Factors, Prevention Guidelines, Diagnostic Tests, Medications and

Surgical Treatments, and Complications of Stroke

Along with Rehabilitation Techniques and Innovations, Tips on Staying Healthy and Maintaining Independence after Stroke, a Glossary of Related Terms, and a Directory of Resources for Stroke Survivors and Their Families

Edited by Amy L. Sutton. 626 pages. 2008. 978-0-7808-1035-8.

"An encyclopedic handbook on stroke that is written in a language the layperson can understand. . . . This is one of the most helpful, readable books on stroke. This volume is highly recommended and should be in every medical, hospital and public library; in addition, every family practitioner should have a copy in his or her office."

—*ARBAonline Dec '08*

SEE ALSO *Hypertension Sourcebook*

Surgery Sourcebook, 2nd Edition

Basic Consumer Health Information about Common Inpatient and Outpatient Surgeries, Including Critical Care and Trauma, Gastrointestinal, Gynecologic and Obstetric, Cardiac and Vascular, Neurologic, Ophthalmologic, Orthopedic, Reconstructive and Cosmetic, and Other Major and Minor Surgeries

Along with Information about Anesthesia and Pain Relief Options, Risks and Complications, Postoperative Recovery Concerns, and Innovative Surgical Techniques and Tools, a Glossary of Related Terms, and a Directory of Additional Resources

Edited by Amy L. Sutton. 645 pages. 2008. 978-0-7808-1004-4.

"Large public libraries and medical libraries would benefit from this material in their reference collections."

—*ARBAonline Aug '08*

SEE ALSO *Cosmetic and Reconstructive Surgery Sourcebook, 2nd Edition*

Thyroid Disorders Sourcebook

Basic Consumer Health Information about Disorders of the Thyroid and Parathyroid Glands, Including Hypothyroidism, Hyperthyroidism, Graves Disease, Hashimoto Thyroiditis, Thyroid Cancer, and Parathyroid Disorders, Featuring Facts about Symptoms, Risk Factors, Tests, and Treatments

Along with Information about the Effects of Thyroid Imbalance on Other Body Systems, Environmental Factors That Affect the Thyroid Gland, a Glossary, and a Directory of Additional Resources

Edited by Joyce Brennfleck Shannon. 573 pages. 2005. 978-0-7808-0745-7.

"Recommended for consumer health collections."

—*American Reference Books Annual, 2006*

"Highly recommended pick for basic consumer health reference holdings at all levels."

—*The Bookwatch, Aug '05*

SEE ALSO *Endocrine and Metabolic Disorders Sourcebook, 2nd Edition*

Transplantation Sourcebook

Basic Consumer Health Information about Organ and Tissue Transplantation, Including Physical and Financial Preparations, Procedures and Issues Relating to Specific Solid Organ and Tissue Transplants, Rehabilitation, Pediatric Transplant Information, the Future of Transplantation, and Organ and Tissue Donation

Along with a Glossary and Listings of Additional Resources

Edited by Joyce Brennfleck Shannon. 610 pages. 2002. 978-0-7808-0322-0.

"Recommended for libraries with an interest in offering consumer health information."

—*E-Streams, Jul '02*

"This is a unique and valuable resource for patients facing transplantation and their families."

—*Doody's Review Service, Jun '02*

Traveler's Health Sourcebook

Basic Consumer Health Information for Travelers, Including Physical and Medical Preparations, Transportation Health and Safety, Essential Information about Food and Water, Sun Exposure, Insect and Snake Bites, Camping and Wilderness Medicine, and Travel with Physical or Medical Disabilities

Along with International Travel Tips, Vaccination Recommendations, Geographical Health Issues, Disease Risks, a Glossary, and a Listing of Additional Resources

Edited by Joyce Brennfleck Shannon. 619 pages. 2000. 978-0-7808-0384-8.

"Recommended reference source."
—Booklist, Feb '01

"This book is recommended for any public library, any travel collection, and especially any collection for the physically disabled."
—American Reference Books Annual, 2001

SEE ALSO *Worldwide Health Sourcebook*

Urinary Tract and Kidney Diseases and Disorders Sourcebook, 2nd Edition

Basic Consumer Health Information about the Urinary System, Including the Bladder, Urethra, Ureters, and Kidneys, with Facts about Urinary Tract Infections, Incontinence, Congenital Disorders, Kidney Stones, Cancers of the Urinary Tract and Kidneys, Kidney Failure, Dialysis, and Kidney Transplantation

Along with Statistical and Demographic Information, Reports on Current Research in Kidney and Urologic Health, a Summary of Commonly Used Diagnostic Tests, a Glossary of Related Terms, and a Directory of Resources for Additional Help and Information

Edited by Ivy L. Alexander. 621 pages. 2005. 978-0-7808-0750-1.

"A good choice for a consumer health information library or for a medical library needing information to refer to their patients."
—American Reference Books Annual, 2006

SEE ALSO *Prostate and Urological Disorders Sourcebook*

Vegetarian Sourcebook

Basic Consumer Health Information about Vegetarian Diets, Lifestyle, and Philosophy, Including Definitions of Vegetarianism and Veganism, Tips about Adopting Vegetarianism, Creating a Vegetarian Pantry, and Meeting Nutritional Needs of Vegetarians, with Facts Regarding Vegetarianism's Effect on Pregnant and Lactating Women, Children, Athletes, and Senior Citizens

Along with a Glossary of Commonly Used Vegetarian Terms and Resources for Additional Help and Information

Edited by Chad T. Kimball. 337 pages. 2002. 978-0-7808-0439-5.

"Organizes into one concise volume the answers to the most common questions concerning vegetarian diets and lifestyles. This title is recommended for public and secondary school libraries."
—E-Streams, Apr '03

"Invaluable reference for public and school library collections alike."
—Library Bookwatch, Apr '03

"The articles in this volume are easy to read and come from authoritative sources. The book does not necessarily support the vegetarian diet but instead provides the pros and cons of this important decision. . . . Recommended for public libraries and consumer health libraries."
—American Reference Books Annual, 2003

SEE ALSO *Diet and Nutrition Sourcebook, 3rd Edition*

Women's Health Concerns Sourcebook, 3rd Edition

Basic Consumer Health Information about Issues and Trends in Women's Health and Health Conditions of Special Concern to Women, Including Endometriosis, Uterine Fibroids, Menstrual Irregularities, Menopause, Sexual Dysfunction, Infertility, Cancer in Women, and Other Such Chronic Disorders as Lupus, Fibromyalgia, and Thyroid Disease

Along with Statistical Data, Tips for Maintaining Wellness, a Glossary, and a Directory of Resources for Further Help and Information

Edited by Sandra J. Judd. 600 pages. 2009. 978-0-7808-1036-5.

SEE ALSO *Breast Cancer Sourcebook, 3rd Edition, Cancer Sourcebook for Women, 3rd Edition, Healthy Heart Sourcebook for Women, Osteoporosis Sourcebook*

Workplace Health and Safety Sourcebook

Basic Consumer Health Information about Workplace Health and Safety, Including the Effect of Workplace Hazards on the Lungs,

Skin, Heart, Ears, Eyes, Brain, Reproductive Organs, Musculoskeletal System, and Other Organs and Body Parts

Along with Information about Occupational Cancer, Personal Protective Equipment, Toxic and Hazardous Chemicals, Child Labor, Stress, and Workplace Violence

Edited by Chad T. Kimball. 610 pages. 2000. 978-0-7808-0231-5.

"As a reference for the general public, this would be useful in any library."

—*E-Streams, Jun '01*

"Provides helpful information for primary care physicians and other caregivers interested in occupational medicine. . . . General readers; professionals."

—*CHOICE, May '01*

■

Worldwide Health Sourcebook

Basic Information about Global Health Issues, Including Malnutrition, Reproductive Health, Disease Dispersion and Prevention, Emerging Diseases, Risky Health Behaviors, and the Leading Causes of Death

Along with Global Health Concerns for Children, Women, and the Elderly, Mental Health Issues, Research and Technology Advancements, and Economic, Environmental, and Political Health Implications, a Glossary, and a Resource Listing for Additional Help and Information

Edited by Joyce Brennfleck Shannon. 597 pages. 2001. 978-0-7808-0330-5.

"Named an Outstanding Academic Title."

—*CHOICE, Jan '02*

"Yet another handy but also unique compilation in the extensive *Health Reference Series*, this is a useful work because many of the international publications reprinted or excerpted are not readily available. Highly recommended."

—*CHOICE, Nov '01*

SEE ALSO *Traveler's Health Sourcebook*

Teen Health Series

Complete Catalog

List price $69 per volume. School and library price $62 per volume.

Abuse and Violence Information for Teens

Health Tips about the Causes and Consequences of Abusive and Violent Behavior

Including Facts about the Types of Abuse and Violence, the Warning Signs of Abusive and Violent Behavior, Health Concerns of Victims, and Getting Help and Staying Safe

Edited by Sandra Augustyn Lawton. 411 pages. 2008. 978-0-7808-1008-2.

"A useful resource for schools and organizations providing services to teens and may also be a starting point in research projects."

—*Reference and Research Book News, Aug '08*

"Violence is a serious problem for teens. . . . This resource gives teens the information they need to face potential threats and get help—either for themselves or for their friends."

—*ARBAonline, Aug '08*

Accident and Safety Information for Teens

Health Tips about Medical Emergencies, Traumatic Injuries, and Disaster Preparedness

Including Facts about Motor Vehicle Accidents, Burns, Poisoning, Firearms, Natural Disasters, National Security Threats, and More

Edited by Karen Bellenir. 420 pages. 2008. 978-0-7808-1046-4.

SEE ALSO *Sports Injuries Information for Teens, 2nd Edition*

Alcohol Information for Teens, 2nd Edition

Health Tips about Alcohol and Alcoholism

Including Facts about Alcohol's Effects on the Body, Brain, and Behavior, the Consequences of Underage Drinking, Alcohol Abuse Prevention and Treatment, and Coping with Alcoholic Parents

Edited by Lisa Bakewell. 400 pages. 2009. 978-0-7808-1043-3.

SEE ALSO *Drug Information for Teens, 2nd Edition*

Allergy Information for Teens

Health Tips about Allergic Reactions Such as Anaphylaxis, Respiratory Problems, and Rashes

Including Facts about Identifying and Managing Allergies to Food, Pollen, Mold, Animals, Chemicals, Drugs, and Other Substances

Edited by Karen Bellenir. 410 pages. 2006. 978-0-7808-0799-0.

"This is a comprehensive, readable text on the subject of allergic diseases in teenagers. 5 Stars (out of 5)!"

—*Doody's Review Service, Jun '06*

"This authoritative and useful self-help title is a solid addition to YA collections, whether for personal interest or reports."

—*School Library Journal, Jul '06*

Asthma Information for Teens

Health Tips about Managing Asthma and Related Concerns

Including Facts about Asthma Causes, Triggers, Symptoms, Diagnosis, and Treatment

Edited by Karen Bellenir. 386 pages. 2005. 978-0-7808-0770-9.

"Highly recommended for medical libraries, public school libraries, and public libraries."

—*American Reference Books Annual, 2006*

"Although this volume is nearly 400 pages long, it is so clearly written and well organized that even hesitant readers will be able to find the facts they need, whether for reports or personal information. . . . A succinct but complete resource."

—*School Library Journal, Sep '05*

Body Information for Teens

Health Tips about Maintaining Well-Being for a Lifetime

Including Facts about the Development and Functioning of the Body's Systems, Organs, and Structures and the Health Impact of Lifestyle Choices

Edited by Sandra Augustyn Lawton. 458 pages. 2007. 978-0-7808-0443-2.

■

Cancer Information for Teens, 2nd Edition

Health Tips about Cancer Awareness, Symptoms, Prevention, Diagnosis, and Treatment

Including Facts about Common Cancers Affecting Teens, Causes, Detection, Coping Strategies, Clinical Trials, Nutrition and Exercise, Cancer in Friends or Family, and More

Edited by Karen Bellenir and Lisa Bakewell. 400 pages. 2009. 978-0-7808-1085-3.

■

Complementary and Alternative Medicine Information for Teens

Health Tips about Non-Traditional and Non-Western Medical Practices

Including Information about Acupuncture, Chiropractic Medicine, Dietary and Herbal Supplements, Hypnosis, Massage Therapy, Prayer and Spirituality, Reflexology, Yoga, and More

Edited by Sandra Augustyn Lawton. 407 pages. 2007. 978-0-7808-0966-6.

"This volume covers CAM specifically for teenagers but of general use also. It should be a welcome addition to both public and academic libraries."

—American Reference Books Annual, 2008

"This volume provides a solid foundation for further investigation of the subject, making it useful for both public and high school libraries."

—VOYA: Voice of Youth Advocates, Jun '07

■

Diabetes Information for Teens

Health Tips about Managing Diabetes and Preventing Related Complications

Including Information about Insulin, Glucose Control, Healthy Eating, Physical Activity, and Learning to Live with Diabetes

Edited by Sandra Augustyn Lawton. 410 pages. 2006. 978-0-7808-0811-9.

"A comprehensive instructional guide for teens. . . . some of the material may also be directed towards parents or teachers. 5 stars (out of 5)!"

—Doody's Review Service, 2006

"Students dealing with their own diabetes or that of a friend or family member or those writing reports on the topic will find this a valuable resource."

—School Library Journal, Aug '06

"This text is directed to the teen population and would be an excellent library resource for a health class or for the teacher as a reference for class preparation. It can, however, serve a much wider audience. The clinical educator on diabetes may find it valuable to educate the newly diagnosed client regardless of age. It also would be an excellent reference and education tool for a preventive medicine seminar on diabetes."

—Physical Therapy, Mar '07

■

Diet Information for Teens, 2nd Edition

Health Tips about Diet and Nutrition

Including Facts about Dietary Guidelines, Food Groups, Nutrients, Healthy Meals, Snacks, Weight Control, Medical Concerns Related to Diet, and More

Edited by Karen Bellenir. 432 pages. 2006. 978-0-7808-0820-1.

"A very quick and pleasant read in spite of the fact that it is very detailed in the information it gives. . . . A book for anyone concerned about diet and nutrition."

—American Reference Books Annual, 2007

SEE ALSO *Eating Disorders Information for Teens, 2nd Edition*

■

Drug Information for Teens, 2nd Edition

Health Tips about the Physical and Mental Effects of Substance Abuse

Including Information about Marijuana, Inhalants, Club Drugs, Stimulants, Hallucinogens,

Opiates, Prescription and Over-the-Counter Drugs, Herbal Products, Tobacco, Alcohol, and More

Edited by Sandra Augustyn Lawton. 468 pages. 2006. 978-0-7808-0862-1.

"As with earlier installments in Omnigraphics' *Teen Health Series, Drug Information for Teens* is designed specifically to meet the needs and interests of middle and high school students. . . . Strongly recommended for both academic and public libraries."

—*American Reference Books Annual, 2007*

"Solid thoughtful advice is given about how to handle peer pressure, drug-related health concerns, and treatment strategies."

—*School Library Journal, Dec '06*

SEE ALSO *Alcohol Information for Teens, 2nd Edition, Tobacco Information for Teens*

Eating Disorders Information for Teens, 2nd Edition

Health Tips about Anorexia, Bulimia, Binge Eating, And Other Eating Disorders

Including Information about Risk Factors, Diagnosis and Treatment, Prevention, Related Health Concerns, and Other Issues

Edited by Sandra Augustyn Lawton. 377 pages. 2009. 978-0-7808-1044-0.

SEE ALSO *Diet Information for Teens, 2nd Edition*

Fitness Information for Teens, 2nd Edition

Health Tips about Exercise, Physical Well-Being, and Health Maintenance

Including Facts about Conditioning, Stretching, Strength Training, Body Shape and Body Image, Sports Nutrition, and Specific Activities for Athletes and Non-Athletes

Edited by Lisa Bakewell. 432 pages. 2009. 978-0-7808-1045-7.

SEE ALSO *Diet Information for Teens, 2nd Edition, Sports Injuries Information for Teens, 2nd Edition*

Learning Disabilities Information for Teens

Health Tips about Academic Skills Disorders and Other Disabilities That Affect Learning

Including Information about Common Signs of Learning Disabilities, School Issues, Learning to Live with a Learning Disability, and Other Related Issues

Edited by Sandra Augustyn Lawton. 400 pages. 2006. 978-0-7808-0796-9.

"This book provides a wealth of information for any reader interested in the signs, causes, and consequences of learning disabilities, as well as related legal rights and educational interventions. . . . Public and academic libraries should want this title for both students and general readers."

—*American Reference Books Annual, 2006*

Mental Health Information for Teens, 2nd Edition

Health Tips about Mental Wellness and Mental Illness

Including Facts about Mental and Emotional Health, Depression and Other Mood Disorders, Anxiety Disorders, Conduct Disorder, Self-Injury, Psychosis, Schizophrenia, and More

Edited by Karen Bellenir. 424 pages. 2006. 978-0-7808-0863-8.

"This excellent overview of the psychological disorders that affect teens provides clear definitions and descriptions, and discusses resources, therapies, coping mechanisms, and medications."

—*School Library Journal Curriculum Connections, Fall '07*

"A well done reference for a specific, often under-represented group."

—*Doody's Review Service, 2006*

SEE ALSO *Stress Information for Teens*

Pregnancy Information for Teens

Health Tips about Teen Pregnancy and Teen Parenting

Including Facts about Prenatal Care, Pregnancy Complications, Labor and Delivery,

Postpartum Care, Pregnancy-Related Lifestyle Concerns, and More

Edited by Sandra Augustyn Lawton. 434 pages. 2007. 978-0-7808-0984-0.

SEE ALSO *Sexual Health Information for Teens, 2nd Edition*

Sexual Health Information for Teens, 2nd Edition

Health Tips about Sexual Development, Reproduction, Contraception, and Sexually Transmitted Infections

Including Facts about Puberty, Sexuality, Birth Control, Chlamydia, Gonorrhea, Herpes, Human Papillomavirus, Syphilis, and More

Edited by Sandra Augustyn Lawton. 430 pages. 2008. 978-0-7808-1010-5.

"This offering represents the most up-to-date information available on an array of topics including abstinence-only sexual education and pregnancy-prevention methods. . . . The range of coverage—from puberty and anatomy to sexually transmitted diseases—is thorough and extensive. Each chapter includes a bibliographic citation, and the three back sections containing additional resources, further reading, and the index are all first-rate. . . . This volume will be well used by students in need of the facts, whether for educational or personal reasons."

—*School Library Journal, Nov '08*

SEE ALSO *Pregnancy Information for Teens*

Skin Health Information for Teens, 2nd Edition

Health Tips about Dermatological Concerns and Skin Cancer Risks

Including Facts about Acne, Warts, Allergies, and Other Conditions and Lifestyle Choices, Such as Tanning, Tattooing, and Piercing, That Affect the Skin, Nails, Scalp, and Hair

Edited by Edited by Kim Wohlenhaus. 400 pages. 2009. 978-0-7808-1042-6.

Sleep Information for Teens

Health Tips about Adolescent Sleep Requirements, Sleep Disorders, and the Effects of Sleep Deprivation

Including Facts about Why People Need Sleep, Sleep Patterns, Circadian Rhythms, Dreaming, Insomnia, Sleep Apnea, Narcolepsy, and More

Edited by Karen Bellenir. 355 pages. 2008. 978-0-7808-1009-9.

SEE ALSO *Body Information for Teens*

Sports Injuries Information for Teens, 2nd Edition

Health Tips about Acute, Traumatic, and Chronic Injuries in Adolescent Athletes

Including Facts about Sprains, Fractures, and Overuse Injuries, Treatment, Rehabilitation, Sport-Specific Safety Guidelines, Fitness Suggestions, and More

Edited by Karen Bellenir. 429 pages. 2008. 978-0-7808-1011-2.

"An engaging selection of informative articles about the prevention and treatment of sports injuries. . . The value of this book is that the articles have been vetted and are often augmented with inserts of useful facts, definitions of technical terms, and quick tips. Sensitive topics like injuries to genitalia are discussed openly and responsibly. This revised edition contains updated articles and defines sport more broadly than the first edition."

—*School Library Journal, Nov '08*

"This work will be useful in the young adult collections of public libraries as well as high school libraries. . . . A useful resource for student research."

—*ARBAonline, Aug '08*

SEE ALSO *Accident and Safety Information for Teens*

Stress Information for Teens

Health Tips about the Mental and Physical Consequences of Stress

Including Information about the Different Kinds of Stress, Symptoms of Stress, Frequent Causes of Stress, Stress Management Techniques, and More

Edited by Sandra Augustyn Lawton. 392 pages. 2008. 978-0-7808-1012-9.

"Understanding what stress is, what causes it, how the body and the mind are impacted by it,

and what teens can do are the general categories addressed here. . . . The chapters are brief but informative, and the list of community-help organizations is exhaustive. Report writers will find information quickly and easily, as will those who have personal concerns. The print is clear and the format is readable, making this an accessible resource for struggling readers and researchers."

—*School Library Journal, Dec '08*

"The articles selected will specifically appeal to young adults and are designed to answer their most common questions."

—*ARBAonline, Aug '08*

SEE ALSO *Mental Health Information for Teens, 2nd Edition*

Suicide Information for Teens

Health Tips about Suicide Causes and Prevention

Including Facts about Depression, Risk Factors, Getting Help, Survivor Support, and More

Edited by Joyce Brennfleck Shannon. 368 pages. 2005. 978-0-7808-0737-2.

"Highly Recommended for libraries serving teenagers as well as those who work with them."

—*E-Streams, Apr '06*

SEE ALSO *Mental Health Information for Teens, 2nd Edition*

Tobacco Information for Teens

Health Tips about the Hazards of Using Cigarettes, Smokeless Tobacco, and Other Nicotine Products

Including Facts about Nicotine Addiction, Immediate and Long-Term Health Effects of Tobacco Use, Related Cancers, Smoking Cessation, Tobacco Use Prevention, and Tobacco Use Statistics

Edited by Karen Bellenir. 440 pages. 2007. 978-0-7808-0976-5.

"A comprehensive resource. Each chapter is written to stand alone, so students can dip in and use the information in each section for reports or to answer personal questions without having to read the entire book. . . . The book is packed full of statistics, with sources to help students look up more."

—*School Library Journal, Sep '07*

"Pulls together a wide variety of authoritative sources to provide a comprehensive overview of tobacco use for this age group. . . . This reasonably priced reference title should be considered a necessary purchase for all public libraries and school media centers, along with academic libraries supporting teacher education."

—*American Reference Books Annual, 2008*

SEE ALSO *Drug Information for Teens, 2nd Edition*

Health Reference Series

Adolescent Health Sourcebook, 2nd Edition
Adult Health Concerns Sourcebook
AIDS Sourcebook, 4th Edition
Alcoholism Sourcebook, 2nd Edition
Allergies Sourcebook, 3rd Edition
Alzheimer Disease Sourcebook, 4th Edition
Arthritis Sourcebook, 2nd Edition
Asthma Sourcebook, 2nd Edition
Attention Deficit Disorder Sourcebook
Autism & Pervasive Developmental Disorders Sourcebook
Back & Neck Sourcebook, 2nd Edition
Blood & Circulatory Disorders Sourcebook, 2nd Edition
Brain Disorders Sourcebook, 2nd Edition
Breast Cancer Sourcebook, 3rd Edition
Breastfeeding Sourcebook
Burns Sourcebook
Cancer Sourcebook, 5th Edition
Cancer Sourcebook for Women, 3rd Edition
Cancer Survivorship Sourcebook
Cardiovascular Diseases & Disorders Sourcebook, 3rd Edition
Caregiving Sourcebook
Child Abuse Sourcebook
Childhood Diseases & Disorders Sourcebook, 2nd Edition
Colds, Flu & Other Common Ailments Sourcebook
Communication Disorders Sourcebook
Complementary & Alternative Medicine Sourcebook, 3rd Edition
Congenital Disorders Sourcebook, 2nd Edition
Contagious Diseases Sourcebook
Cosmetic & Reconstructive Surgery Sourcebook, 2nd Edition
Death & Dying Sourcebook, 2nd Edition
Dental Care & Oral Health Sourcebook, 3rd Edition
Depression Sourcebook, 2nd Edition
Dermatological Disorders Sourcebook, 2nd Edition
Diabetes Sourcebook, 4th Edition
Diet & Nutrition Sourcebook, 3rd Edition
Digestive Diseases & Disorder Sourcebook
Disabilities Sourcebook
Disease Management Sourcebook
Domestic Violence Sourcebook, 3rd Edition
Drug Abuse Sourcebook, 2nd Edition
Ear, Nose & Throat Disorders Sourcebook, 2nd Edition
Eating Disorders Sourcebook, 2nd Edition
Emergency Medical Services Sourcebook
Endocrine & Metabolic Disorders Sourcebook, 2nd Edition
Environmental Health Sourcebook, 2nd Edition
Ethnic Diseases Sourcebook
Eye Care Sourcebook, 3rd Edition
Family Planning Sourcebook
Fitness & Exercise Sourcebook, 3rd Edition
Food Safety Sourcebook
Forensic Medicine Sourcebook
Gastrointestinal Diseases & Disorders Sourcebook, 2nd Edition
Genetic Disorders Sourcebook, 3rd Edition
Head Trauma Sourcebook
Headache Sourcebook
Health Insurance Sourcebook
Healthy Aging Sourcebook
Healthy Children Sourcebook
Healthy Heart Sourcebook for Women
Hepatitis Sourcebook
Household Safety Sourcebook
Hypertension Sourcebook
Immune System Disorders Sourcebook, 2nd Edition
Infant & Toddler Health Sourcebook
Infectious Diseases Sourcebook
Injury & Trauma Sourcebook